Psychiatry

ton, Merrill T.
  Textbook of psychiatry.

  Rev. ed. of: Psychiatry, 4th ed. 1981.
  1. Psychiatry. I. Peterson, Margaret H. II. Davis,
mes Allan (date-   ). III. Eaton, Merrill T.
ychiatry. IV. Title. [DNLM: 1. Mental Disorders.
M 100 E15p]
C454.E18 1985   616.89   84-29596
3N 0-87488-838-7

pyright © 1985 by
EDICAL EXAMINATION PUBLISHING CO., INC.
03 New Hyde Park Road
w Hyde Park, New York

inted in the United States of America

Te

Textbook Series

Psychiatr

Fifth Edition

Merrill T. Eaton, Jr., M.D., F.A.P.A.
Professor of Psychiatry
University of Nebraska College of Medicine
Omaha, Nebraska

Margaret H. Peterson, M.D., F.A.P.A.
Associate Clinical Professor of Psychiatry
University of California, Irvine
California College of Medicine
Irvine, California

James A. Davis, M.D., F.A.P.A.
Associate Professor of Psychiatry
University of Nebraska College of Medicine
Omaha, Nebraska

MEDICAL EXAMINATION PUBLISHING CO., INC.

Contents

About the Authors

MERRILL T. EATON, JR., M.D., interned at St. Elizabeth's Hospital in Washington, D.C. after obtaining his Bachelor of Arts and Doctor of Medicine degrees from Indiana University. Following military service he obtained residency training in psychiatry at the Colorado State Hospital in Pueblo and at the Sheppard and Enoch Pratt Hospital in Towson, Maryland. From 1949 to 1960 he was a member of the faculty of the University of Kansas School of Medicine. Since 1960 he has taught at the University of Nebraska College of Medicine where he is now Professor and Chairman of the Department of Psychiatry and Director of the Nebraska Psychiatric Institute. Dr. Eaton is a Fellow of the American Psychiatric Association and the American College of Physicians. He is a member of the Board of Directors of the Group for the Advancement of Psychiatry and was formerly Chairman of the Publications Board of that organization.

MARGARET H. PETERSON, M.D., holds degrees of Bachelor of Arts, Master of Arts, and Doctor of Medicine from the University of Nebraska. After interning at Immanuel Hospital in Omaha she served as a resident in psychiatry at the Nebraska Psychiatric Institute and was then on the faculty of the University of Nebraska College of Medicine for nine years. She is now in private practice in Newport Beach, California, and is an Associate Clinical Professor of Psychiatry at the University of California, Irvine, California College of Medicine.

JAMES A. DAVIS, M.D., attended the University of Iowa as an undergraduate and completed his medical education at the University of Nebraska Medical Center in 1968. After internship at Immanuel Hospital in Omaha he obtained psychiatric residency training at the Nebraska Psychiatric Institute where he is now an Associate Professor of Psychiatry and the Director of Psychiatric Liaison Service. In 1974 a Distinguished Teacher Award was presented to him at the College of Medicine Commencement.

Preface

Psychiatry was first published in 1967 as part of the Medical Outline Series. It was intended as a concise overview of clinical psychiatry for use as an introduction to the subject or for review. In subsequent editions it became more a textbook than an outline, and with this, the fifth edition, it becomes part of the Textbook Series.

For the medical student it is intended for use as a beginning text in basic psychiatry and then later as a review of those things that have been learned during clerkship and from journals, lectures, and more comprehensive texts. It is hoped that it will continue to be useful to house officers and practicing physicians when a brief review of general psychiatry or of a specific topic is desired, whether as part of preparation for licensing or specialty board examination, or simply to help maintain current clinical knowledge and competence.

For the convenience of beginning medical students and readers from other disciplines the language has been kept as simple as possible and technical terms are defined as they are introduced. The diagnostic terminology and the grouping of diagnostic categories is based on DSM III, the third edition of the *Diagnostic and Statistical Manual of Mental Disorders* published by the American Psychiatric Association.

To assist the person who is reviewing, questions have been placed at the end of each chapter. Some of these call for factual information which the authors consider to be important, others for original thinking about mental health problems. Most can be answered after reading the chapter they accompany; a few require the use of references.

Selected references at the end of each chapter offer source material, more detailed discussions, and, sometimes, alternate points of view to those presented here.

The revision of this book has been influenced by comments from readers of previous editions: medical students and their teachers, resident physicians, persons preparing for board examinations, and members of colleague professions in the health fields and related disciplines, including law. It is hoped that suggestions and comments will continue to be received from those readers, who, as fellow students with the authors, join in the continual striving for a better understanding of mental health and illness.

notice

The authors and the publisher of this book have made every effort to ensure that all therapeutic modalities that are recommended are in accordance with accepted standards at the time of publication.

The drugs specified within this book may not have specific approval from the Food and Drug Administration in regard to the indications and dosages that may be recommended by the authors. The manufacturer's package insert is the best source of current prescribing information.

Part I

PSYCHODYNAMICS, PERSONALITY DEVELOPMENT,
EXAMINATION, AND CLASSIFICATION

Chapter 1

INTRODUCTION TO DYNAMIC PSYCHIATRY

PREVALENCE OF MENTAL DISORDERS

A knowledge of psychiatry, the branch of medicine that deals with mental, emotional, and behavioral disorders, is needed not only by the mental health specialist, but also by most other health professionals. The prevalence of psychiatric disorders makes this necessary.

It has been estimated that at any given time, one person in four is experiencing discomfort as a result of mental or emotional symptoms such as anxiety or depression. Almost everyone has had these symptoms at one time or another. This is not to say that all of us are, or have been, mentally ill, but it is also estimated that at any one time 15 percent of the population needs mental health service, and at least one person in 10 is hospitalized at some time in life for mental illness. One thinks of mental illness as a cause of distress and disability rather than death, but the life expectancy of persons with major mental illnesses is decreased, and there are 27,000 known suicide victims in the United States each year.

Other indices of human maladaptation and emotional suffering could be listed, and it is clear that despite the apparent advances of civilization, there is a vast amount of human misery, a major portion of which stems from mental illness. To understand the reasons for this and to prepare to alleviate it, one·must look first at the basic nature of human activities.

THE NATURE OF HUMAN BEHAVIOR

The understanding of human behavior in health and disease is facilitated by a biopsychosocial orientation. One must understand the function of the brain, the organ of the mind, its neurotransmitters, and the other systems that influence it, including the endocrine and circulatory. One must also understand the social milieu and the demands and stresses it places upon the individual through its expectations and values. In addition, one must understand the psychology of the individual, the ways in which behavior patterns and responses are learned or acquired. Most of all, one must be aware of how these three elements, the biological, psychological, and social, interact. One way of conceptualizing this interaction is through dynamic psychiatry.

The first assumption of psychodynamics is that behavior is purposeful (motivated and goal directed). The components of goal-directed behavior which cannot be further reduced or simplified are referred to as instincts. Of the attempts to classify instincts, the most widely utilized is that proposed by Freud, who postulated a life instinct, Eros, and a death instinct, Thanatos. The life instinct has two components:

1. Survival of the individual
2. Survival of the species (reproduction)

The death instinct may be turned on the self, or it may be externalized in the form of hostile, sadistic, or destructive behavior.

Freud viewed the instincts as being accompanied by energy. The energy attached to the life instinct he termed libido, and that to the death instinct, morbido.

That survival and reproduction are basic biological functions and account for many activities is obvious. Also, that living organisms die is a statement of fact; but the idea that there is an innate striving toward self-destruction is less readily acceptable; though, if true, it might help to account for a variety of risk-taking phenomena ranging from reckless driving to nuclear warfare. There may be a certain paradox in human society that makes the death instinct necessary for the survival of the species. Though Malthus' prediction that unchecked reproduction would exhaust food supplies may not be literally correct, unchecked trends in population growth can prove a major problem to society in that if food supplies are not exhausted, space may be. Already, population growth has created numerous environmental problems.

Those things which appear to meet the goals of the life instinct are perceived as pleasurable (e.g., eating, sexual activity), and those which threaten its goals are generally painful. Hence, the Pleasure Principle, which offers a basic statement about the goals of behavior: The organism tends to seek the greatest possible pleasure and to avoid pain. The terms satisfaction and security, which Sullivan used to designate the basic human operations, are similar, though not identical, in meaning to pleasure and avoidance of pain. Long before modern psychiatric theories were formulated, Napoleon observed: "Men are moved by two levers only: fear and self-interest."

The Pleasure Principle is modified by experience. One learns to defer a small immediate pleasure in order to attain a greater pleasure later; one learns to accept some pain to avoid greater pain (e.g., one permits a dentist to drill a tooth), or accepts discomfort in the hope of subsequent satisfaction. This modification of the Pleasure Principle is called the Reality Principle.

The operation of instincts for survival and reproduction, the working of the Pleasure Principle, and to an extent the application of the Reality Principle can be observed also in animals, both in the laboratory and in their natural habitat. In fact, these concepts are more difficult to study in man than in most species because of our complex social organizations.

There are other animals which form societies: herds, packs, colonies, or flocks. It is generally believed that our tendency to form social groups rather than to live in isolation is biologically determined. This tendency can be viewed as a separate herd instinct or as a component of the life instinct. The alternate possibility that formation of tribes and of more complex social units was forced upon humans by population growth, shortage of food supplies, and a need for common defense against enemies cannot be rejected completely.

When one gets food from the supermarket rather than hunting for it in the forest, though more diverse sources of satisfaction for hunger are to be found, the total process is infinitely more complicated. Societies do, and probably must, impose numerous restrictions on instinctually determined behavior. The individual has to accept some regulations and modify behavior to conform with them. That is, one must to some extent adjust to society. More than this, one must develop a competence in dealing with it. Cooperative effort, sharing, compromise, division of labor, and specialization are characteristic of group living. Cooperative endeavor requires a medium of communication, language, which becomes more elaborate the more complex the cooperation. With division of labor and specialization comes the need for a medium of exchange, money.

As one conforms to and/or masters the intricacies of social living, there is a direct interaction with significant people in the immediate environment. For an adult, the nature of relationships with specific people (e.g., spouse, employer, coworkers, friends) influences the extent to which satisfaction and security are attained.

THE THEORY OF THE UNCONSCIOUS

A second basic assumption of dynamic psychiatry is that the human being is not always aware of the purposes of actions. Subjective efforts to account for mistakes, the observation of illogical and self-defeating human behavior, and on a more scientific level, experimental studies of motivation and decision making, provide evidence for this. One explanation for this may be found in Freud's Theory of the Unconscious, which depends in part upon the concept of repression.

Repression is best understood if the personality is divided somewhat arbitrarily into id, ego, and superego.

The id is composed of basic instinctual drives and operates on the Pleasure Principle.

The ego describes the portion of the personality that deals with the external world; it is roughly synonymous with self or at least with those aspects of self of which one is more or less aware. The ego operates on the Reality Principle. Ego functioning is influenced by:

1. Impulses from the id
2. Superego
3. Social environment

The superego represents a system of values, including some of the restrictions on instinctual behavior made necessary by society, acquired at an early age by identification with parents, and assimilated into the personality so as to function automatically. The demands of the social environment are most likely to differ from the superego values when the individual:

1. Acquires the superego from socially deviant parents
2. Lives in a rapidly changing society
3. Is socially mobile and moves into a group whose standards differ from those of the parents

The effect of the social environment on the ego is not limited to ways in which instinctual activity is curtailed by social custom and regulation but also includes the actual opportunities or impediments for instinctual satisfaction and the threats to survival within it.

Since multiple forces impinge upon the ego, conflicts occur. Instinctual impulses may be in conflict with one another (e.g., sex and survival — the desire to court a woman whose husband owns a shotgun); instinctual impulses may conflict with superego values; superego values may be in conflict themselves when a situation poses two different problems (e.g., loyalty versus honesty). There are conflicts between environmental demands and all portions of the personality.

Conflict produces discomfort and dysfunction; it is often resolved by excluding one of the conflicting elements from consciousness. This is the process of repression. The mechanism of repression is also used to exclude painful memories from consciousness. The levels of consciousness are as follows:

1. *Conscious:* Awareness of the self and the environment — limited to one thought at a time.
2. *Preconscious:* Thoughts, memories, and impulses which can readily be brought to consciousness.
3. *Subconscious:* Thoughts, memories, and impulses repressed or partly repressed, capable of producing conflict or discomfort, but also relatively capable of verbal representation. Thoughts which are usually subconscious may come into awareness spontaneously under special circumstances.
4. *Unconscious:* Deeply repressed thoughts, memories, and impulses which are essentially incapable of verbal representation and id impulses which have never attained verbal representation.

The removal of an impulse from conscious awareness by repression does not stop its influence on activity. The failure of repression resulting in disturbing thoughts or impulses approaching consciousness is a psychological factor in the production of anxiety. Anxiety is an unpleasant feeling, similar to fear, with many of the physical concomitants of fear. Fear signals an external danger and is proportionate to that danger. Anxiety either has no external cause or is disproportionate to the danger involved. Thus, anxiety is a signal or warning of internal danger.

A number of phenomena are used to aid in the maintenance of repression. These are termed Ego Defense Mechanisms (the terms Mental Mechanisms and Defense Mechanisms are essentially synonymous with this). The primary functions of these mechanisms are:

1. To minimize anxiety
2. To protect the ego
3. To maintain repression

Repression is useful to the individual since:

1. It prevents discomfort.
2. It leads to some economy of time and effort.

In regard to the latter, the exclusion of conflictual material from conscious thought simplifies decision making, since some alternate courses of action are automatically excluded from consideration. This unconscious economy can be illustrated by an analogy to a conscious process, prejudice. (Prejudice is often conscious, though the reasons for it may be outside awareness.) Suppose a man is in a restaurant. He knows that he does not like seafood. There is a part of the menu he need not read; some options he need not consider. The disadvantages of repression include:

1. Interference with rational decision making
2. Complications in living resulting from defense mechanisms used to maintain it
3. Utilization of energy

The last point is based upon the Libido Theory. This theory is less widely accepted than is the Theory of Instincts and the Theory of the Unconscious. Libido is described as the energy associated with the life instinct. This energy is utilized in attaining instinctual goals; that is, portions of it may be "cathected" to the objects by which an instinctual need may be satisfied.

According to the Libido Theory, some of this energy may be diverted in order to maintain repression. The more that is repressed, the less energy there is for goal-seeking activity. It has not been possible to identify and measure the energy component of repression, and the theory remains unproven. However, the concept of repression, per se, and of the defense mechanisms, does not require this particular construct anyway. Ego Defense Mechanisms are:

1. Unconscious (i.e., the person utilizing them is not aware of doing so; however, most of them have conscious analogs).
2. Not in themselves pathological (most of them are used regularly by healthy people; desirable or undesirable consequences depend on the circumstances, manner, and extent of use).

Exceptions to these two generalizations will be noted. A listing of defense mechanisms is an attempt to classify complex patterns of activity. The infinite varieties of human behavior make any classification, by necessity, incomplete. Definitions of various mechanisms overlap. The same observed behavior may apparently be explained by more than one mechanism, and often several mechanisms are used in combination. In addition, the mechanisms may serve other purposes besides the primary ones. Ego Defense Mechanisms include:

Repression

Repression is the involuntary exclusion of a painful or conflictual thought, impulse, or memory from awareness. This is the primary ego defense mechanism; others reinforce it.

Suppression

Suppression is usually classified as an ego defense mechanism, but it is actually the conscious analog of repression; intentional exclusion of material from consciousness. At times suppression may lead to subsequent repression. Examples: (1) A young man at work finds that he is letting thoughts about a date that evening interfere with his duties; he decides not to think about plans for the evening until he leaves work. (2) A student goes on vacation worried that she may be failing; she decides not to spoil her holiday by thinking of school. (3) A woman makes an embarrassing *faux pas* at a party; she makes an effort to forget all about it.

In the first example, suppression was probably a desirable mechanism, since it permitted concentration on work and deferred dealing with plans for the evening until a more appropriate time. In the second instance, suppression would have been undesirable if failing work could have been corrected during vacation or if a realistic appraisal of probable consequences of the school situation would have permitted better planning.

Introjection

Introjection involves the assimilation of the object into one's own ego and/or super-ego. This is one of the earliest mechanisms utilized. The parent becomes almost literally a part of the child. Parental values, preferences, and attitudes are acquired.

Identification

Identification is similar to introjection, but it is of less intensity and complete-ness. It involves the unconscious modeling of one's self upon another person. One may also identify with values and attitudes of a group. Examples: (1) Without be-ing aware that he is copying his teacher, a house officer assumes a similar mode of dress and manner with patients. (2) A school girl wants her mother to buy her the same kind of shoes her classmates are wearing; she angrily rejects the idea that she is trying to be like the other girls and insists that the shoes are truly the best available and the style she has always wanted. Conscious analogs of identification are intentional imitation of others and volitional efforts to conform to a group.

Displacement

Displacement involves changing the object by which an instinctual drive is to be satisfied or shifting the emotional component from one object or idea to another. Examples: (1) A woman is abandoned by her fiance; she quickly finds another man about whom she develops the same feelings. (2) A salesman is angered by his supe-rior but suppresses his anger; later, on return to his home, he punishes one of his children for misbehavior that would usually be tolerated or ignored.

Displacements are often quite satisfactory and workable mechanisms; if one can-not have steak it is comforting to like hamburger equally well. As the March Hare observed, "I like what I have is the same as I have what I like." However, the exam-ple of displaced anger illustrates a situation which, if often repeated, could cause serious complications in the person's life. Conscious acceptance of a substitute with full recognition that it is a substitute for something one wants is an analog of dis-placement.

Aim Inhibition

In aim inhibition a limitation is placed upon instinctual demands; partial or modified fulfillment of desires is accepted. Examples: (1) A person is conscious of sexual desire but finding the desire frustrated "decides" that all that is really wanted in the relationship is companionship. (2) A student who originally wanted to be a physician decides to become a physician's assistant.

Aim inhibition, like the other mechanisms, is neither healthful nor pathologi-cal, desirable nor undesirable in itself. It may be better to have half a loaf than no bread, but an unnecessary aim inhibition may rob one of otherwise attainable satisfactions.

Projection

In projection one's thoughts or impulses are attributed to another person. In com-mon use, the term is limited to unacceptable or undesirable impulses. Examples:

(1) A man unable to accept that he has competitive or hostile feelings about an acquaintance says, "He doesn't like me." (2) A woman denying to herself that she has sexual feelings about a coworker accuses him, without basis, of flirting, and describes him as a "wolf."

This defense mechanism is commonly overutilized by the paranoid.

A broader definition of projection includes certain operations that allow for empathy and understanding of others. Recognition that another person is lonely or sad may be based not upon having seen other examples of loneliness or sadness and learning the outward manifestations, but upon having experienced the feelings and recognizing automatically that another person's situation would evoke them.

Reaction Formation

Reaction formation goes to the opposite extreme; overcompensation for unacceptable impulses. Examples: (1) A man dislikes an employee violently; without being aware of doing so, he bends over backward not to criticize the employee and gives him special privileges and advancements. (2) A person with strong antisocial impulses leads a crusade against vice. (3) A married woman who is disturbed by feeling attracted to one of her husband's friends treats the friend rudely.

Intentional efforts to compensate for conscious dislikes and prejudices are sometimes analogous to this mechanism.

Undoing

Undoing is an act or communication which partially negates a previous one. Examples: (1) Two close friends have a violent argument; when they next meet each acts as if the disagreement had never occurred. (2) Asked to recommend a friend for a job, a man makes derogatory comments which prevents the person's getting the position; a few days later he drops in to see the friend and brings him a small gift.

In a conscious analog of this, Napoleon made it a practice after reprimanding any officer to find some words of praise to say at their next meeting.

Sublimation

In sublimation the force of an instinctual drive is attenuated by using the energy in other, usually constructive, activities. This definition implies acceptance of the Libido Theory; the examples do not require it. Sublimation is often combined with other mechanisms, among them aim inhibition, displacement, and symbolization. Examples: (1) A married man who is dissatisfied with his sex life, but who has not had an extramarital affair, becomes very busy repairing his house while his wife is out of town. Thus, he has no time for social activities. (2) A woman is forced to undertake a restrictive diet; she becomes interested in painting and does a number of still life pictures, most of which include fruit.

The conscious use of work or of hobbies to divert one's thoughts from a problem or from a rejected wish is an analog of this. Sublimation is often a desirable mechanism; however, the consequences may, in addition to preventing instinctual satisfaction, interfere with the person's life in other ways if disproportionate time, money, or effort is used in the activity.

Compensation

Compensation is a mechanism in which encountering failure or frustration in some sphere of activity, one overemphasizes another. The term is also applied to the process of overcorrecting for a handicap or limitation. Examples: (1) A physically unattractive adolescent becomes an expert dancer. (2) An adolescent who as a child was asthmatic becomes a long-distance runner on the track team. (3) Demosthenes, who overcame stuttering to become a great orator.

Rationalization

Rationalization offers a socially acceptable and apparently more or less logical explanation for an act or decision actually produced by unconscious impulses. The person rationalizing is not intentionally inventing a story to fool someone else, but instead is misleading self as well as the listener. Examples: (1) A man buys a new car, having convinced himself that his older car will not make it through the winter. (2) A woman with a closet full of dresses buys a new one because she does not have anything to wear.

Idealization

Idealization is the overestimation of the desirable qualities and underestimation of the limitations of a desired object. Examples: (1) A lover speaks in glowing terms of the appearance and intelligence of an average-looking person who is not very bright. (2) A purchaser having finally decided between two items, expounds upon the advantages of the one chosen.

Note that the first example could include the mechanism of displacement, and the second, rationalization. Up to a point, mutual idealization can make for a happy relationship; however, unrealistic expectations of another person based upon this mechanism can lead to serious disappointment.

Isolation

Isolation is the splitting off of the emotional components from a thought. Example: A medical student dissects a cadaver without being disturbed by thoughts of death. Isolation may be temporary (affect postponement). Examples: A bank teller appears calm and cool while frustrating a robbery, but afterward is tearful and tremulous.

The mechanism of isolation is commonly overutilized by patients with Obsessive Compulsive Disorder and other persons with compulsive personalities.

Denial

Denial is failure to recognize obvious implications or consequences of a thought, act, or situation. Examples: (1) A person having an extramarital affair gives no thought to the possibility of pregnancy. (2) People living near a volcano disregard the dangers involved. (3) A handicapped person plans to return to former activities without planning a realistic program of rehabilitation.

Denial is undesirable when it prevents appropriate action. If denial by a cancer patient interferes with treatment, the patient is harmed, but if only the prospect of death is denied, the benefit and comfort to the patient may outweigh such failures to act as not reviewing one's will. Denial also reduces or eliminates stress in situations in which nothing can be done.

Dissociation

Dissociation is the splitting off of a group of thoughts or activities from the main portion of consciousness; compartmentalization. Example: A politician works vigorously for integrity in government, but at the same time engages in a business venture involving a conflict of interest without being consciously hypocritical and seeing no connection between the two activities.

Some dissociation is helpful in keeping one portion of one's life from interfering with another (e.g., not bringing problems home from the office). However, dissociation is responsible for some symptoms of mental illness; it occurs in hysteria (certain somatoform and dissociative disorders) and schizophrenia. The dissociation of hysteria involves a large segment of the consciousness, while that in schizophrenia is of numerous small portions. The apparent splitting of affect from content often noted in schizophrenia is usually spoken of as dissociation of affect, though isolation might be a better term.

Splitting

Splitting is the dissociation or denial of some elements of a situation, or things about a person, so as to prevent ambivalent feelings. This results in the situation or person being seen as all good or all bad.

This elimination of ambivalence may be an effective defense in some situations in which complete reliance on another person is temporarily necessary, but in most cases splitting is unrealistic and undesirable. Splitting is likely to lead to sudden reversals of attitude. A person who is seen as all good is almost certain at some time or other to do something that offends. In most relationships such a lapse by a person who is viewed positively would be excused, or at most would lead to some slight modification in the attitude toward that person. Where splitting is involved, such a lapse may turn love into hate, respect into contempt. This mechanism, in its pathological form, is common in patients with Borderline Personality Disorder.

Symbolization

In symbolization an object or act represents a complex group of objects and acts, some of which may be conflictual or unacceptable to the ego; or objects or acts stand for a repressed desire. Examples: (1) A solider, asked why he volunteered, says, "To defend the flag." He rejects as irrelevant a question about the purpose of the war. (2) A boy asks for a girl's hand (in marriage).

As in the second illustration, symbolization is often combined with displacement. It is one of the mechanisms usually involved in phobias.

Condensation

Condensation is the reaction to a single idea with all of the emotions associated with a group of ideas; or the expression of a complex group of ideas with a single word or phrase. This mechanism is closely related to symoblization. Examples: (1) A man in a tavern utters a single four-letter word; a fight ensues. (2) A slogan doubles the sale of an otherwise unremarkable detergent.

Complex Formation

In complex formation a number of related or apparently unrelated ideas are associated in the unconscious in such a way that anything which threatens to bring any one of them into consciousness evokes the feeling associated with the entire group. This mechanism is closely related to the mechanisms of symbolization and condensation. Conditioning may also account for some apparent complex formations.

Fantasy

Fantasy involves daydreaming. Daydreams usually represent wishes, but they are not bound by the Reality Principle. They can provide pleasure, escape from the stresses of daily living, a partial gratification of otherwise unattainable desires, and on occasion may contribute to creative activities. Daydreams can be harmful if they occupy a disproportionate amount of time and attention, if they tantalize the person so that he or she becomes tempted to act them out in a detrimental way, or if they become substitutes for real efforts to seek goals. Examples: (1) A man spends much of his spare time daydreaming of being a millionaire, but he neglects to do a small amount of additional work that would win him a modest increase in salary and open the way to further advancement. (2) A girl daydreams about the perfect romance; she refuses to have dates with boys she knows because they do not measure up to her fantasy of the ideal man. (3) A woman with a responsible but relatively routine job sometimes at the end of a busy day reads science fiction stories and imagines exploring the planets. This takes her mind away from the day's problems and she goes to bed relaxed.

The first and second examples show fantasy as a potentially undesirable mechanism; the third as advantageous.

Dreaming

Repressed material appears and conflicts may be worked through in dreams; various mechanisms disguise the content of the dream. Among these are displacement, symbolization, and condensation.

Conversion

In conversion conflicts are represented by physical symptoms involving portions of the body innervated by sensory or motor nerves. This mechanism and somatization are the only ones that are always pathological. Example: A man's arm becomes paralyzed after impulses to strike another are repressed.

Somatization

In somatization conflicts are represented by physical symptoms involving parts of the body innervated by the sympathetic and parasympathetic systems. Example: A highly competitive and aggressive person whose life situation requires that such behavior be restricted develops hypertension.

In addition to the ego defense mechanisms which are unconscious devices that ward off anxiety, a person uses a variety of conscious activities to avoid or cope with anxiety-provoking situations and to lessen feelings of anxiety once they appear.

Ineffectual attempts to meet instinctual needs in a complex society, interference of unconscious processes with successful adaptation, anxiety arising from intrapsychic conflict, the development of maladaptive mechanisms, and the failure of effective ego defense mechanisms are contributing factors in the etiology of some psychiatric disorders.

REVIEW QUESTIONS

1. What is the prevalence of psychiatric impairment in the general population?
2. What is an instinct? What are the components of the life instinct, Eros?
3. What is the Pleasure Principle? The Reality Principle?
4. Would you expect mental illness to be more or less prevalent in lower socio-economic groups? Why?
5. What is the ego? What forces influence its function?
6. How does anxiety differ from fear?
7. How does repression differ from suppression?
8. What do ego defense mechanisms do?
9. Name several common ego defense mechanisms. Define them and give original examples.

SELECTED REFERENCES

1. Akhtar, Salman, and Jessica Price Byrne: The concept of splitting and its clinical relevance. *Am J Psychiatry* 140(8):1013-1016, 1983.

2. Betz, Barbara J.: Some neurophysiologic aspects of individual behavior. *Am J Psychiatry* 126(10):1251-1256, 1979.

3. Cousins, Norman: Denial. *JAMA* (2):210-212, 1982.

4. Freud, Anna: *The Ego and the Mechanisms of Defense.* New York, International Universities Press, 1946.

5. Freud, Sigmund: *The Ego and the Id.* London, Hogarth Press, 1949.

6. Grant, Igor, Joel Yager, Hervey L. Sweetwood, and Richard Olshen: Life events and symptoms. *Arch Gen Psychiatry* 39:598-605, 1982.

7. Gregory, Ian, and Donald J. Smeltzer: *Psychiatry: Essentials of Clinical Practice.* 2nd ed. Boston, Little, Brown, 1983, pp. 1-14.

8. Mullahy, Patrick: *Oedipus Myth and Complex.* New York, Hermitage Press, 1948.

9. The President's Commission on Mental Health: *Report to the President from the President's Commission on Mental Health,* Volume I. Washington, D.C., U.S. Government Printing Office, 1978.

10. Srole, Leo and Anita K. Fisher (Eds.): *Mental Health in the Metropolis: The Midtown Manhattan Study,* revised edition. New York, New York University Press, 1978.

11. White, Robert B., and Robert M. Gilliland: *Elements of Psychopathology: The Mechanisms of Defense.* New York, Grune & Stratton, 1975.

Chapter 2

PERSONALITY DEVELOPMENT

LEARNING TO MEET INSTINCTUAL NEEDS

The ability to meet basic human needs in a complex society is acquired gradually. The child is helpless at birth and is dependent on adults. It is many years before he or she is ready to function as an independent and responsible member of society.

Children are not alike at birth. Heredity and congenital factors influence adaptive capacities. Some of these factors, not yet specifically identified, may partially determine differences in intelligence, temperament, and the intensity of certain internal drives as they influence the functioning of various organs, endocrine glands, and the brain, and as they determine physical strength and stature. However, despite these differences at birth, most children have the capacity for a healthy adaptation to living.

Most mental disorders are not inherited. Some types of mental retardation such as Down's syndrome and the syndromes associated with inborn errors of metabolism (e.g., phenylketonuria) are congenital or inherited. The only adult psychosis that is definitely inherited is the brain syndrome associated with Huntington's chorea.

There is evidence that a predisposition to some other mental illnesses (e.g., Manic and Bipolar Affective Disorders; some Schizophrenic Disorders) may be inherited. This predisposition represents only one factor in the etiology of the illness.

Heredity factors may affect life experiences indirectly (e.g., life will be different for a little girl who inherits a face and figure considered beautiful in her culture than for one not similarly endowed; an inherited alopecia could be a source of embarrassment affecting emotional growth and development).

Not all inherited characteristics are present at birth. Some emerge with general physical maturation. The relation of life experiences to the maturation of certain learning capacities may be important.

The observations of ethology (that branch of biology which studies animals in their natural habitats) offers some interesting possibilities concerning the significance of some very early experiences in life. The process of imprinting is one of

14

these. At an early age, a duckling, for example, will follow a mature duck. A process analogous to identification occurs. The duckling starts to behave as a duck and subsequently relates to ducks. However, if the duckling follows a member of another species, it will apparently identify with that species.

There may be brief periods during maturation in which certain skills (e.g., language, music) are developed very rapidly. If something interferes with acquiring them at the critical age (e.g., an illness) they may never be fully developed.

While heredity and maturation play some part in the acquisition of skill in dealing with the environment, the demands and opportunities of the social environment itself have much to do with the development of successful adaptive patterns. Diagnosable psychiatric disorders together with such related manifestations of maladaptation as delinquency and educational failure are vastly more prevalent in lower socioeconomic groups. Statistically, one's chances of achieving mental health as an adult correlate more directly with socioeconomic status than any other factor. There is reasonable evidence that poverty and a high incidence of mental disorders are not simply coexisting results of constitutional factors. The role of socioeconomic factors in mental health is an important consideration in community mental health planning.

Important as they are, the combination of hereditary and social factors does not alone determine personality structure and adaptive capacity. Much of this is acquired through individual experience, individual learning.

There is much that is not yet known about how learning takes place. Some learning results from trial and accidental success. If something works, one does it again. The model of the conditioned reflex (i.e., Pavlov's experiment in which a dog is offered food at the same time another stimulus, the ringing of a bell, occurs. After a time the dog will salivate at the ringing of the bell even if food is not forthcoming) can be used to account for some learning. An experience that offers pleasure or pain sets up a reaction to associated factors; this, if reinforced by subsequent experiences, produces a conditioned response. Extinction of the response occurs if the anticipated reward ceases to appear, but if rewards are given intermittently the response will continue to occur at a stable rate (e.g., people continue to play slot machines even though the rewards appear at irregular intervals). B. F. Skinner has noted that attention, affection, and approval may act as general reinforcers. His term operant conditioning refers to the process by which spontaneous activities are reinforced (intentionally, as by a parent, teacher, or therapist; or unintentionally).

In an attempt to evaluate factors which may produce deviant behavior, Harlow and others have set up experimental situations with baby monkeys to study the effects of various forms of social deprivation. Isolation or lack of mothering in the first 6 months produces behavioral abnormalities in monkeys similar to those observed in disturbed humans. Interactions between infant monkeys partially compensate for lack of mothering during the critical first few months of life. To what extent inferences about monkey behavior can be applied to human behavior remains to be seen.

There are various other ways of looking at the way character traits develop, coping mechanisms are acquired, and ego defenses established. These various approaches are not necessarily contradictory. Among those who proposed that cultural pressures are of importance in molding the personality, producing conflict and anxiety, and contributing to the etiology of mental disorders were Karen Horney, Erich Fromm, and H. S. Sullivan. Horney proposed that hostile impulses were the main source of neurotic anxiety, and in coping with these hostile impulses, three general ways of reacting could be employed: moving toward, moving against, and moving away from the source or object of the hostility. Fromm felt that the interaction of the child and parent was important in the development of basic attitudes toward other people. He labeled these basic attitudes receptive, exploitative, and hoarding. Sullivan believed that habitual attitudes exhibited in interactions with other people were traits which had met with the approval of significant people in the past, especially in childhood, and he stressed the importance of interpersonal relations in emotional illness and health.

Whatever frame of reference one uses, the psychiatrist and the layman as well agree with the poet Wordsworth, who said, "The child is father of the man," and with the forgotten originator of the proverb "As the twig is bent, so the tree is inclined."

The student of personality development must have a thorough understanding of the normal growth and maturation of the child. One should be familiar with the stages of development, milestones, described by Gesell, and with the intellectual developmental stages described by Jean Piaget, and the characteristics of each.

At 1 to 2 weeks a normally developing infant smiles; at 2 to 4 weeks follows an object with his or her eyes; at 4 to 8 weeks smiles meaningfully at a person ("social smiling"); at 16 to 18 weeks vocalizes; by 6 to 8 months sits; by 9 to 12 months stands; and by 12 to 15 months walks and talks.

Piaget observed four stages in the development of intelligence: a sensorimotor stage, birth to 18 months, which, though preverbal, includes the acquisition of some practical basic knowledge; a preoperational stage, 18 months to 7 or 8 years, with the beginning of organized language; a stage of concrete operations, 7 to 8 through 11 to 12 years, in which thinking is concrete rather than abstract; and a propositional or formal operations phase in which the capacity for abstract thought develops.

Still another aspect of human development which is reviewed in detail because of its continuing direct and indirect influence on contemporary psychiatry is Freud's description of psychosexual development.

PSYCHOSEXUAL OR PSYCHOSOCIAL DEVELOPMENT

The concept of psychosexual development relates to the maturation of the components of the life instinct, Eros, which are involved in reproduction and preservation of the species. It takes into account both a biological sequence of maturative processes and the influence of environmental factors on growth and development.

The meeting of instinctual needs is experienced as pleasurable; the pleasure associated with sexuality is described as erotic. The maturational sequence presumed to occur in psychosexual development is one of shifting erotogenic zones, beginning in infancy at the mouth. According to this concept, the sucking of the infant at breast, bottle, or for that matter, thumb, is properly regarded as sexual. This in no way implies that the infant experiences genital sexual satisfaction from nursing, since the genitals do not become primary erogenous zones until much later in the maturation process.

Evidence for this theory is found in the failure of persons who have marked difficulties in passing through early development phases to acquire adequate adult sexual adjustment. Utilization of various erogenous zones in foreplay and in variant sexual activity, though it may be explained in other ways, is also suggestive of possible validity of the concept.

Alternatively, one may recognize, for example, the infant's pleasure and preoccupation in oral activities, without viewing this as an early stage of the sexual maturation. It is, after all, essential to individual survival. Since difficulties in any area of personality function are likely to interfere with other adjustments, oral problems could interfere with sexual maturation without orality being itself a step in the maturation process.

Accordingly, some psychiatrists prefer a less than literal interpretation of Freudian ideas of psychosexual behavior. If psychosexual is a figure of speech, not a designation of a maturation process, then the term psychosocial is a less ambiguous one. While the implications of the terms psychosexual development and psychosocial development are by no means identical, many observations concerning the stages of development and their consequences are.

STAGES OF PSYCHOSEXUAL DEVELOPMENT

The stages of psychosexual (psychosocial) development generally recognized are:

1. Oral stage
2. Anal stage
3. Phallic stage
4. Latency period
5. Genital stage

The oral stage is sometimes subdivided into a passive (sucking, dependent) stage and an active (biting, aggressive, sadistic) stage. The anal stage may be divided into expulsive and retentive phases. A urethral stage is sometimes described as separate from and prior to the phallic.

CHARACTER DEVELOPMENT, FIXATION, AND REGRESSION

Each stage of development has an influence on the subsequent personality. The precise effect is determined in part by the relative amounts of satisfaction and frustration encountered during each stage. At any time of life and in any sphere of activity, experiences modify expectations. During the experiences in early stages of development, the child learns what to expect from the environment, from other people, and from his or her own activities and efforts. He or she acquires likes and dislikes, and learns to approach certain situations with hope, others with fear, and still others with uncertainty (which is sometimes more uncomfortable even than fear).

In a successful satisfactory sequence of development, the passing of a stage does not end the gratifications associated with it, but they are supplanted in intensity and urgency by those of the next. A specific activity associated with any stage may persist in its original form. This is likely to occur if it has been quite gratifying, even though other gratifications partly take its place, unless it becomes subject to environmental pressure (e.g., "you are too old to do that any more"), or gets involved in conflicts with other instinctual drives or superego values. Modification of the original activity may eliminate the external or internal pressure.

An activity that has led to more frustration than gratification is likely to be dropped, or indeed, reaction formation may cause an activity opposite to the original one to appear. Reaction formation also occurs against gratifying activities if external or internal pressures are too great for modification to permit their being continued.

Fixation

Psychosexual development may be arrested or partially arrested at any stage. This is termed fixation. Fixation sometimes occurs when the activities of a given phase of development are particularly rewarding themselves and are encouraged and prolonged by significant people in the child's environment. Fixation may also occur when experiences in a particular phase of development are relatively unsatisfactory. With some reinforcement by occasional rewarding experiences, the individual continues beyond the normal development period to seek a satisfaction partially denied him or her by environment or circumstances. Dependent upon degree, fixation may prevent satisfactory progress in subsequent developmental periods, or may merely lead to the perpetuation of a number of character traits associated with the developmental period in which the fixation occurred.

Regression

Under stress at any time in life or during development when frustrations are encountered in a developmental phase, one may return to the activities that previously gave greatest satisfaction. This is regression; it may be transitory or prolonged. Example: During physical illness, many people become demanding and dependent. Some degree of regression usually occurs with illness.

THE ORAL STAGE OF DEVELOPMENT

During the first few months of life, goal-directed behavior is largely limited to sucking. In the beginning, the activity is quite passive. The breast or bottle is offered to the infant. The baby indicates hunger by crying, and if fed on a demand or modified demand schedule, learns in time to cry more purposefully and may stop crying before the actual feeding begins if mother's presence and behavior, or if another cue such as the sound of a bottle warmer, announces that food is soon forthcoming.

During feeding, the infant is held and is handled, cuddled, or stroked. This is apparently almost as essential to normal development as is the food itself. Marasmus, a progressive emaciation, has been observed to occur in the absence of other causes in hospitalized infants who are not handled during feeding or otherwise, and is reversed when handling takes place. The nursing infant is passive, dependent, and presumably experiences feelings of security while receiving affection and tenderness.

Frustrations can be encountered during the early oral stage of development. The infant can fail to get enough food (even though there is enough for survival and some growth). There can be mechanical difficulties in nursing, food intolerance, or a lack of some of the physical contact, tenderness, and affection that accompanies normal development at this age.

As the oral stage progresses, more purposeful activity appears. Objects other than food (e.g., toys, the thumb) are put in the mouth. Later, food is taken from a cup or spoon and soon solid foods can be eaten. The child begins to understand a few words, then to speak a little. Before long, a few steps are taken.

As the child becomes more active and gets new gratifications, the first one, sucking at breast or bottle, is lost. The weaning may be gradual or abrupt; it may be a stormy period for the mother and child or may take place easily.

The early efforts at independence, accepting some foods offered and rejecting others, reaching for things that are wanted, attempts at locomotion, and attempts at communication may result in a wide variety of satisfactions and frustrations.

The choices between breast and bottle feeding, between feeding on schedule and on demand, and between relatively early or late introduction of cup feeding, of solid foods, and weaning have some bearing on psychosexual development. However, though their consequences are worthy of consideration, the real questions of importance concerning an infant's progress through this stage of development are:

1. Is eating a satisfying experience? Is there enough food? Is feeding frequent enough to prevent long periods of hunger and discomfort? Is the food well tolerated? Are frustrating mechanical difficulties during nursing and/or cup and spoon feeding avoided?
2. Is eating accompanied by physical contact, feelings of security, and the experience of being treated with affection and tenderness?
3. Is the normal progress from passive dependence to active independence facilitated? Is the infant frustrated by attempts to get him or her to do things beyond his or her physical capacities? Is he or she held back, for example, in efforts at self-feeding, because it is easier and less messy for mother to do the feeding? Is he or she so overprotected as to fail to have the experience of succeeding in overcoming minor difficulties and frustrations?

During the oral phase the infant becomes increasingly aware of the environment; ego function begins to develop in dealing with the environment; the superego begins to develop through introjection and identification. Character traits derived from the oral stage of development include:

1. Those directly related to food intake and the use of the mouth. The infant who has passed through the oral phase comfortably, without marked frustration, fixation, or subsequent regression, will probably always enjoy eating and like a wide variety of foods. Overeating, undereating, peculiar eating habits, and unusual food preferences may stem from difficulties in this period. The attitude toward a variety of mouth activities not directly related to eating itself (smoking; use of coffee, tea, and alcoholic beverages; chewing gum; use of lipstick; kissing; and even talking and singing) are influenced by this stage of development.
2. Those related to infantile dependency, passivity, or early strivings toward autonomy. The healthy person can enjoy having things done for him or her, being taken care of, and depending on others. At the same time there is confidence in the ability to act independently and do things alone. Too great a need to depend on others, or at the opposite extreme, an unwillingness to accept help, may stem from experiences in early infancy.
3. Those associated with physical contact, tenderness, and affection. Feelings about being touched and touching, likes and dislikes for various tactile sensations, and feelings about being in close physical proximity to others are influenced by early experiences. The capacity for giving and receiving affection is affected.
4. Those derived from the total experience of security and comfort in this stage of development. Optimism or pessimism, representing the general expectations one has of the environment, gets a start in early development. Indirectly, the balance between optimism and pessimism has much to do with one's ability to tolerate frustration and with tendencies toward depression. Other expectations of the environment, including ideas of its consistency or predictability, and the influence of one's own behavior upon it and the significant people in it are also acquired early.

In studying character traits it is important to avoid hasty value judgments. Most traits are in themselves neither desirable nor undesirable. Their consequences vary with the degree to which they are present, the circumstances in which they are present, the circumstances in which they become manifest, and the actions they produce. A trait is desirable or undesirable in terms of its contribution, direct or indirect, to satisfaction and security; to meeting basic needs; and to effectiveness in dealing with the environment. A trait that is useful in one situation may be maladaptive in another.

The interrelationship between various character traits from this stage of growth may lead to complex formation, symbolization, and displacement. Examples: (1) An adult who feels insecure or lonely may turn to food or drink for comfort. (2) A feeling of tenderness or affection may be expressed by a gift of food: chicken soup for the sick or candy for the beloved. (3) The executive's dyspeptic grasp for antacid tablets accompanies a reaction formation against dependent needs.

Clinically, events of the oral stage of development are often etiological factors in obesity and anorexia, psychophysiological disturbances of the upper gastrointestinal tract, and some of the Personality Disorders. At times, at least, they contribute to alcohol problems and depressions. A role in the etiology of Schizophrenic Disorders has been postulated.

THE ANAL STAGE OF DEVELOPMENT

As maturation progresses, the chief erotogenic zone ceases to be the mouth. The beginning of the anal stage occurs in the range of time during which the infant acquires some physical capacity to control defecation. In the early phase, pleasure is thought to be associated with the ability to expel feces; this represents an added control over the self and the environment. The fact that adults do not usually regard a soiled diaper with enthusiasm offers the infant a possible means of expressing hostility or resentment.

Parental efforts to train the child to defecate in a designated receptacle at a designated time give the infant one of his or her first experiences with external compulsion, with authority, and, at times, with punishment. Some external compulsion occurs earlier with, for example, efforts at spoon feeding (and the infant may display some reaction to this by blowing food). Soon the infant acquires the ability to retain feces as well as to control expulsion. This provides a way to please or to disturb parents.

Thanks in part to the psychiatric insights of modern society, and in part to diaper services and disposable diapers, many infants go through the anal stage with minimal discomfort. However, efforts at habit training before the infant has the sphincter control to cooperate, unduly prolonged periods of enforced sitting on the potty, or punishments associated with bowel activity are potential sources of difficulty. Parental preoccupation with bowel function (sometimes extending far beyond the normal termination of this stage) can also influence the personality. Character traits derived from the anal stage of development include:

1. Those directly related to bowel function, including attitudes toward defecation, excrement, and rest rooms. A number of slang expressions related to anal function are used to express hostility or disgust; however, there are some that are used to express pleasure. The mouth is more frequently used in adult sexual practices than is the anus; however, anal masturbation and anal stimulation in both heterosexual and homosexual relations is not unusual. Though the buttocks of movie stars are not photographed as often as their breasts, they do not escape attention. The viewer, depending on attitudes acquired early, may be attracted, repelled, ambivalent, selectively inattentive, or disinterested.

2. Those related to neatness, cleanliness, and orderliness. The connection with this stage of development is apparent. Practices of cleanliness may be consistent or inconsistent. A person may be consistently untidy and enjoy it as a way of life (e.g., Pigpen); or may be untidy and feel perpetually guilty about it. One may be neat and find cleanliness a source of pleasure (perhaps there are even housewives as well as advertising executives who can be thrilled by an improved detergent); or may keep clean and tidy out of grim determination and a sense of duty (just as another "duty" is done precisely on time each morning). A person who is made uncomfortable by dirt or clutter in the home may be delighted by getting dirty outdoors or may enjoy finger painting.
3. Those related to time and schedule. This includes attitudes toward promptness, waiting, and completion of tasks by fixed deadlines.
4. Those related to authority and external compulsion. This stage has much to do with whether one can be compliant and conforming, either happily or begrudgingly. It affects the degree to which one resists the demands of others and the nature of resistance, overt or covert.
5. Those related to hostility, aggression, and destructiveness.
6. Those related to money and possessions. This includes stinginess or generosity. There is ample evidence that the attitudes toward money are interrelated with other attitudes derived from the anal stage of development. The usual and probably correct explanation lies in the fact that the feces itself is a material thing which can be given or withheld; that is, the parental demands that the potty be used are more than a little akin to the requests that one gets later in life, say, from the Internal Revenue Service. An alternate and noncontradictory explanation lies in the fact that much required in the handling of money and material possessions is closely related to orderliness and scheduling (keeping budgets and accounts; paying bills and installments when they are due). Also, the person who works to obtain money is often under the authority or subject to the demands of others. At any rate, in the patois, a person who accumulates enough "filthy lucre" has a certain kind of pot full of money.

Clinically, events in the anal stage of development may have some bearing on the development of psychophysiological disorders of the lower gastrointestinal tract, some Personality Disorders, Obsessive Compulsive Disorders, and certain addictions (Substance Use Disorders with dependence).

THE PHALLIC STAGE OF DEVELOPMENT

Shortly after bowel control is established and habit training is completed, the genital organs themselves become the principal erotogenic zone. The child manifests an interest in the sexual organs and becomes aware of pleasurable sensations from them. Curiosity about the sexual organs of other children and of adults of both sexes is present. Tendencies to display the genitals or engage in autoerotic practices meet with varying degrees of parental disapproval, restriction, or punishment.

The Oedipus Situation

The term Oedipus Situation, or Oedipus Complex, refers to the child's presumed sexual attraction to the parent of the opposite sex. (Technically, the term, taken from Sophocles' tragedy, *Oedipus Rex,* which was based on a Greek legend, applies to a boy's sexual feelings toward his mother. In general usage, the term is applied to a girl's feelings toward her father as well, in preference to the less frequently used term, Electra Complex.) The child's curiosity about parents' sexual organs is to a greater or lesser degree rebuffed. Overtly erotic behavior is rebuffed gently by the understanding parent and harshly by the parent who is alarmed by it. The child's tendency to get into bed with the parents encounters some setting of limits by the parent of the opposite sex and by the parent of the same sex as well.

The child may behave in a way which suggests jealousy of the parent of the same sex and competition for the other parent's love and attention. Competing with a grown-up who is larger and more powerful can lead to fear of reprisals or punishments. (Another interpretation of the Oedipal Situation is that it symbolizes the son's rebellion against the strength and authority of the father rather than implying a sexual attraction for the mother). Parental attitudes often may evoke vague or specific feelings of guilt.

The Primal Scene

The phrase primal scene is used to describe the child's first observation of intercourse by the parents, or at least the first observation of this that occurs during the phallic stage. Most children do observe parental intercourse during this stage of development; some because they are still sleeping in the parents' bedroom; others inadvertently or because of curiosity come into the parents' room at the appropriate (or inappropriate?) time. If the man is in the superior position, this together with the movements and facial expression of the person approaching orgasm may be readily misinterpreted as aggressive, i.e., as an attack on the mother by the father. This impression is sometimes augmented by parental quarrels over sex.

Castration Fears

An interpretation of the primal scene as aggressive and/or fears arising from competition with the parent of the same sex contribute to fears of genital injury or loss, spoken of as castration fears. Castration fears may also arise in connection with punishments for autoerotic behavior or frustration of sexual advances by the parent of the opposite sex. A boy's awareness that girls and women do not have penises lends some credence to his fear.

Penis Envy

The little girl may fear genital injury. However, she does not have any basis for fear of losing a penis, though she may get some idea that one has already been taken from her, perhaps as a punishment. She is likely to feel that she lacks something desirable. A tendency of some women to envy men may have its onset in envy of the penis; however, if one rejects the hypothesis of psychosexual maturation in favor of a concept of psychosocial development, one might attribute the early emergence of jealousy of the male to his social role, involving, even in childhood, somewhat greater freedom, than to his anatomical appurtenances.

The little boy may have feelings of inferiority or inadequacy as he compares his penis with those of older siblings and adults.

Resolution of the Oedipal Situation

Sexual desires for the parent, or even the desires to monopolize the parent's attention, are doomed to frustration. Identification with the parent of the same sex, giving up competition, and displacing sexual interest to others, can contribute to the resolution of the Oedipus Situation. However, the subsequent process of maturation itself leads to a lessening of phallic eroticism, and in that sense, one grows out of the Oedipus Situation.

The development of sexual identity, beginning to see oneself as a boy or a girl, progresses rapidly during this stage of development. The attitude toward this role is influenced by events directly related to the phallic stage, but other factors are involved. Parental attitudes toward the child's sex (e.g., a mother's delight in having a little girl or, conversely, her wish that she had a son instead), toward the child as a representative of that sex (e.g., pride in the little girl's being pretty and "so feminine" versus disappointment in her appearance; viewing the son as a real boy or viewing him as a sissy, or worse, because he wants a doll or cries at minor hurt), and the parent's own feelings about being a man or woman, including attitudes toward persons of the opposite sex, all influence a child's feelings about sexual identity. Character traits derived from the phallic stage of development include:

1. Those directly related to sexuality. While the patterning of sexual interest and activities usually takes place in adolescence, some attitudes which govern it develop in this stage. As the oral stage influences the enjoyment of food, the phallic influences the enjoyment of sex. Fears of sexuality and guilt feelings concerning it influence subsequent behavior. The view of sexual activity as affectionate or aggressive is also governed by events during this period.
2. Those related to sexual organs, secondary sex characteristics, and the body generally. These include some traits related to modesty and to exhibitionism. Displaying accomplishments or possessions may be substituted for displaying the body.
3. Those related to sexual identity. This includes the way one feels about being a man or woman, about activities generally associated with one's own sex, and one's attitudes toward persons of the same and of the opposite sex. One may view successful members of the same sex as objects for admiration, identification, and emulation; as dangerous rivals; or even as objects of contempt. Likewise, members of the opposite sex may be viewed as generally desirable, admirable, worthy of respect, potentially dangerous, or a trifle revolting; one may expect them to be warm and affectionate or hostile and punitive.
4. Those associated with competition. Most directly involved are feelings about competing for the attentions of a person of the opposite sex. For example, a boy may be reluctant to ask a popular girl for a date, or he may regard her popularity as a special incentive. The girl who has a pattern of breaking up friends' engagements or marriages may be acting out impulses from the Oedipal Situation. The amount of jealousy, fear, and/or hostility felt for rivals stems from this phase of development. Tendencies to avoid or seek competition with members of the same sex in other spheres represent derivatives of the attitudes toward sexual competition. The extent of feelings of inferiority experienced is also related to events of this period of development.
5. Those derived from sexual curiosity. To some extent this may influence attitudes toward learning, research, and experimentation, exploration, and in general toward the unknown and unfamiliar.

Clinically, events in the phallic stage are believed to play some part in the etiology of Psychosexual Dysfunctions, Paraphilias, homosexuality, Somatoform Disorders, and Anxiety Disorders (with the probable exception of the Obsessive Compulsive Disorders).

THE LATENCY PERIOD

By about the time the child is ready to begin school, the maturing sexual drive enters a period of quiescence. This latency period lasts until puberty. There may be continued curiosity about sex and some sex play, but erotic activities are usually of minimal significance in daily life. Many of the feelings of the phallic stage are repressed.

Childhood masturbation, Oedipal strivings, and the primal scene, together with such knowledge of sexuality as was acquired, are "forgotten": A well-known teacher illustrates these changes with the story of the 10-year-old, the 8-year-old, the 6-year-old, and the 4-year-old child observing the activities of two dogs. The 10 year old says, "They're fighting"; the 8 year old replies, "They're not fighting, they're playing"; the 6 year old says, "They're having intercourse"; and the 4 year old adds, "They're having intercourse, and from behind, too."

Though this is a period in which psychosexual development is at a relative standstill, psychosocial development is not. Experiences in the first years of school influence attitudes toward subsequent education. The child makes rapid progress in learning to interact with others. Preschool children playing together are largely occupied with individual interests; they may share play equipment or fight over a toy, but they do not spend much time in group projects or games. In school the child learns to share, to take turns, to cooperate, to compromise, and to take a part in group and team activities. One also learns to compete as an individual and as part of a team, to play fair, and to follow established rules in competition.

Some efforts have been made in recent years to deemphasize competition in the school room and on the playgrounds so that everyone wins and children do not experience feelings of failure. To an extent this can reduce stress and contribute to a child's having a more positive self-image. On the other hand, if carried to an extreme, it can interfere with learning competitive skills essential in adult life. As an adult, one competes with others for one's mate (unless no one else *wants* him or her) and with other candidates for jobs. One needs to learn to accept both victory and defeat ("you can't win 'em all") without being overwhelmed by either. It is as unfortunate to be unable to be assertive and competitive as it is to be unable to collaborate or to feel a pressure to compete in situations that do not call for competition.

Many factors determine the degree to which the group experiences during grammar school are rewarding or frustrating. These include: character traits derived from earlier developmental stages, intellectual and physical capacities and the rate of their maturation (e.g., poor muscular development and coordination may cause a child to be chosen last or excluded from some playground games), previous experiences in playing with other children, availability of playmates in the neighborhood in addition to those at school, parental attitudes toward playmates, differences in ethnic or cultural background which tend to set the child apart from the group, and the skills of teachers and playground supervisors in helping children acquire competence in group activities. The character traits derived from these experiences include:

1.   Those related to participation in relatively structured social activities, sports, games, and clubs. Variations are encountered in the amount of participation, the energy and enthusiasm accompanying it, satisfaction or dissatisfaction with the amount of participation, the relative emphasis on cooperation or competition in the activities chosen, and the roles taken in groups (e.g., leader, follower, loyal opposition).

2.   Those related to vocational activities. A blending of skills in cooperation, compromise, and competition is necessary in many vocational settings. Some occupations require one skill more than another. The attitudes toward group participation affect vocational aptitudes and interests.

During preadolescence, toward the end of the latency period, the youngster
usually develops a close friendship with a person of the same sex. This peer relationship influences the pattern of subsequent relationships with persons of the
same sex.

THE GENITAL PERIOD

Puberty, the acquisition of secondary sex characteristics, and the beginning of the
capacity for procreation marks the beginning of adolescence and of the genital
phase of psychosexual development. The genital organs again become active erogenous zones. Most boys and some girls begin to masturbate again between the ages
of 11 and 13. An active awareness of sexual attraction to members of the opposite
sex manifests itself. The important events, tasks, and often problems of adolescence include:

1.   Establishing a pattern for adult sexual activity
2.   Choosing an occupation
3.   Emancipating oneself from parents (resolving conflicts over dependence and
independence)
4.   Developing a personal identity

Adolescence is probably more a social phenomenon than a developmental one.
In primitive times children passed quickly from puberty into adulthood. Adolescent
dependence is extended in modern society with the prolongation of education and
the long period between the time one becomes an adult physically and the time
when he or she can actually be independent and self-supporting.

There are three stages of adolescence which overlap and blend together.
They are: early (11-14), middle (15-16), and late (17-18).

1.   Early adolescence is characterized by an increase in sexual drive. Physical
appearance is important during this stage. While in the fifth through the
eighth grade in school new sexual roles are practiced. Initially, the child is
strongly attracted to a member of the opposite sex. This relationship may be
idealized and romanticized. On the other hand, manifestations of sexuality
are often primitive and aggressive (e.g., "goosing," pulling hair, teasing, and
using deletable expletives). Groups begin to form, but they have a chaotic
and ephemeral quality.
2.   Middle adolescence, when one is usually in the ninth and tenth grades, is the
period in which heterosexual roles are practiced. Dating is formalized, as is
social protocol. Group (peer) behavior is intense; not to belong is devastating.
The adolescent will assume a negative identity (biggest "acid head," class
clown, drop-out, etc.) rather than have no identity at all. In the adolescent's
social environment there are various peer groups with which he or she may
affiliate and identify. Adolescents recognize and stereotype these groups.
They vary from time to time and from setting to setting. Though some, such
as the studious and conforming "straights" and the athletically oriented
"jocks," are relatively enduring, at a given place and time one may or may not
find "freaks," "angels," "Valley girls," or "punks." For a current local listing

and descriptive profiles, consult any alert adolescent. Group participation helps the adolescent find an identity separate from the parentally prescribed one and makes it possible to challenge and question the values of adult society. This stage terminates about the time one get's a driver's license (an important puberty rite in our society).

3. Late adolescence is the period in which an autonomous identity separate from parents and adaptable to the adult world is acquired. Vocational choice becomes important. Adolescents frequently change their vocational plans; however, this is rarely a problem if the youth continues to follow an educational program compatible with a variety of career choices within his or her capacity (taking into account intellectual, physical, and personality factors). Parental pressure to choose a career incompatible with interests or abilities can create serious problems. Loneliness, as one moves away from the peer groups, can be a problem if a partner is not found. Romances occur and sometimes end stormily with feelings of depression and suicidal thoughts. Separation and individuation may progress smoothly as the adolescent begins to be away from home more, possibly to earn more of his or her own spending money, and to make more independent decisions. This is facilitated as parents show appropriate confidence in the young person's judgment and impose fewer rules and restrictions. However, dependence-independence conflicts can be manifested by arguments with parents or runaway behavior. Alcohol or other drug misuse can be used to flout parental authority as well as to establish an identity.

Character traits derived (in part) from adolescent experiences include:

1. Those related to adult sexual activity. This includes the degree to which one is able to find a suitable object for satisfaction of the sexual drive in a member of the opposite sex. In terms of Libido Theory, success lies in the outward direction of libido and its cathexis to an appropriate sexual object, the marriage partner. Libido may be partly or totally directed toward the self. (The term *narcissism,* derived from the Greek legend of the youth who fell in love with his own reflection, is applied to this.) Libido may be directed toward a parent, with failure to resolve a reactivated Oedipus Complex. (Usually, aim inhibition and other repressive mechanisms conceal its true nature; e.g., the girl who cannot marry because she has to stay home and keep house for her widowed father, a healthy business executive who would likely marry his secretary if he could get his daughter "out of his hair.") Libido may be directed to a member of the same rather than the opposite sex, or may find outlet in deviant sexual activity. Factors in the choice of a mate, the roles occupied by marriage partners, and the patterns of marital and extramarital sex behavior are influenced.

2. Those related to vocational adjustment, including career preferences, ambitions, and job satisfaction.

3. Those related to emancipation from parental control and assumption of adult responsibilities. The traits and attitudes derived from this stage of development tend to enhance or modify the attitudes toward dependence and independence developed in the oral phase and the attitudes toward authority formed in the anal phase.

BEYOND ADOLESCENCE

Though the stages of development beginning in infancy and culminating with the resolution of adolescent conflicts prepare one for the assumption of adult roles (vocational, marital, and parental), the experiences in assuming these roles as a young adult further shape the personality. One has a new occupational peer group with its values and expectations. One relates to supervisors and employees, and to a spouse. Techniques that have been effective with previous groups and individuals are used and mechanisms of displacement and projection are employed, but these new relationships are different from the old and can modify existing character traits or contribute to the development of new ones.

The successes and failures of early adult life contribute or detract from one's sense of security and self-esteem. This leads to changes in the need for various defense mechanisms. In middle life, some of the pressures encountered by the young adult in getting and holding employment, making a home, and raising children are reduced, and if one has achieved some of one's occupational goals, obtained a degree of financial security, and raised one's family, one begins to have more time for new activities and relationships. On the other hand, one may encounter midlife crises with feelings of loss of purpose and that one's energies have been misdirected.

As one, reluctantly or otherwise, becomes a senior citizen, one finds one has new roles and new problems in living (among the greatest of these are the identity problems, along with the economic problems, associated with retirement). If health is maintained, sexual activity continues into late life, though opportunities for its expression may be reduced. However, the intensity of the sex drive is often reduced. New concerns about sexual function and attractiveness replace some of the conflicts of earlier life.

For better or worse, character traits and the ways that defense mechanisms manifest themselves continue to change. Too often, if the older person fails to find new interests and to receive intellectual stimulation, a contraction of the personality with a narrowing of interest occurs. This is by no means an inevitable manifestation of aging.

INTERRELATIONSHIPS BETWEEN
DEVELOPMENTAL STAGES

The transition from each stage of psychosexual development to the next is gradual. Even in the absence of significant fixation or regression the experiences at each level influence subsequent levels. Thus, the personality evolves gradually. Attitudes from earlier stages influence the way the experiences of subsequent stages are perceived. For example, the optimism or pessimism resulting from the oral stage and the attitudes toward authority derived from the anal stage influence the way the child reacts to efforts of parents to curb sex play during the phallic stage. Also, behavior patterns, major and minor, from each stage of development, modify the way the child is treated by others. For example, a child who has a capacity for giving and receiving affection will as a result of his or her behavior be treated differently by significant adults than one who does not.

Traits derived from different stages blend and combine in various ways. They govern to a large extent the choice of adaptive patterns by which the individual seeks to meet basic instinctive goals. Adults have traits derived from each stage, but in many persons, traits from one stage or another predominate, so that one may speak of the "oral character," the "anal character," etc. These may represent highly adaptive personality patterns or maladaptive ones.

Some of the interests and desires from each stage of development must subsequently be inhibited, modified, or given up, and this, both as it occurs from environmental pressure and from the development of the superego, requires repression and the development of the ego defense mechanisms. As the child leaves the passive oral stage he or she must give up the desire to suck the breast, and later, even the desire to suck the thumb; still later, any pleasure in playing with feces must be abandoned, and then some of the desires of the phallic phase must be driven from awareness.

The developmental stages described should not be taken too literally. They are constructs, and as such are helpful in understanding the evolution of behavior. Practically every author who has studied personality development since Freud has introduced his or her own list of developmental stages. Among the more helpful of these are the ones described by Sullivan and those described by Erik Erikson. Each of these authors recognized, as Freud apparently did not, that growth and development goes on throughout life. Though much of one's personality is developed in the first few years of life, personality is never completely static.

Sullivan's stages are: infancy (birth to the appearance of articulate speech), childhood (up to the need for compeers), the juvenile era (up to the period of chum relationships), preadolescence (to puberty), early adolescence, and late adolescence.

Erik Erikson described eight developmental stages, in each of which there is a psychosocial crisis: (1) oral sensory (basic trust versus mistrust), (2) muscular-anal (autonomy versus shame and doubt), (3) locomotor-genital (initiative versus guilt), (4) latency (industry versus inferiority), (5) puberty and adolescence (identity versus role confusion), (6) young adulthood (intimacy versus isolation), (7) adulthood (generativity versus stagnation), and (8) maturity (ego integrity versus despair).

INFLUENCE OF SPECIFIC EXPERIENCES
AT VARIOUS LEVELS OF DEVELOPMENT

There are some events which are not directly related to psychosexual maturation but which may influence it. These can occur at any stage of development. They include:

1. Maternal absences
2. Birth of sibling(s)
3. Deaths in the immediate family
4. Individual traumatic experiences

Maternal Absences

The absence of the mother for a period of days or weeks is likely to be disturbing to the small child. Absences may result from vacations, illnesses, or other reasons. Before the child has sufficient ability to grasp verbal communications concerning reasons for absence and anticipated return, and a concept of time so as to know when to expect the parent's return, the absence of the parent may be viewed as an abandonment. One would expect this to have the greatest impact during the oral stage. However, guilt feelings concerning rebellion against authority in the anal stage as well as guilt feelings from the phallic stage may complicate the child's reaction to absences in these later periods. The duration of absences, previous experience with brief absences (a 3-day absence would be less likely to affect a working mother's child who has learned early that mother goes away and comes home after a time than it would for a child who had never been separated from the mother for more than an hour or so), character development prior to the time of absence, and whether or not the child is well cared for during the absence and has familiar people around would all modify the possible impact of absences.

There is some evidence that such absences may have some bearing on later feelings of insecurity, fears of abandonment, and tendencies toward depression.

Personality Development 29

Birth of Siblings

A sibling arriving during the early stages of development probably involves a period of maternal absence beyond the comprehension of the child. Then, when the mother returns, there is a loss of attention. To some degree, one would expect the sibling to be blamed for this, and would expect rivalry to occur. Some regression often occurs; e.g., the newly-weaned child wants the bottle again, or the child who has been trained to use the potty begins to soil. Changes in feeding patterns, new steps in habit training, moving the child out of the parents' bedroom, or other changes in the child's routine are best undertaken well before or considerably after the new baby arrives. Setting aside times for the child to receive undivided attention is also helpful.

Deaths in the Immediate Family

The small child does not understand death nor the reaction of others to it. If there have been hostile feelings to the person who dies, guilt feelings may be experienced. One may even believe that thoughts or wishes caused the death. The permanent loss of either parent by death or otherwise creates some problems in working through the phallic and subsequent stages of development. This may influence character development in a variety of ways, but apparently in itself does not predispose to maladjustment in adult life except as a contributing factor in some depressions.

Individual Traumatic Experiences

A variety of frightening or hurtful experiences may occur. These may create feelings of insecurity or cause particular complex formations. On the basis of material obtained from patients, it was at one time thought that sexual experiences, often assaults by adults, were frequently significant in the etiology of those mental disorders then known as neuroses. However, many of these "memories" are spurious and result from fantasies and distortions of feelings experienced in the phallic stage. A single traumatic experience may leave its mark, but recurring frustrations and recurring unsatisfactory experiences in association with certain settings or types of activities are likely to have more profound results.

REVIEW QUESTIONS

1. Name the phases of psychosexual development.
2. What is the difference between fixation and regression?
3. What is a normally developing child able to do at 4 weeks of age? At 8 weeks? At 24 weeks?
4. What character traits would you expect to be derived from the anal stage of development? Give original examples.
5. What character traits would be expected to be derived from the phallic stage of development? Give original examples?
6. What major problems are common in adolescence, and how does the outcome of attempts to solve them affect the adult personality?

7. What effects do later stages of development have on the character traits derived from early life?

SELECTED REFERENCES

1. Blos, Peter: *On Adolescence.* New York, Free Press of Glencoe, 1962.

2. Chittenden, Edward A.: Piaget and elementary science. *Science and Children* 8(4):9-17, 1970.

3. Erikson, Erik: *Childhood and Society.* New York, Norton, 1963.

4. Erikson, Erik: *Identity, Youth, and Crisis.* New York, Norton, 1968.

5. Harlow, H. F., and M.K. Harlow: Social deprivation in monkeys. *Sci Am,* November, pp. 136-146, 1962.

6. Hollingshead, A. B., and F. C. Redlick: *Social Class and Mental Illness.* New York, Wiley, 1958, pp. 194-250, 357-382.

7. Knoblock, Hilda, and Benjamin Pasamanick, (Eds.): *Gesell and Amatruda's Developmental Diagnosis.* 3rd ed. New York, Harper & Row, 1974.

8. Kolb, Lawrence C, and H. K. H. Brodie: *Modern Clinical Psychiatry.* 10th ed. Philadelphia, Saunders, 1982, pp. 58-79.

9. Lidz, Theodore: *The Person: His and Her Development Through the Life Cycle.* 2nd rev. ed. New York, Basic Books, 1976.

10. McKinney, William T.: Primate social isolation. *Arch Gen Psychiatry* 31(3):422-426, 1974.

11. Mullahy, Patrick: *Oedipus, Myth and Complex.* New York, Hermitage Press, 1948.

12. Neugarten, Bernice L.: Time, age, and the life cycle. *Am J Psychiatry* 136(7): 887-894, 1979.

13. Piaget, Jean: *The Origins of Intelligence in Children.* Translated by Margaret Cook. New York, International Universities Press, 1952.

14. Piaget, Jean: The relationship of affectivity to intelligence in the mental development of the child. *Bull Menninger Clin,* 26:129-137, 1962. Reprinted in S. I. Harrison and J. F. McDermott: *Childhood Psychopathology: An Anthology of Basic Readings.* New York, International Universities Press, 1972, pp. 167-175.

15. Vaillant, George E., and Eva Milofsky: Natural history of male psychological health: IX. Empirical evidence for Erikson's model of the life cycle. *Am J Psychiatry* 137(11):1348-1359, 1980.

16. Wilson, Edward O.: *On Human Nature.* Cambridge, Massachusetts, Harvard University Press, 1978.

17. Zegans, Leonard S.: An appraisal of ethological contributions to psychiatric theory and research. *Am J Psychiatry* 124(6):729-739, 1967.

Chapter 3

PSYCHIATRIC EXAMINATION

THE NATURE OF THE PSYCHIATRIC
EXAMINATION AND THE INTERVIEW SITUATION

Most patients who consult psychiatrists do so voluntarily in hope of obtaining relief from troublesome symptoms or help in solving personal problems. When a patient is seen for other reasons (e.g., an examination for insurance or legal purposes) or has not personally sought help (e.g., a patient on a general medical ward whose physician suspects that emotional problems are contributing to another illness) modifications of the usual examination procedures may be necessary.

The fact that a patient elects to see a physician about personal problems rather than someone else (e.g., a friend, bartender, social worker, or minister) implies that the patient believes that he or she may be sick, or at least that the problems are health related. This imposes certain obligations on the doctor (e.g., differential diagnosis) that a psychologist in a counseling bureau, for example, might not have. To fulfill these obligations, the physician must take a history and perform other examinations similar to those done for patients with other types of illness. Nevertheless, the physician must remember that *the patient is not there to be examined, but to be helped.*

The interview consists of the patient communicating personal information so that the examiner can understand the nature and extent of the problems, make a tentative diagnosis, and reach conclusions which lead to recommendation of a course of action.

Whenever possible the interview is conducted in privacy. The room should be arranged so that the patient (and the examiner) can be comfortable. Things that the patient might need during an interview (e.g., a box of tissues; an ashtray) should be in easy reach. Chairs are arranged so that the patient can make eye contact easily, but can also avoid it. Because of some associations which one may have with such an arrangement, interviewing across a desk is best avoided. Some people feel trapped and uncomfortable in any room from which an abrupt departure would be difficult or awkward; accordingly, the examiner's chair should be located so as not to appear to block the exit.

After introducing oneself, one may begin by asking the patient the reason the appointment has been requested, or focusing on the expectation of benefit, one may ask, "What can I do for you?" If the patient has already given the reason for the appointment when he or she called to arrange it, or if information has been received from the person who referred the patient, the interview can begin with a brief summary of what one understands the purpose of the interview to be together with a request for verification. Example: "Dr.____ told me you have recently been having marital problems which have caused you to be depressed. Is this correct?" This allows the patient to disagree or redefine the problem in his or her own words. Following this opening, the patient is asked to explain the problem, including: onset, duration, frequency, intensity, fluctuation (daily, weekly, monthly), what makes it worse (better), what solutions have been attempted or considered (including any recommendations that have been rejected), and what other symptoms or problems are being experienced.

Though the examiner may wish to take some notes during the interview, detailed note-taking is best avoided. Note-taking may interfere with the spontaneity of an interview, cause the patient to slow down and dictate, or cause the patient to have concern about personal things becoming a matter of record. Also, it is difficult to take legible notes and observe the patient at the same time. One may, however, want to jot down significant factual information which might be difficult to recall accurately such as dates, amounts of medication that have previously been used, or the exact order in which a sequence of events occurred.

After the presenting complaint and present illness is discussed, the examiner directs the interview toward the past life of the patient. Example: "Now that we have discussed the present problem, in order to understand it better, I need to know about your past life, beginning with date and place of your birth, and giving your life history or autobiography up to the present time."

As the patient proceeds with this, or after it is finished, one may supplement the spontaneous biographical sketch with specific questions so that one may have an adequate grasp of the patient's background and life history. Past difficulties are identified but are not explored in depth at this point unless this is really necessary for differential diagnosis or treatment planning. In questioning about potentially embarrassing subjects it is important to observe the patient's level of anxiety and to phrase questions tactfully.

At the end of the interview the examiner should be prepared to summarize what he or she has been told, and to make recommendations for further studies or treatment, if indicated, or for a course of action that a patient may undertake in dealing with the problem. It is important that the patient understand what is being recommended and why the recommendation is being made, and the examiner should know whether or not the patient concurs in the recommendation and will follow it, or if not, what the reasons for this are.

ORGANIZING THE PSYCHIATRIC HISTORY

Though the skilled interviewer asks questions systematically and in logical sequence, the information obtained during history-taking is usually somewhat disorganized. The patient has been given the opportunity to describe symptoms and problems in his or her own way, and to furnish biographical materials spontaneously. The information furnished is often not in chronological sequence. Frequently the examiner must deviate from a systematic line of questioning to follow up something the patient has introduced about another subject. Neglecting to follow such leads can result in failure to obtain clinically important information. After the examination, one reorganizes this information together with one's observations, following a standard form. This helps in diagnosis and in arriving at an understanding of the patient as a person, and it serves as a temporary medical record. How much is then placed in permanent hospital, clinic, or office records depends on several factors.

Hospitals strive for simplified records and may use specific outlines, or even check lists, if records are computerized. Also, in preparing permanent records, one remembers that these may be subpoenaed in court proceedings, that a patient may exercise the right to see the chart, and that there are other situations in which records are not solely for the use of the physician and staff. Some information which is helpful in understanding a patient and in case formulation, but is not necessary for diagnosis and treatment planning may be excluded for these reasons. For example, anecdotal material about persons who play a part in the patient's life may not need to be included in the permanent record unless directly related to the illness.

Examining the psychiatric patient is not basically different from examining other medical patients. As a matter of fact, any complete medical examination includes a mental status examination in abbreviated form. The usual recording procedure for the psychiatric examination includes noting the chief complaint, history of the illness, past history, family history, mental examination, and general physical examination.

The chief complaint is recorded briefly, usually in the form of a quotation except when paraphrasing makes the meaning more clear.

For the history of present illness, the examiner organizes the history elicited from the interview in chronological sequence and discusses the significant features, e.g., onset, duration, frequency, etc. In preparing this section, the description of the problem is placed in a logical sequence so that a person unfamiliar with the patient can understand the situation. Next, the past history is recorded as follows:

1. Birth and early development
2. Childhood (age 5 to puberty)
3. Adolescence
4. Adult life

Concerning birth and early development, one records available information including the date and place of the patient's birth; whether there were siblings and, if so, the patient's place in the birth order; any complications in pregnancy or delivery that the patient has been told occurred; health as an infant; whether breast or bottle fed, and whether there were feeding problems; and any developmental difficulties or signs of emotional distress that the patient recalls or believes to have occurred from what she or he has been told, such as difficulties in toilet training, delay in walking or talking, head banging, temper tantrums, nightmares or night terrors, and any other signs of nervousness that may have been noted. Some examiners make a point of recording the patient's two or three earliest recollections in the belief that these may sometimes provide significant clues about the patient's personality structure.

About childhood, one records information about school adjustments, peer interaction, and relationships with siblings and parents. The examiner also notes special problems such as enuresis (bed-wetting), encopresis (soiling), school phobia, nightmares, or sleepwalking. The record should also include significant events that the patient recalls from this stage of development, and whether these events are recalled as pleasant or unpleasant. Events such as a move from one town to another, the birth of a sibling, an illness, the illness of a family member, a change in the parent's economic circumstances, or a marriage or divorce in the family are recorded in chronological order, and any apparent correlation with changes in the patient's adjustment is noted.

During adolescence most patients experience some turmoil. Included here is: peer group behavior, school performance, authority conflicts (with parents; with police), sexual behavior, drug history, vocational experiences, and outside interests (music, sports, etc.).

Experiences in adult life are also recorded in chronological order and, in addition to illnesses and to events which the patient has stressed as being particularly important in his or her life, one makes note of any further education obtained after adolescence, experiences in and reactions to military service, job changes, including reasons why they were made, and the development (and severance) of close relationships, including love affairs and marriages.

In taking the history, one has inquired about the extent of the use of various chemical substances, including prescription medicines, nonprescription medications, alcohol, and other drugs used for nonmedical purposes. Details concerning any significant use of alcohol or other drugs are noted even if this has no apparent bearing on the presenting complaint. One notes the circumstances under which the substance was first used, quantities, frequency, apparent effects, and, if the use of the psychoactive drug has been discontinued, the time that this occurred and the circumstances. This information may be introduced chronologically in the history or summarized separately.

Likewise, information about sexual history beginning with the patient's first awareness of sexual feelings, sex instruction, and various types of sexual feelings and activities has been elicited and may be recorded in chronological sequence or as a separate section of the history.

Next, the family history is recorded, including the medical and psychiatric history of the parents, grandparents, uncles, aunts, siblings, spouse, and children. Though many medical histories record only the causes of death of deceased relatives and the health status of the living, the psychiatric history usually includes some description of the personalities of significant family members as perceived by the patient. The education and occupation of significant family members may also be relevant.

THE MENTAL STATUS EXAMINATION

The mental status examination is the objective recording of the observations the examiner has made concerning the patient. One usually does not perform a mental examination as a separate procedure. Most observations are made during history-taking, and when one needs to ask specific questions or perform tests they are introduced in context of the interview (e.g., "Along with your nervousness, have you noticed any trouble with memory? Just to make sure, let me ask a few questions to test your memory"). There are numerous ways to record the mental status examination. The following outline method is often used.

1. *General Appearance, Attitude, and Behavior:* It is not easy to describe a person's appearance in two or three sentences without using vague or stereotyped language or introducing value judgments, but such a description, with well-chosen adjectives, is essential. Ordinary language is usually more effective in conveying the picture of the patient than is technical jargon. The description, of course, includes facial expression and grooming. After describing the patient, one makes note of the attitude toward the examination and the examiner (e.g., hostile, suspicious, friendly, ingratiating). Is the patient

courteous? Cooperative? Is attention easily gained and retained, or is the patient distractable? At this point, and throughout the mental examination, one does not attempt to explain what one observes nor is an attempt made to indicate its relevance to the illness. These explanations and inferences are recorded later as a part of a formulation.

While noting the patient's attitude toward being examined may later be helpful in assessing the validity of certain portions of the history and subjective data from the patient that figures in the mental examination, the patient's prevailing attitudes toward life and toward significant people (e.g., optimism, pessimism, cynicism) should also be noted because of their possible bearing on the illness.

One notes the amount of motor activity, mentioning decreased activity or psychomotor retardation, restlessness, hyperactivity, or agitation, if present. One also notes gestures, mannerisms, tics (brief, recurrent, small movements which are apparently involuntary and inappropriate), athetoid movements (irregular, slow, apparently purposeless movements which seem to follow a pattern), posturing, cerea flexibilitas (the waxy flexibility of the catatonic states in which a patient will maintain unnatural postures in which he or she has been placed), echopraxia (the pathological repetition of movements made by others), or any other unusual motor activity. It is more important to describe what one observes accurately than to label it with the correct (?) technical term.

Lastly, one records outward signs of anxiety such as tremor, hyperhidrosis (excessive perspiration), pupillary dilatation, apparent tension or startle reaction (e.g., jumping at a slight noise or an unexpected movement).

2. *Stream of Mental Activity:* Note the amount of spontaneous speech, indicating if it is overproductive or underproductive. Then indicate if the reaction time in replying to specific questions is quicker or slower than average and state whether replies are relevant, coherent, logical, and reach goal ideas. Describe or give examples of anything unusual about the speech or stream of thought, including speech defects; blocking (a sudden interruption of speech or train of thought usually resulting from unconscious factors); mutism (refusal or inability to speak); echolalia (meaningless repetition of words spoken by the examiner); perseveration (involuntary repetition of the answer to a previous question in response to a new question); neologisms (new words formed to express symbolic or condensed ideas; neologisms must be differentiated from technical words, slang, and other words with which the examiner may not be familiar); looseness of associations or derailment (a loss of continuity and speech in which the patient seems to move from one subject to another in a haphazard, disconnected, unrelated manner); flight of ideas (rapidly skipping from one idea to another in a series of ideas which appear to have some continuity though connecting links are missing); rhyming; punning; rambling; circumstantiality, or failure to reach goal ideas.

3. *Affect and Mood:* Affect is the feeling tone accompanying expressed ideas, while mood refers to a more pervasive overall emotional state. In this portion of the mental examination one records both subjective material from the patient (e.g., what is said in response to such questions as "How are you feeling?", "How are your spirits?", or "To what extent are you troubled by feelings of depression?") and the examiner's own observations of how the patient appears to feel. Tone of voice, facial expression, and posture may reveal mood. One tries to determine whether the range of emotion the patient experiences is broad or restricted. One indicates whether the prevailing mood is depressed, and, if so, to what extent, within normal limits, or elevated. The normal mood shows some fluctuation in the course of an interview, but frequent

marked fluctuations are noted as lability of affect. The term flatness of affect is applied when no fluctuations are observed; though this term could be applied to a depressed or elevated mood that remained constant, in customary use it is restricted to an apathy or apparent lack of feeling.

One notes specific emotions that may accompany certain ideas (anger, amusement). One also notes any inappropriate affect or apparent dissociation of affect from content (appearing sad when discussing a pleasant occurrence; laughing when discussing a misfortune; expressing anger when reporting something someone said which was apparently a compliment). A specific type of inappropriate affect sometimes seen is la belle indifference (a bland attitude toward symptoms and disability produced by them) frequently seen in Conversion Disorders. (Example: An attractive 20-year-old woman who is suddenly paralyzed from the waist down does not appear depressed or express concern about her future, but instead discusses her situation in a cheerful and unconcerned manner.)

4. *Thought Content:* Under the heading Thought Content one may record some of the patient's major preoccupations. One also records any abnormal types of thought content such as phobias (intense unrealistic fears), obsessions (recurring unwanted thoughts which cannot voluntarily be excluded from consciousness), compulsions (repetitive unwanted urges to perform some act or engage in some type of behavior; recurring irresistible impulses), hallucinations (false sensory perceptions without external stimulus), illusions (distorted perceptions), delusions (false beliefs that are not amenable to logical persuasion nor a part of the person's culture) or ideas of reference (incorrect interpretation of incidents as having reference to one's self such as observing other people talking and believing that one is being talked about; believing without cause that something a minister says in a sermon is a personal criticism; or seeming to find a personal message in a television program).

If, in evaluating affect and mood, one has noted depression or elation, one indicates whether there is concomitant ideational content. One indicates whether a depressed person has guilt feelings, ideas of unworthiness, feelings of hopelessness, and to what extent thoughts of suicide are present. If elation is noted, one indicates whether grandiose ideas are expressed.

Sometimes one encounters thought content which may or may not be pathological or which one does not know quite how to categorize. In that case it is best to give illustrative examples. If someone claims to be the Messiah, you are fairly safe in calling it a delusion, but if someone claims to be the guru of a prominent political figure, it might be best merely to record the statement without labeling (or libeling?) it as delusional pending further information. If someone hears a song about "the old masterpainter" as "the old masturbator" one may not be sure whether this is an illusion or an idea of reference.

As in recording an evaluation of mood, recording of thought content includes both objective material from the patient and one's clinical observations. A patient may express abnormal thought content spontaneously, or only in response to specific questions. On the other hand, a patient may deny the presence of a particular symptom, but the examiner may nevertheless have reason to believe that it may be present. In that case, one records the questions that were asked, the answers, and the observations that gives rise to the doubt. In asking about delusions, one may ask if the patient has experienced delusions or anything that other people regarded as delusional (if it is reasonable to believe that the word would be in the patient's vocabulary), or one may ask about imagination or unusual mental experiences. In asking about hallucinations, one may use the word itself, or may ask about whether one had ever had the experience of hearing or seeing things that were unreal or that other people did not hear or see (questions such as "What are the voices saying to you?" are best avoided, since, at the least, they are likely to be offensive to patients who are not hallucinating and, at worst, they may be anti-therapeutic in that they imply that the examiner "believes in" voices). A patient may deny hallucinations but appear to be listening to something and/or may appear to be talking to himself. While one certainly cannot categorize such behavior as being proof that the patient is hallucinating, it should be described.

5. *Sensorium and Mental Capacity:* In recording observations about sensorium and mental capacity, it is important to indicate whether these are based solely upon the interview or whether a detailed sensorium examination has been done, which is necessary only if the history or symptoms suggest the possibility of an organic mental disorder. One notes whether the patient is oriented to time, place, and person (knows the date, where one is, and to whom one is speaking). One indicates whether the patient's intelligence is apparently within normal limits (based on vocabulary, grasp of concepts, and problem solving ability). If a brief oral or pencil and paper screening test of intelligence is used (as one might if there appeared to be a discrepancy between the patient's apparent intellectual functioning and past attainments, or if one suspected mental retardation), the name of the test and the result is indicated. One notes any apparent difficulty in recollection and immediate recall (remembering something that one has just been told), recent memories (events in the few days prior to examination), or remote memory. One may check the patient's ability to read and understand a test paragraph or a newspaper clipping and may obtain a sample of handwriting. Simple arithmetical ability may be checked. One may also test the number of digits a patient can recall, forward and in reverse, and may evaluate the ability to maintain a mental set by doing serial additions or subtractions. Whether the patient's thinking tends to be concrete or abstract and whether there is a capacity for good conceptual thinking may be apparent from the interview or may be tested by asking the patient to interpret a series of proverbs or give the similarities and differences between various objects. One may also wish to comment on the patient's fund of general information.
6. *Insight and Judgment:* Insight refers specifically to the extent to which the patient recognizes that he or she is ill, and generally to one's degree of self-understanding. Judgment includes the ability to make a critical assessment of various possible courses of action and make a prudent choice among them. It can be impaired by difficulties in processing information, by impulsivity, or by a variety of other factors, including low self-esteem. One can assess this quality on the basis of the ways in which the patient deals with various problems in living, or may evaluate responses to a series of test situations. If test questions are used, note both the patient's responses and his or her reasons for choosing them.

PSYCHOLOGICAL TESTING

A variety of standardized tests and rating scales may be used to supplement clinical evaluation. Some of these are useful in diagnosis, others in treatment planning, and others simply help give one a better understanding of the patient's personality. There are a number of tests and rating scales that are relatively easy to administer and score. Some of these have only limited validity but may still be of use for screening purposes. They may help identify a need for more elaborate testing. There are some pencil and paper tests which patients may do while awaiting an appointment and which can be scored by clerical personnel or be sent away for scoring. There are other verbal tests that the clinician may do during the examination, if they appear indicated.

Other tests require special training and skill in administration, scoring, or interpretation. The psychiatrist should have a thorough familiarity with a number of these, and the primary physician should know the uses and limitations of the more commonly used ones. These tests should be administered, scored, and interpreted by or under the direction of a qualified clinical psychologist. A qualified clinical psychologist will usually have a doctoral degree from a graduate training program in clinical psychology approved by the Education and Training Board of the American Psychological Association and have had an internship in clinical psychology, board certification by the American Board of Professional Psychology, licensure or certification in the state in which he or she practices, and listing in the National Register of Health Service Providers in Psychology.

The four types of tests most widely used are:

1. Intelligence tests
2. Tests for organic brain impairment
3. Projective tests
4. Personality inventories

Intelligence Tests

Intelligence tests attempt to measure the basic intellectual capacities and problem-solving abilities of the individual. Despite attempts to measure basic intelligence, these tests are influenced to a greater or lesser degree by cultural background and educational opportunities. One of the problems in evaluating intelligence lies in its definition. It is sometimes facetiously defined as that quality measured by a standard test of intelligence. It is the quality that enables the ape to put two jointed sticks together to reach the banana.

Probably the most frequently used tests of intelligence are the two Wechsler scales, the Wechsler Adult Intelligence Scale (WAIS) and the Wechsler Intelligence Scale for Children (WISC). These tests are grouped into subtests involving both verbal and performance skills, and they can be helpful not only in the general assessment of intelligence, but also in detecting to some extent the presence of organic factors, psychotic deterioration, or emotional difficulties. The WAIS contains 11 subtests, six for the verbal scale (information, comprehension, arithmetic, similarities, digit span, and vocabulary) and five for the performance scale (digit symbol, picture completion, block design, picture arrangement, object assembly). This test is individually administered. Scoring is according to a standardization schedule, so that the person is being compared with other persons of the same age. The WISC consists of 12 subtests, of which 10 are usually used. The verbal scale includes general information, general comprehension, arithmetic, similarities, vocabulary, and digit span. The performance scale subtests are picture completion, picture arrangement, coding and mazes, block designs, and object assembly.

The Stanford-Binet scale is an individually administered examination which involves performance of tasks ranging from simple manipulation or identification of common objects to complex abstract reasoning. It consists of graded problems which can be solved successfully by persons of average intelligence at each age level from ages 2 through adult, and some problems which can only be solved by superior adults. To obtain the IQ (the intelligence quotient), the person's score on the test, or Mental Age is compared with the Chronological Age (up to age 15 years, 9 months), and the results of the MA, divided by the CA, multiplied by 100 equals a standard score, the IQ. For subjects under 2 and over 16 years of age, the test requires special interpretation because of the difficulties inherent in testing infants, and the assumption that maximum mental capacity is reached by age 15 years, 9 months.

Both the Wechsler scales and the Stanford-Binet should be administered and interpreted by persons with special training. There are, however, a number of simpler screening tests, some of which only take a few minutes to administer, which may be useful if one keeps their limitations in mind.

Tests for Organic Brain Impairment

Although there may be some indications of organic impairment in variations of performance on different subtests of the WAIS, a number of other individual tests and batteries of tests may be used. One of the most widely used is the Bender-Gestalt Test in which the subject is asked to copy nine simple designs. Other single tests include the Benton Visual Retention Test, the Perceptual Maze Test, and various block design tests. Such single tests are probably no more than 70 percent accurate in detecting brain damage, but in many cases are helpful when used as part of a complete case study. Groups of tests such as the Luria-Nebraska Neuropsychological Battery or the Halstead-Reitan Battery are more accurate, but their use requires special training and is quite time consuming. They can make an important contribution in cases in which there is difficulty in differential diagnosis, but they are not suitable for routine use.

Projective Tests

Projective methods provide a stimulus situation sufficiently unstructured that the response reflects the subject's underlying personality or psychopathology. Among these are word association tests, sentence completion tests, picture arrangement tests, the Rorschach Test, the Thematic Apperception Test, and the Draw-A-Person Test.

In the Rorschach test, the subject is shown a series of 10 cards on which are printed bilaterally symmetrical ink blots, five in black and gray only, two with additional bright red, and three in pastel shades. In telling what one sees in these ink blots, the subject gives clues to internal functioning. Scoring of each response takes into account the portion or area of the blot used (whole, large detail, small detail, etc.), the factors determining the response (form, movement, color, etc.), the content of the response, and some additional factors (popular responses, original responses, etc.). Some indices may then be calculated from the total scores, but more often interpretation is more subjective, taking into account not only the actual scores but other factors less easy to quantify.

In the Thematic Apperception Test (TAT), the subject is shown pictures of persons in various situations, and is asked to make up a story about each picture. It is assumed that in this, as in the other projective tests, the subject's responses are determined by previous emotional experiences and characteristic ways of reacting, and that these will be revealed during the test.

In the Draw-A-Person Test, the patient is asked to draw a person and then to draw someone of the opposite sex. Inferences may be drawn from the size of the figures, the dress, details, symmetry, etc.

Personality Inventories

There are a number of self-report or self-assessment questionnaires on which a patient may indicate the presence or absence of certain symptoms, attitudes, feelings, or preferences. Some of these are useful for screening and others for following the progress of a patient under treatment. The most popular and widely used is the Minnesota Multiphasic Personality Inventory (MMPI). It contains 550 statements to be answered "True," "False," or "Cannot say." The subject's attitudes are assessed in 26 areas, including religious, social, sexual, educational, and occupational spheres, and indications of neurotic or psychotic traits may be revealed. Scores on the individual clinical scales are used to construct a profile which can be compared with standardized profiles. One of the values of the MMPI is that it has been standardized against clinical diagnostic categories.

PHYSICAL AND NEUROLOGICAL EXAMINATION

A physical and neurological examination is recorded as part of the data base for any hospitalized psychiatric patient and is required for many outpatients. In some cases, if an outpatient has had a recent physical examination elsewhere, or is under the care of a primary physician, and has no symptoms or complaints suggestive of organic brain disease or of diseases of other systems, this may be omitted. Laboratory tests, x-rays, electroencephalograms, and other diagnostic procedures are included in the data base if needed.

DIAGNOSTIC IMPRESSION, SUMMARY, AND FORMULATION

After completing the psychiatric examination and entering one's diagnostic impression on the record, it is helpful to record a brief summary and formulation. The summary serves to highlight those things in the history and the findings on examination which the clinician believes to be of most relevance to the illness. An attempt is made to explain or account for unusual findings and to call attention to circumstances which may influence the meaning or validity of certain observations (e.g., the observation that a patient's shirt is dirty has a different significance if he came directly from work at a filling station than if he came from a bank).

After identifying and interpreting the key elements in the history and the significant findings on examination, one proceeds with the formulation.

The formulation utilizes data to construct hypotheses about the origin of the patient's difficulties. The formulation answers, tentatively, as many of these questions as possible:

1. What sort of person is the patient?
2. What factors contributed to the development of a mental illness?
3. What caused the illness to occur when it did?
4. What factors contributed to the form taken by the illness (both its general type and specific symptoms)?
5. What led the patient to seek treatment when and where he or she did?

In order to answer these questions, the formulation utilizes an evaluation, not merely enumeration or recapitulation, of all of the biopsychosocial factors contributing to the disorder, including genetic and constitutional predisposing factors;

significant events from the developmental history, traits derived from various stages of psychosocial development, character structure, prevailing ego defense mechanisms; and intrapsychic, interpersonal, and environmental stresses.

Following formulation, one is ready to discuss differential diagnosis and treatment plan.

PROBLEM-ORIENTED MEDICAL RECORDING

Problem-oriented medical recording has several advantages in psychiatric practice. Among these, it takes into account all of the patient's problems and not merely the presenting complaint (which may be only a "ticket of admission" to the clinic or hospital and not one of the things that is really most troublesome) or the symptoms of a particular disease or syndrome. The problem-oriented medical record has four main elements:

1. The data base (including the components of the psychiatric examination already described).
2. The problem list.
3. The problem plan.
4. Progress notes; these include: (a) subjective data, (b) objective data, (c) assessment, (d) plans. The acronym for the components of each progress note is SOAP.

The problem list includes the problems of the patient labeled and in numerical order. The purpose of the problem plan is to project patient management item by item.

The progress notes reflect a continuous summary of the problems from the initiation of treatment to conclusion. If a new problem occurs (e.g., a side effect from a medication), it is added to the problem list and described in the progress notes. When writing progress notes one lists the problem by name and by number. Then, under the heading Subjective, one describes the patient's view of the problem, usually as a quotation. Under the Objective heading one describes any new or pertinent findings, e.g., results from psychological testing, x-rays, or the laboratory, etc. Next, the recorder interprets the subjective and objective findings under the heading Assessment. The final section of the progress notes includes the plan of treatment for the specific problem.

On discharge from treatment, a final summary is done problem by problem in numerical sequence. Thus, problem number one is discussed first, number two second, etc. The format is the same for the Discharge Summary as for the progress notes, e.g., Subjective, Objective, Assessment, Plan.

An example for the use of a problem-oriented medical record in psychiatry is: A 14-year-old adolescent and his parents come to the psychiatrist because he ran away the previous weekend.

1. Data Base includes: Psychiatric history (personal and family), mental status examination
2. Problem List: #1 Runaway behavior
3. Problem Plan: #1 Runaway behavior — psychiatric evaluation
4. Progress Note: #1 Runaway behavior
   a. Subjective: "I can't get along with my parents."
   b. Objective: During the interview the parents and the patient expressed much anger, both verbally and nonverbally, toward each other.

   c. Assessment: The dependence–independence conflict of adolescence is being manifested by authority conflicts with the parents and runaway behavior.
   d. Plan: (1) Admit to an inpatient adolescent unit for cooling-off period of 1 week, (2) Psychological testing, (3) Physical and neurological examination, (4) Family counseling.

On discharge, the summary might look like this:

   a. Subjective: "I ran away because I can't get along with my parents."
   b. Objective: No runaway behavior occurred while on the inpatient unit
   c. Assessment: Psychiatric history, mental status examination, and psychological testing suggest a Conduct Disorder, Undersocialized Nonagressive, manifested by authority conflicts between the adolescent and his parents. Physical and neurological examination and routine laboratory studies were normal.
   d. Plan: (1) Discharge patient to his parents (by mutual consent), (2) Weekly family counseling for six sessions, (3) Reevaluate in 6 weeks.

In a modification of problem-oriented recording known as goal-oriented recording, each goal-oriented progress note is linked to a correspondingly numbered goal in the treatment plan.

EXAMINATION OF THE UNCOOPERATIVE PATIENT

Examination of a patient who either cannot or will not cooperate would appear to be a difficult and unprofitable task. However, much can be discovered in a careful examination of an unwilling or even a comatose patient.

General Appearance and Behavior

Does the patient appear comatose or alert? What spontaneous movements are noted? Describe facial expression and posture. Does the patient appear to look at the examiner? Do the eyes follow movement within the room?

Speech

Is the patient consistently mute, or is there some spontaneous speech? If so, is it meaningful? Does it give any clues about mood? Thought content? In the absence of speech, are there any apparent attempts at speech or other communication?

Response to Stimuli

Does the patient appear aware of the presence of the examiner? Does he or she react to things that the examiner says? Is there any emotional reaction to what is said (e.g., a change of facial expression when a family member is mentioned)? What is the response to a request such as asking the patient to raise a hand or open his or her mouth? Is there any reaction to sudden noises or other unexpected stimuli? Is there echopraxia or echolalia? If the patient is unable or unwilling to respond verbally, will he or she write answers to questions?

    If one attempts to move the patient's arm to a different position, is there active cooperation? Passive cooperation? Are muscles relaxed or tense? Is waxy flexibility present? Is there resistance? Movement in the opposite direction? A show of anger?

REVIEW QUESTIONS

1. In a psychiatric examination, what general areas are investigated?
2. What is the value of the patient's past history in the assessment of current complaints?
3. In what periods of the patient's past life would you expect to find early evidence of difficulties in socialization?
4. Under what circumstances would you be likely to examine the patient's sensorium in detail? What psychological tests would be helpful in your assessment of this patient?
5. Define delusion, hallucination, ideas of reference.
6. Name and describe some commonly used psychological tests. What are their uses and limitations?
7. What is meant by a projective test? Name and describe two projective tests.
8. In what portion of the psychiatric examination would you note that the patient commonly used rationalization and denial? What psychological tests would be helpful in your assessment of this patient?
9. Do you think it is important to communicate your impression of the nature of the problem and your recommendations to the patient? Why?

SELECTED REFERENCES

1. Anastasi, Anne: *Psychological Testing.* 5th ed. New York, Macmillan, 1982.

2. Andreasen, Nancy C.: Thought, language, and communication disorders: Clinical assessment, definition of terms, and evaluation of their reliability. *Arch Gen Psychiatry* 36:1315-1321, 1979.

3. Chandrasena, R.: Schneider's first rank symptoms: A review. *Psychiatr J Univ Ottawa* 8(2):86-95, 1983.

4. Golden, Charles J.: *Clinical Interpretation of Objective Psychological Tests.* New York, Grune & Stratton, 1979.

5. Golden, Charles J.: *Diagnosis and Rehabilitation in Clinical Neuropsychology.* Springfield, Illinois, Thomas, 1978.

6. Katzman, Robert, Theodore Brown, Paula Fuld, Arthur Peck, Ruben Schechter, and Herbert Schimmel: Validation of a short orientation-memory-concentration test of cognitive impairment. *Am J Psychiatry* 140(6):734-739, 1983.

7. Ketai, Richard: Affect, mood, emotion, and feeling: Semantic considerations. *Am J Psychiatry* 132(11):1215-1217, 1975.

8. Levy, Joshua, and K.A. Grigg: Early memories. *Arch Gen Psychiatry* 7(1): 57-69, 1962.

9. Meldman, Monte Jay, D. Harris, R. J. Pellicore, and E. L. Johnson: A computer-assisted, goal oriented psychiatric progress note system. *Am J Psychiatry* 134(1):38-41, 1977.

10. Muecke, Lee N., and David W. Krueger: Physical findings in a psychiatric out-patient clinic. *Am J Psychiatry* 138(9):1241-1242, 1981.

11. Robins, Lee N., John E. Helzer, Jack Croughan, and Kathryn S. Ratcliff: National Institute of Mental Health Diagnostic Interview Schedule. *Arch Gen Psychiatry* 38:381-389, 1981.

12. Ryback, Ralph S., and Johanna S. Gardner: Problem formulation: The problem oriented record. *Am J Psychiatry* 130(3):312-316, 1973.

13. Vickar, Garry M., and Marijan Herjanic: The use of problem oriented medical records in community mental health centers. *Am J Psychiatry* 133(3):340-341, 1976.

14. Weed, Lawrence L.: Medical records that guide and teach. *N Engl J Med* 278: 600, 625-657, 1968.

Chapter 4

CLASSIFICATION OF MENTAL ILLNESS

THE PURPOSE OF CLASSIFICATION

The human tendency to classify and categorize things is so ubiquitous and so natural that any attempt to explain or justify a particular classification may have the elements of rationalization. However, there are some specific uses for the classification of mental illness.

1.   For brevity in communication
2.   For research
3.   For data storage and retrieval

In addition, a standard nomenclature is needed, not only so that terms used in medical records and scientific articles can be understood by all readers, but also so that utilization review committees, accreditation agencies, and insurance carriers can evaluate reports. The needs of the latter go beyond classification itself in requiring diagnostic criteria for each entity and bases for estimating appropriate durations of treatment.

OBJECTIONS TO CLASSIFICATION

Many human problems do not lend themselves to classification. They are too diverse and too specific to the life of the individual. Giving the problem a name and category may seem a little like cutting it up to fit a Procrustean bed. This, among other reasons, has led some authorities to raise a serious question as to whether the values of classification are really sufficient to justify its use.

An objection to current nomenclature is that much of psychiatric classification is descriptive rather than etiological. It is said, in effect, that you cannot learn much about febrile illness by studying a group of fevers unless you are able to separate them on the basis of cause. From this point of view, the diagnostic groupings may interfere more with meaningful research than help it. This objection may not be altogether valid, since it is based on the assumption that it might be possible to classify psychiatric disorders on the basis of specific etiological factors; the evidence suggests, on the other hand, that most psychiatric disorders result from multiple causative factors rather than from a single main one.

Another objection to classification is that labeling a patient may be harmful. This objection is valid to the extent that the diagnosis is viewed as a stereotype by the clinician, to the extent that it is disturbing to the patient if furnished without adequate interpretation, and to the extent that society, including prospective employers, may discriminate against a person who has had a particular diagnosis, if such information is made available.

Recent research fails to support the contention that a psychiatric label unduly influences others' perceptions of an individual and studies of social distance reactions to the mentally ill patient suggest that these are more influenced by the degree of impairment than by the diagnosis. Nevertheless, persons who have had a psychiatric diagnosis do sometimes encounter discrimination (e.g., by prospective employers; by insurance companies on other than a sound actuarial basis). It would seem better to combat this through public education and political action by professional organizations than to avoid the issue by not making appropriate diagnoses or pretending that mental illness does not exist.

Problem-oriented recording with its emphasis on recognizing all of a patient's problems and not just those referable to a chief complaint or to a specific illness may eliminate some of the concerns about classification.

INCREASING THE COMMUNICATION VALUE
OF CLASSIFICATION

In the first *Diagnostic and Statistical Manual of Mental Disorders,* published by the American Psychiatric Association in 1952, and in the 1968 edition, DSM-II, the emphasis was largely on naming disorders, grouping them appropriately, and furnishing brief definitions or descriptions of each. The new *Diagnostic and Statistical Manual of Mental Disorders* (DSM-III), published in 1980, has enhanced the communication value of classification in several ways. It supplies more detailed descriptions of the disorders and lists diagnostic criteria for each. In addition, it supplies components of classification that go beyond simply identifying illnesses.

Naming a disease has limited communication value. Knowing a diagnosis does give one a general idea of the illness, its main symptoms, and possibly some of the special problems that are most likely to arise in its treatment. It does not give one much of an idea of severity or prognosis, nor does it give many clues to the life situation and personality of the patient. It offers only limited help in planning treatment. In order to supply more relevant information, DSM-III utilizes what is called *multiaxial* diagnoses. Each patient's diagnosis includes an evaluation of five components (called axes) of his or her condition. Axis I represents the identification of a clinical psychiatric syndrome, an acute or chronic mental illness, if present. Axis II identifies the Personality Disorders, essentially life-long maladaptive behavior patterns, in adults. It may also be used to indicate prominent personality features if no Personality Disorder is present. For children and adolescents, Axis II is used to record specific developmental disorders. A person may have a diagnosis on Axis I, Axis II, or both.

Axis III identifies any nonpsychiatric disorder that may be present which is relevant to the understanding or management of the case. Axis IV records psychosocial stressors that may be relevant to the development or exacerbation of psychiatric illness. It indicates the nature of the stresses (e.g., marital, occupational, legal) and their severity (rated on a seven-point scale from None to Catastrophic).

Finally, Axis V is used to indicate the highest level of adaptive functioning achieved by the person during the year prior to evaluation. It utilizes a seven-point scale ranging from Superior to Grossly Impaired.

By indicating the presence or absence of relevant information on all five axes, one is able to convey a much more comprehensive picture of the patient's condition than is possible by just naming his or her disease. However, the recording of Axes IV and V evaluations is optional. It was made optional because it is sometimes necessary to furnish, with the patient's consent, diagnoses to third-party payers (insurors) or to employers. The information conveyed by Axes IV and V goes beyond the needs of such persons, could interfere with a patient's right to privacy, and might be misused. Accordingly, these axes will be used for the most part in teaching and research settings in which adequate safeguards for confidentiality can be maintained. The current diagnostic terms are as follows[1]:

All official DSM-III codes and terms are included in ICD-9-CM. However, in order to differentiate those DSM-III categories that use the same ICD-9-CM codes, unofficial non-ICD-9-CM codes are provided in parentheses for use when greater specificity is necessary.

The long dashes indicate the need for a fifth-digit subtype or other qualifying term.

DISORDERS USUALLY FIRST EVIDENT IN INFANCY, CHILDHOOD OR ADOLESCENCE

Mental retardation
(Code in fifth digit: 1 = with other behavioral symptoms [requiring attention or treatment and that are not part of another disorder], 0 = without other behavioral symptoms.)
317.0(x) Mild mental retardation, _____
318.0(x) Moderate mental retardation, _____
318.1(x) Severe mental retardation, _____
318.2(x) Profound mental retardation, _____
319.0(x) Unspecified mental retardation, _____

Attention deficit disorder
314.01 with hyperactivity
314.00 without hyperactivity
314.80 residual type

Conduct disorder
312.00 undersocialized, aggressive
312.10 undersocialized, nonaggressive
312.23 socialized, aggressive
312.21 socialized, nonaggressive
312.90 atypical

Anxiety disorders of childhood or adolescence
309.21 Separation anxiety disorder
313.21 Avoidant disorder of childhood or adolescence
313.00 Overanxious disorder

Other disorders of infancy, childhood or adolescence
313.89 Reactive attachment disorder of infancy
313.22 Schizoid disorder of childhood or adolescence
313.23 Elective mutism
313.81 Oppositional disorder
313.82 Identity disorder

---

[1]Reprinted from the *Diagnostic and Statistical Manual of Mental Disorders,* Third edition. Published by the American Psychiatric Association, Washington, D.C., 1980, by permission of the copyright owners.

Eating disorders
307.10 Anorexia nervosa
307.51 Bulimia
307.52 Pica
307.53 Rumination disorder of
         infancy
307.50 Atypical eating disorder

Stereotyped movement disorders
307.21 Transient tic disorder
307.22 Chronic motor tic disorder
307.23 Tourette's disorder
307.20 Atypical tic disorder
307.30 Atypical stereotyped move-
         ment disorder

Other disorders with physical manifestations
307.00 Stuttering
307.60 Functional enuresis
307.70 Functional encopresis
307.46 Sleepwalking disorder
307.46 Sleep terror disorder
         (307.49)

Pervasive developmental disorder
Code in fifth digit: 0 = full syndrome present, 1 = residual state.
299.0x Infantile autism, _____
299.9x Childhood onset pervasive
         developmental disorder,

299.8x Atypical, _____

Specific developmental disorders
Note: These are coded on Axis II.
315.00 Developmental reading
         disorder
315.10 Developmental arithmetic
         disorder
315.31 Developmental language
         disorder
315.39 Developmental articula-
         tion disorder
315.50 Mixed specific develop-
         mental disorder
315.90 Atypical specific develop-
         mental disorder

ORGANIC MENTAL DISORDERS
Section 1, Organic mental disorders whose etiology or pathophysiological process is listed below (taken from the mental disorders section of ICD-9-CM).

Dementias arising in the senium and presenium

Primary degenerative dementia, senile onset,
290.30 with delirium
290.20 with delusions
290.21 with depression
290.00 uncomplicated
Code in fifth digit:
1 = with delirium, 2 = with delusions,
3 = with depression, 0 = uncomplicated.
290.1x Primary degenerative dementia, presenile onset, _____
290.4x Multi-infarct dementia, _____

Substance-induced

Alcohol
303.00 intoxication
291.40 idiosyncratic intoxication
291.80 withdrawal
291.00 withdrawal delirium
291.30 hallucinosis
291.10 amnestic disorder
Code severity of dementia in fifth digit: 1 = mild, 2 = moderate, 3 = severe, 0 = unspecified.
291.2x Dementia associated with alcoholism, _____

Barbiturate or similarly acting sedative or hypnotic
305.40 intoxication (327.00)
292.00 withdrawl (327.01)
292.00 withdrawal delirium (327.02)
292.83 amnestic disorder (327.04)

Opioid
305.50 intoxication (327.10)
292.00 withdrawal (327.11)

Cocaine
305.60 intoxication (327.20)

Amphetamine or similarly acting sympathomimetic
305.70 intoxication (327.30)
292.81 delirium (327.32)
292.11 delusional disorder (327.35)
292.00 withdrawl (327.31)

Phencyclidine (PCP) or similarly acting arylcyclohexylamine
305.90   intoxication (327.40)
292.81   delirium (327.42)
292.90   mixed organic mental disorder (327.49)

Hallucinogen
305.30   hallucinosis (327.56)
292.11   delusional disorder (327.55)
292.84   affective disorder (327.57)

Cannabis
305.20   intoxication (327.60)
292.11   delusional disorder (327.65)

Tobacco
292.00   withdrawl (327.71)

Caffeine
305.90   intoxication (327.80)

Other or unspecified substance
305.90   intoxication (327.90)
292.00   withdrawal (327.91)
292.81   delirium (327.92)
292.82   dementia (327.93)
292.83   amnestic disorder (327.94)
292.11   delusional disorder (327.95)
292.12   hallucinosis (327.96)
292.84   affective disorder (327.97)
292.89   personality disorder (327.98)
292.90   atypical or mixed organic mental disorder (327.99)

Section 2. Organic brain syndromes whose etiology or pathophysiological process is either noted as an additional diagnosis from outside the mental disorders section of ICD–9–CM or is unknown.

293.00   Delirium
294.10   Dementia
294.00   Amnestic syndrome
293.81   Organic delusional syndrome
293.82   Organic hallucinosis
293.83   Organic affective syndrome
310.10   Organic personality syndrome
294.80   Atypical or mixed organic brain syndrome

SUBSTANCE USE DISORDERS

Code in fifth digit: 1 = continuous, 2 = episodic, 3 = in remission, 0 = unspecified.

305.0x   Alcohol abuse, _____
303.9x   Alcohol dependence (Alcoholism), _____
305.4x   Barbiturate or similarly acting sedative or hypnotic abuse,_____
304.1x   Barbiturate or similarly acting sedative or hypnotic dependence, _____
305.5x   Opioid abuse, _____
304.0x   Opioid dependence, _____
305.6x   Cocaine abuse, _____
305.7x   Amphetamine or similarly acting sympathomimetic abuse, _____
304.4x   Amphetamine or similarly acting sympathomimetic dependence, _____
305.9x   Phencyclidine (PCP) or similarly acting arylcyclohexylamine abuse, _____ (328.4x)
305.3x   Hallucinogen abuse, _____
305.2x   Cannabis abuse, _____
304.3x   Cannabis dependence, _____
305.1x   Tobacco dependence, _____
305.9x   Other, mixed or unspecified substance abuse, _____
304.6x   Other specified substance dependence, _____
304.9x   Unspecified substance dependence, _____
304.7x   Dependence on combination of opioid and other nonalcoholic substance, _____
304.8x   Dependence on combination of substances, excluding opioids and alcohol, _____

SCHIZOPHRENIC DISORDERS

Code in fifth digit: 1 = subchronic, 2 = chronic, 3 = subchronic with acute exacerbation, 4 = chronic with acute exacerbation, 5 = in remission, 0 = unspecified.

Schizophrenia,
295.1x disorganized, _____
295.2x catatonic, _____
295.3x paranoid, _____
295.9x undifferentiated, _____
295.6x residual, _____

PARANOID DISORDERS

297.10 Paranoia
297.30 Shared paranoid disorder
298.30 Acute paranoid disorder
297.90 Atypical paranoid disorder

PSYCHOTIC DISORDERS NOT ELSEWHERE CLASSIFIED

295.40 Schizophreniform disorder
298.80 Brief reactive psychosis
295.70 Schizoaffective disorder
298.90 Atypical psychosis

NEUROTIC DISORDERS: These are included in Affective, Anxiety, Somatoform, Dissociative, and Psychosexual Disorders. In order to facilitate the identification of the categories that in DSM–II were grouped together in the class of Neuroses, the DSM–II terms are included separately in parentheses after the corresponding categories. These DSM–II terms are included in ICD–9–CM and therefore are acceptable as alternatives to the recommended DSM–III terms that precede them.

AFFECTIVE DISORDERS
Major affective disorders

Code major depressive episode in fifth digit: 6 = in remission, 4 = with psychotic features (the unofficial non-ICD-9-CM fifth digit 7 may be used instead to indicate that the psychotic features are mood-incongruent), 3 = with melancholia, 2 = without melancholia, 0 = unspecified.

Code manic episode in fifth digit: 6 = in remission, 4 = with psychotic features (the unofficial non-ICD-9-CM fifth digit 7 may be used instead to indicate that the psychotic features are mood-incongruent), 2 = without psychotic features, 0 = unspecified.

Bipolar disorder,
296.6x mixed, _____
296.4x manic, _____
296.5x depressed, _____

Major depression,
296.2x single episode, _____
290.3x recurrent, _____

Other specific affective disorders
301.13 Cyclothymic disorder
300.40 Dysthymic disorder
(or Depressive neurosis)

Atypical affective disorders
296.70 Atypical bipolar disorder
296.82 Atypical depression

ANXIETY DISORDERS

Phobic disorders (or Phobic neuroses)
300.21 Agoraphobia with panic attacks
300.22 Agoraphobia without panic attacks
300.23 Social phobia
300.29 Simple phobia

Anxiety states (or Anxiety neuroses)
300.01 Panic disorder
300.02 Generalized anxiety disorder
300.30 Obsessive compulsive disorder (or Obsessive compulsive neurosis)

Post-traumatic stress disorder
308.30 acute
309.81 chronic or delayed
300.00 Atypical anxiety disorder

SOMATOFORM DISORDERS
300.81 Somatization disorder
300.11 Conversion disorder (or Hysterical neurosis, conversion type)
307.80 Psychogenic pain disorder
300.70 Hypochondriasis (or Hypochondriacal neurosis)
300.70 Atypical somatoform disorder (300.71)

DISSOCIATIVE DISORDERS (OR HYSTERICAL NEUROSES, DISSOCIATIVE TYPE)
300.12 Psychogenic amnesia

300.13   Psychogenic fugue
300.14   Multiple personality
300.60   Depersonalization disorder
(or Depersonalization neurosis)
300.15   Atypical dissociative disorder

PSYCHOSEXUAL DISORDERS
Gender identity disorders
Indicate sexual history in the fifth digit
of Transsexualism code: 1 = asexual,
2 = homosexual, 3 = heterosexual, 0 =
unspecified.
302.5x   Transsexualism, _____
302.60   Gender identity disorder of
childhood
302.85   Atypical gender identity
disorder

Paraphilias

302.81   Fetishism
302.30   Transvestism
302.10   Zoophilia
302.20   Pedophilia
302.40   Exhibitionism
302.82   Voyeurism
302.83   Sexual masochism
302.84   Sexual sadism
302.90   Atypical paraphilia

Psychosexual dysfunctions

302.71   Inhibited sexual desire
302.72   Inhibited sexual excitement
302.73   Inhibited female orgasm
302.74   Inhibited male orgasm
302.75   Premature ejaculation
302.76   Functional dyspareunia
306.51   Functional vaginismus
302.70   Atypical psychosexual dysfunction

Other psychosexual disorders

302.00   Ego-dystonic homosexuality
302.89   Psychosexual disorder not
elsewhere classified

FACTITIOUS DISORDERS

300.16   Factitious disorder with psychological symptoms
301.51   Chronic factitious disorder
with physical symptoms
300.19   Atypical factitious disorder
with physical symptoms

DISORDERS OF IMPULSE CONTROL NOT ELSEWHERE CLASSIFIED

312.31   Pathological gambling
312.32   Kleptomania
312.33   Pyromania
312.34   Intermittent explosive disorder
312.35   Isolated explosive disorder
312.39   Atypical impulse control disorder

ADJUSTMENT DISORDER
309.00   with depressed mood
309.24   with anxious mood
309.28   with mixed emotional features
309.30   with disturbance of conduct
309.40   with mixed disturbance of emotions and conduct
309.23   with work (or academic)
inhibition
309.83   with withdrawal
309.90   with atypical features

PSYCHOLOGICAL FACTORS AFFECTING PHYSICAL CONDITION
Specify physical condition on Axis III.
316.00   Psychological factors affecting physical condition

PERSONALITY DISORDERS
Note: these are coded on Axis II.
301.00   Paranoid
301.20   Schizoid
301.22   Schizotypal
301.50   Histrionic
301.81   Narcissistic
301.70   Antisocial
301.83   Borderline
301.82   Avoidant
301.60   Dependent
301.40   Compulsive
301.84   Passive–Aggressive
301.89   Atypical, mixed or
other personality disorder

**V CODES FOR CONDITIONS NOT
ATTRIBUTABLE TO A MENTAL
DISORDER THAT ARE A FOCUS
OF ATTENTION OR TREATMENT**
V65.20   Malingering
V62.89   Borderline intellectual
           functioning (V62.88)
V71.01   Adult antisocial behavior
V71.02   Childhood or adolescent
           antisocial behavior
V62.30   Academic problem
V62.20   Occupational problem
V62.82   Uncomplicated bereavement
V15.81   Noncompliance with medical
           treatment
V62.89   Phase of life problem or other
           life circumstance problem
V61.10   Marital problem
V61.20   Parent-child problem
V61.80   Other specified family cir-
           cumstances
V62.81   Other interpersonal problem

ADDITIONAL CODES
300.90   Unspecified mental disorder
           (nonpsychotic)
V71.09   No diagnosis or condition on
           Axis I
799.90   Diagnosis or condition deferred
           on Axis I

V71.09   No diagnosis on Axis II
799.90   Diagnosis deferred on
           Axis II

MODIFICATIONS OF OFFICIAL NOMENCLATURE

In addition to using the diagnostic terms from DSM-III, the physician may use other
terms from the ninth edition of the *International Classification of Diseases:
Clinical Modifications (ICD-9-CM)*. While DSM-III is compatible with ICD-9-CM,
the latter does include some terms which do not appear in DSM-III. These include
simple schizophrenia, latent schizophrenia, and neurasthenia, among others.
     One can also use more detailed subclassification, add qualifying phrases, or
utilize additional axes to help describe a patient's condition. DSM-III has a five-
digit coding system, but for purposes of data retrieval a sixth digit may be added
to code a subclassification, qualifying terms, or rating on an additional axis.

DISCUSSION OF OFFICIAL NOMENCLATURE

The definitions and descriptions of the disorders listed in the classification will be included in the chapters devoted to clinical entities, Chapters 6 through 18. However, some general comments can be made at this point.

The first main heading in the classification is Disorders Usually First Evident in Infancy, Childhood or Adolescence. Note that the conditions in the first subgroup under this heading, Mental Retardation, and several of the disorders (e.g., stuttering) listed under the other subheadings may be identified in adult patients even though they are first manifested in early life. There are other conditions listed under some of these subheadings that can be diagnosed only in infants, children, or adolescents. On the other hand, children and adolescents can have "adult" illnesses which are listed in other parts of the classification system.

The next main heading is Organic Mental Disorders. The word organic is unfortunate here because it implies a dualism, a separation between mind and body. What it actually refers to is a group of conditions in which there is reversible or irreversible brain damage.

The Organic Mental Disorders are divided into two sections. In the first, there is a subheading for Dementias Arising in the Senium and Presenium. Following this, the next subheading is for Substance-Induced Disorders. At a glance this looks long and complicated, but it really is not. It is simply a list of substances (chemicals; drugs), used or misused for recreational purposes, and under each of these is a list of the types of brain syndromes that the substance may produce.

In the second section under the heading of Organic Mental Disorders, one finds those in which the etiology or pathogenesis is either noted as an additional diagnosis from some other section of ICD-9-CM or is unknown. For these, there is one list of the different types of brain syndromes that may be produced.

The heading Substance Use Disorders comes next. Here again is a list of recreational drugs which can be misused (abused) or upon which one may become dependent.

The next four main headings are:

1.   Schizophrenic Disorders
2.   Paranoid Disorders
3.   Psychoses Not Elsewhere Classified
4.   Affective Disorders

Though the word psychosis appears only in the third of these headings, all of the conditions in these four groups except Cyclothymic and Dysthymic Disorders are conditions that would have formerly been called psychoses, and are still identified that way in ICD-9-CM.

A psychosis is a mental condition that:

1.   Is usually severe
2.   Involves the total personality
3.   Is usually accompanied by some difficulties in reality testing

The term psychosis is imprecise. A person may have a mild case of a disease that would generally be classified as a psychosis, but not actually be psychotic. On the other hand, a person may have a disorder that is usually mild but may actually be quite severely ill, show involvement of the total personality, and have impaired reality testing. Nevertheless, when one designates a condition as a psychosis, or a patient as being psychotic at a particular time, the word has communication value.

After the psychoses the next group of main headings includes:

1. Anxiety Disorders
2. Somatoform Disorders
3. Dissociative Disorders

These represent groups of conditions formerly termed neuroses and currently listed in ICD-9-CM as Neurotic Disorders. The neuroses:

1. Have an acute onset (in contradistinction to Personality Disorders)
2. Are usually mild
3. Do not involve the total personality
4. Are not accompanied by disturbances in reality testing
5. Are manifested by anxiety or its derivatives

After the neuroses one finds the Psychosexual Disorders. Subclassifications under this heading include:

1. Gender Identity Disorders
2. Paraphilias (formerly referred to as Sexual Deviations)
3. Psychosexual Dysfunctions
4. Other Psychosexual Disorders

Among the Psychosexual Dysfunctions listed is Inhibited Sexual Excitement. This includes various types of impotence and frigidity. Listed under Other Psychosexual Disorders is Ego-dystonic homosexuality.

Factitious Disorders are listed next, and following them are Disorders of Impulse Control Not Elsewhere Classified. This is essentially a new classification. In the past, the first three disorders listed under it, Pathological Gambling, Kleptomania, and Pyromania, would have been classified with the neuroses as forms of Obsessive Compulsive Neurosis. Patients with Intermittent Explosive Disorder would have been diagnosed as having a Personality Disorder, Explosive Personality.

The next major classification, Adjustment Disorders, includes conditions formerly referred to as Transient Situational Disturbances. These are conditions in which maladaptive behavior is attributed to identifiable environmental stresses.

Psychological Factors Affecting Physical Condition is the next category. It is here that one would classify psychophysiological (psychosomatic) disorders. The category of Psychological Factors Affecting Physical Condition is not in itself a diagnosis but is entered on Axis I along with the Axis III diagnosis of the disease of another system in which psychological factors probably, or definitely, play an important role.

Personality Disorders, recorded on Axis II, come next. These are:

1. Essentially life-long processes
2. Manifested by habitual or recurring patterns of maladaptive behavior rather than subjective symptoms

Finally, the classification has a place for Conditions Not Attributable to a Mental Disorder. These are also recorded on Axis I. They represent human problems (e.g., occupational problems; marital problems) about which a patient may wish to consult a physician and for which he or she may need psychiatrically oriented counseling, and also behavioral problems (e.g., noncompliance with medical treatment; adult antisocial behavior in the absence of a diagnosable Personality Disorder) about which others involved in the patient's situation may seek consultation.

Finally, there are Additional Codes under which one finds a place for Unspecified Mental Disorders (nonpsychotic), a residual category for conditions not included in the nomenclature.

DIAGNOSTIC TERMS NOT FOUND IN DSM-III

In psychiatric literature, one will encounter a number of diagnostic terms that are not included in the current nomenclature. Some of these are older terms that are still in use and some are new ones that have not yet been generally accepted. There are certainly no objections to the use in research of terms that are not standard so long as the researcher defines them. If a term is defined and then used consistently, no confusion results. In addition to research usage, older and newer terms may be valuable in a given setting for communication because of specific differences in meaning assigned to them. In keeping statistical records, and in formal presentations in the literature, it is helpful if authors will translate these terms into the most closely applicable official terminology.

Among the older classifications was one prepared by Adolf Meyer, based upon his concept of ergasia. This term is derived from a Greek word meaning work, or energy. When the energies of the whole person were involved in a psychiatric disorder, Meyer spoke of it as an holergasia. The term holergasia, or holergastic reaction, then, is essentially synonymous to the term psychosis. In the same way, the term merergasia, referring to a syndrome that causes only partial impairment of personality functioning is roughly synonymous with neurosis.

Dementia praecox is an older term for the conditions now classified as Schizophrenic Disorders. Patients at present classified as having an Antisocial Personality Disorder would formerly have been called Sociopathic Personalities or Psychopathic Personalities. However, the latter term was somewhat broader in its application than is the present classification of Antisocial Personality and included some of the other Personality Disorders. In older clinical records and articles, one finds diagnoses such as Schizophrenic reaction or Paranoid reaction. In current usage these would be Schizophrenic Disorders and Paranoid Disorders. The word reaction used in that way is not to be confused with reactive disorders such as the Adjustment Disorders. Involutional Melancholia (Involutional Psychosis) was used to describe a depressive syndrome seen in persons in late middle life. This condition would now be classified under the Affective Disorders as a Major Depressive Disorder. The terms Character Disorder or Character Neurosis indicate disturbances that could usually be classified among the Personality Disorders.

DEFINITIONS OF DIAGNOSTIC TERMS

For more information about the meaning of any of the diagnostic terms included in the DSM-III outline reproduced in this chapter, one may turn to the third edition of the *Diagnostic and Statistical Manual of Mental Disorders* itself. There one will find definitions, brief descriptions, and diagnostic criteria. If one needs more information than is provided in DSM-III, one then may turn to this or any other current edition of a standard textbook of psychiatry. The more important conditions, or groups of conditions, merit separate chapters, but if an inspection of chapter headings does not indicate where the discussion of a particular condition is to be found, the index will. For the meaning of older terms not listed in this chapter, one may find cross references to official diagnoses in the indices of current textbooks, or may find definitions in psychiatric glossaries or dictionaries.

Newer diagnostic terms encountered in books and journals are usually defined in context, or if not, references are usually given in the bibliographies. However, if one encounters a diagnosis that is not included in DSM–III in a clinical record, and does not find it defined in textbooks or psychiatric dictionaries, one may need the help of a medical librarian to see if there is a description of the condition in the current literature.

DSM–III OPERATIONAL CRITERIA

For each diagnosis, the *Diagnostic and Statistical Manual of Mental Disorders* provides a list of criteria. These criteria are potentially helpful to accrediting agencies, utilization committees, and Professional Standards Review Organizations in determining whether a hospital's or clinic's admissions are appropriate, whether standard treatments are being used, and whether durations of hospitalizations for various conditions are excessive. Likewise, they can be used by government agencies and insurance carriers in determining whether to pay claims for care or to require further justification. While specific criteria serve a useful purpose, it should be remembered that patients are individuals and that diagnosis and treatment cannot always come from a cookbook or a computer. At least not yet.

The DSM–III criteria are of several types. Among them are:

1.   Duration of symptoms
2.   Symptoms or findings which must be present
3.   Lists of symptoms or findings of which a certain number must be present
4.   Symptoms or findings which must not be present

Even if one cannot record an official diagnosis unless the patient has been sick for a certain number of days, one may be able to anticipate the diagnosis and institute an appropriate treatment plan sooner. From the practical clinical point of view, the other types of criteria, at best, admit of some exceptions. A symptom nearly always present in a given disorder may be absent in a particular case. A patient may have two findings from group A and three from group B instead of the reverse. A single symptom not characteristic of the disorder and usually present in another illness may still be found. Moreover, not all well-qualified clinicians accept certain of the DSM–III criteria.

The foregoing problems are of little consequence if the criteria are used only as guidelines. If one is required to apply them literally, there is still a way out. Under almost every heading there are categories for atypical cases, and in addition, one has available the classification of Atypical Psychosis and Unspecified Mental Disorder (Nonpsychotic).

In the chapters in this book describing various disorders, we are *not* listing DSM–III criteria. These criteria are not used in all settings, and the student, house officer, or practitioner who needs them should refer either to the Manual or to the *Quick Reference to Diagnostic Criteria from DSM–III,* a pocket-sized book of 267 pages, available from the American Psychiatric Association.

REVIEW QUESTIONS

1.   Why is a classification system for mental illness necessary?
2.   Discuss objections to the current method of classification.
3.   Are there situations in which labeling a patient might be helpful to him or her?

4. How does a Psychosis differ from a Neurosis?
5. How would the following disorders be classified using standard nomenclature: Psychasthenia? Dementia praecox? Involutional melancholia? Sociopathic personality?
6. What is meant by multiaxial diagnosis? Discuss its advantages and disadvantages.
7. Under what circumstances would you use the diagnosis of Atypical Psychosis? Unspecified Mental Disorder (Nonpsychotic)?
8. Read a description of Cycloid Psychosis (cf. Selected Reference No. 8). If you saw this diagnosis in a clinical record, would it communicate anything to you about the patient that would not be indicated by any of the diagnostic terms in DSM-III? If a record librarian asked you for help in coding the diagnosis, what DSM-III codings might you suggest?

SELECTED REFERENCES

1. Charney, Dennis S., and J. Craig Nelson: Delusional and nondelusional unipolar depression: Further evidence for distinct subtypes. *Am J Psychiatry* 138(3):328-333, 1981.

2. *Diagnostic and Statistical Manual of Mental Disorders,* 3rd ed. Prepared by the Committee on Nomenclature and Statistics of the American Psychiatric Association, Washington, D.C., American Psychiatric Association, 1980.

3. Grove, William M., Nancy C. Andreasen, Patricia McDonald-Scott, Martin B. Keller, and Robert W. Shapiro: Reliability studies of psychiatric diagnosis. *Arch Gen Psychiatry* 38(4):408-413, 1981.

4. Fisher, Lawrence: On the classification of families. *Arch Gen Psychiatry* 34:424-433, 1977.

5. Karasu, Toksoz B., and Andrew E. Skodol: VIth axis for DSM-III: Psychodynamic evaluation. *Am J Psychiatry* 137(5):607-610, 1980.

6. Lindsay, William R.: The effects of labeling: Blind and nonblind ratings of social skills in schizophrenic and nonschizophrenic control subjects. *Am J Psychiatry* 139(2):216-219, 1982.

7. Looney, John G., Martin R. Lipp, and Robert L. Spitzer: A new method of classification for psychophysiologic disorders. *Am J Psychiatry* 135(3):304-308, 1978.

8. Perris, Carlo: Morbidity suppressive effect of lithium carbonate in cycloid psychosis. *Arch Gen Psychiatry* (35):328-331, 1978.

9. Schwarts, Carol C., Jerome K. Myers, and Boris M. Astrachan: Psychiatric labeling and the rehabilitation of the mental patient. *Arch Gen Psychiatry* 30(3):329-334, 1974.

10. Spitzer, Robert L.: More on pseudoscience in science and the case for psychiatric diagnosis. *Arch Gen Psychiatry* 33:459-470, 1976.

Part II

THE CLINICAL ENTITIES

Chapter 5

THE MENTALLY HEALTHY ADULT

WHAT IS "NORMAL"?

A meaningful concept of mental health is important in differential diagnosis, in evaluating candidates for certain occupations, and in setting treatment goals. In a broader sense it is also important to parents who hope to help their children become mentally healthy adults, and to school systems and other social institutions that have a role in facilitating personality development.

Mental examination techniques together with standardized personality tests are designed more to identify illnesses than to measure health. The lack of measures of mental health may in part reflect a lack of consensus as to its definition. Some of the possible concepts of mental health are discussed below.

1. Normality represents being average, feeling and functioning as well as most other people, measuring up to the standard of one's society. This is a concept that is usually dismissed, though in some settings it could have a limited usefulness in screening. The high prevalence of mental illness as shown both in the surveys of the general population mentioned in Chapter 1 and in studies of selected groups would make it more normal in this sense to have some psychiatric symptoms than to be free of them.
2. Health is the absence of disease. A person who does not have a diagnosable mental disorder and is free of troublesome psychiatric symptoms and grossly maladaptive behavior patterns can be said to be mentally healthy.
3. Mental health is more than the absence of disease; it implies a feeling of well-being and an ability to function at full capacity physically, intellectually, and emotionally. The last part of this definition suggests an individual standard for the patient, taking biological potential into account.
4. Mental health is part of a continuum. There are degrees of mental health just as there are degrees of mental illness. Symptoms (e.g., anxiety; depression) and maladaptive behavior patterns (e.g., alcohol misuse; passive-

aggressive behavior) occurring in individuals with relatively good mental health differ from those of the mentally ill only in intensity, frequency, and duration. Differences are quantitative, not qualitative

5. Being adjusted is being mentally healthy. Adjustment refers to a relationship with the physical and social environment which allows the person to meet basic biological needs. One survives, reproduces, and is generally successful in seeking pleasure and avoiding pain. A well-adjusted person is not necessarily creative, productive, socially useful, or a stimulating companion. From some clinical viewpoints this might be an adequate concept of mental health. One might add that it does not deemphasize the importance of creativity (or for that matter, genius, beauty, or the ability to run a mile in under 4 minutes), but considers it a separate quality from that of mental health. There would be some question in many cases as to whether adjustment could be an appropriate treatment goal. It cannot be the goal of social institutions involved in personality development. The progress of civilization requires more than an aggregate of adjusted individuals. Without creativity a society would remain primitive as long as food supplies were ample. With tranquil, well-adjusted people who follow a line of least resistance in meeting basic needs, necessity is indeed the only mother of invention.

6. Competence in dealing with the environment offers a broader basis for an operational definition of mental health than does adjustment. Competence is relative; it includes some ability to alter the environment rather than simply accommodating to it. A person competent in dealing with the social environment achieves something more than mediocrity; he or she achieves satisfactions beyond those required for most basic needs and does not require the stimulus of challenge, discomfort, or pain to exercise originality and creativity.

7. Ego strength may be closely related to a capacity for either adjustment or competence. The strong ego has a high ability to tolerate stress. The person with good ego strength can cope effectively with a wide variety of environmental situations. One might ask if it is appropriate to view a person of limited ego strength as mentally unhealthy if that person is free of symptoms, happy, functioning well, and apparently making a satisfactory adjustment. One may never have to tolerate the stresses he or she is least prepared to meet and may never need to deal effectively with environmental situations outside one's capacities. However, the person with limited ego strength might be a poor candidate for certain occupations. Such a person's prognosis for maintaining the present state of well-being is less good than that of a person with better ego strength.

Unless otherwise indicated, in the remainder of this chapter reference to the mentally healthy adult indicates a person who is free of psychiatric disease, has a general feeling of well-being (most of the time), functions at or near full biological capacity, is competent in dealing with the environment, and has good ego strength.

A mentally healthy person, while free of gross symptoms and usually feeling well, is not always happy. Life, after all, is never altogether smooth and easy; it presents everyone with some sources of discomfort and sorrow. The healthy adult may at times have some minor psychiatric symptoms. He or she functions on the Reality Principle as well as the Pleasure Principle and, to attain goals, defers some satisfactions and tolerates some stresses, and while being well equipped to tolerate stress, may show some effects from it. However, the ability and willingness to tolerate discomfort is rewarded by the achievement of objectives more often than not, and in a balance sheet of satisfactions and discomforts, the balance would be on the credit, not the debit side.

CHARACTER TRAITS
OF THE MENTALLY HEALTHY ADULT

In discussing character traits derived from the various stages of psychosexual development, it was emphasized that caution should be used in making value judgments concerning them. A variety of different character traits can be adaptive, can contribute to meeting basic needs, and are useful in the pursuit of satisfaction and security. However, some character traits offer more of a contribution to competence in dealing with a wider range of environmental situations than do others. Often these are traits that are near the midpoint in a continuum between two opposite characteristics. They are often marked by flexibility and a capacity for modification to meet changing environmental situations. Some character traits as they appear in most healthy adults are discussed below.

Optimism and Pessimism

Optimism, a cheerful expectation that things will turn out well (that one will indeed be fed), is up to a point an asset in most environmental situations. It helps a person tolerate stress; it makes others like and have confidence in him or her. However, the optimism should not be so great as to support unreasonable expectations, prevent constructive efforts to attain objectives and solve problems, or prevent the exercise of reasonable precautions.

Dependence and Independence

Both persons who are highly dependent and those who are generally quite independent can make successful adjustments. However, a capacity to function in both dependent and independent roles, to be taken care of or take care of oneself, to follow or to lead, depending upon the circumstances, is most adaptive. One must distinguish facultative, elective dependence from obligatory helplessness. One must also distinguish genuine independent behavior from that which is a reaction formation, an attempt at denial of dependent needs.

Organization and Systematization

To a degree the anal character traits producing neatness, cleanliness, promptness, and orderliness, are highly adaptive. The healthy person employs related traits in organizing knowledge and experience so as to draw meaningful conclusions from it. One approaches tasks and problems in living systematically but, optimally, is able to deviate from the systems when it is expedient or desirable to do so, and does not oversystematize.

Curiosity

Curiosity, partially scopophilic in origin, is useful not only to scientists, explorers, and inventors, but to almost anyone. The interest in identifying things in one's environment, finding out what they are, how they work, and why they are there, provides a great deal of useful data. Unless balanced by caution, it may lead one into dangerous situations.

Sexual Identity

The healthy man or woman is usually well satisfied with being his or her sex (despite some interpretations of feminine castration complex to the contrary). He likes being a boy; she, a girl — up to the end of adolescence, when hopefully he begins to like being a man and she a woman. The mentally healthy adult is relatively free from fears and complexes involving sexuality and is able to enjoy an active and satisfactory sex life.

Competition, Collaboration, and Compromise

Though able to pursue objectives alone, the healthy person works effectively with others. One is able to compete comfortably and aggressively, if necessary, with others, but he or she is competitive only when the situation calls for it. One is able to share and to compromise.

Relationship to Authority

The healthy person can accept the authority possessed by individuals and institutions (i.e., can accept an employer's orders and obeys the law). One does not feel compelled to rebel, but on the other hand is not afraid of authority and can oppose it, if necessary accepting consequences when indicated.

Emotional Expression and Emotional Control

The ability to tolerate strong emotions is a part of having good ego strength. Certain emotions are productive of satisfactions and others lead to constructive activity. The healthy person does not need to avoid situations which can arouse strong emotions or need to use mechanisms of isolation and dissociation to keep from feeling. One does not repress emotion but can inhibit or defer action based on the emotion. The emotions are free; the behavior is under control.

Capacity for Intimacy

An ability to form close and lasting relationships with persons of both sexes is characteristic of the mentally healthy person.

Satisfaction and Security

Most healthy people show a balanced approach to satisfaction and security. Their energies and activities are about equally divided between those productive of satisfaction and those contributing to security. The balance can be shifted with circumstances (i.e., the healthy person does not feel a compulsion to work during a vacation but can give up many satisfactions during a crisis). Similarly, there is a balance between long- and short-range planning.

THE EGO DEFENSES OF THE HEALTHY ADULT

The healthier the person, the stronger the ego, the less need there is for repression. Everyone represses painful memories, unacceptable impulses, and some elements of intrapsychic conflict. Repression protects the ego, but repressed material continues to exert some effect on behavior and it may rob decision making of some of its logical components. Also, according to the Libido Theory, it utilizes energy. It is preferable to be able to face a painful memory, to learn what one can from it, and to suppress it voluntarily than to repress it. It is better to reject an unacceptable impulse consciously than to bury it in the unconscious from whence it may lead to unintentional and unexpected behavior.

When the emotional component in a situation interferes with objective handling of it the healthy person does not employ isolation, denial, or dissociation. One does, however, attempt to control feelings and to separate them from the needs of the situation. In a difficult interpersonal situation one does not use projection so as to justify blaming the other person, but one does try to empathize with the other person, to see the situation as that person sees it, and to grasp the other person's feeling. One suspects one's rationalizations and checks them for objectivity. As reason is substituted for rationalization, one may at times elect to give others a reason that is actually oversimplified but acceptable, but rarely fools oneself.

Certain mechanisms (e.g., sublimation, identification, and sometimes aim inhibition and displacement) are often regarded as healthy, but even these mechanisms are not as healthy as are their conscious analogs.

SELF-ESTEEM AND MENTAL HEALTH

A healthy person has self-respect. In part because of the role of projection in interpersonal relationships, it is not easy to respect, admire, or trust others unless one can respect and trust oneself. The healthy person is relatively free of feelings of inadequacy and inferiority. However, the self-concept is not based upon denial of limitations, but on accepting them, correcting them if possible and desirable, and utilizing the most adaptive capacities available. The healthy person's self-esteem and, closely related to it, the parts of the personality used in obtaining various objectives, is based upon multiple rather than single qualities, at least some of which are of a relatively enduring character. Beauty or physical strength can be a source of self-esteem and are useful, but they do not last. Other qualities and abilities must be there to take their place in maintaining self-esteem when they go.

INTERPERSONAL RELATIONSHIPS
AND MENTAL HEALTH

Since man is a social being, skill in dealing with others, particularly but not exclusively with the significant people in one's life, is an essential adaptive capacity. The healthy person does not need to be an extrovert, to have a large number of friends, or to like an extensive social life, but does need to work and get along with others and to maintain some rewarding intimate relationships. Several of the character traits listed as typical of the mentally well contribute to smooth interpersonal relationships.

In studying the relationships of healthy people, one finds a consideration for others and an ability to collaborate. A person interacting with one or more others may be collaborating to meet a common need or may be meeting reciprocal needs. Along with finding healthy relationships, one finds a relative absence of destructive or disintegrative tendencies in interpersonal relationships. Relationships are not destroyed by efforts to exploit or by useless competition, power struggles, and jealousies. Eric Berne, in *Games People Play,* lists a number of interpersonal transactions, verbal and nonverbal, that have ulterior motives and are used to manipulate others. These maladaptive patterns often appear to be defenses against intimacy.

DECISION MAKING

The healthier the person, the more decisions and choices he or she is likely to make consciously. In choosing between two or more options, one must recognize that each carries with it consequences, not all of which may be desirable. However, not making a decision, or postponing one, also has predictable consequences. Not choosing is a choice (e.g., the woman who cannot decide whether she wants another child and postpones pregnancy indefinitely 'eventually reaches the menopause; the person who cannot decide whether to take a new job eventually loses the opportunity).

Indecision is generally uncomfortable, but the person with a strong ego resists the urge to decide impulsively. One may defer a decision long enough to study alternatives or to give a trial to a course of action, but he or she does not evade the decision. Certain minor decisions in everyday life (e.g., how to use the time available for recreation; how to use money for luxuries) may appear to be on whim and may not make sense to others, but one knows what one is doing and evaluates the satisfactions resulting from it.

Major decisions (e.g., career choice; marriage) are made on the basis of conscious determinants, recognized needs, and predicted consequences. They may not work out well, but they are based on sound reasons. This does not imply that most decisions on such matters are rational; the average person, in this sense, is not mentally healthy and is influenced in decision making by unconscious factors.

The healthy person chooses work within his or her range of capacities that will afford maximum satisfaction and security. A marriage choice blends anaclitic and narcissistic factors. This results in marriage, usually, to someone whose interests and values are similar to one's own (the narcissistic element) and on whom one can at times depend, and with whom one can meet reciprocal needs (the anaclitic element).

Once a person, healthy or otherwise, makes a decision, there is some tendency to suppress or repress consideration of other courses of action and to rationalize the choice. One finds reasons why it "had to be" or "was the best thing after all" even if it is not turning out well. This is adaptive to the extent that it conserves energy and eliminates the discomfort of uncertainty. It facilitates a full effort to make a decision work. The healthy person, however, while not ruminating on a decision once it is made, not vacillating, is still able to reevaluate it. One can recognize a mistake, account for it, and learn how to avoid repeating it. One can rectify a bad decision because one has suppressed rather than repressed factors that entered into the choice and has not overutilized rationalization to justify the course of action.

DEALING WITH STRESS

The strong ego can accept and cope with stress. When gratifications are denied, substitutes are found. These are consciously selected. The person recognizes a need for satisfactions. One does not sublimate unconsciously in a way that conceals the underlying need and may prevent gratifications under more opportune circumstances. Neither does one seek gratifications in ways that are essentially self-destructive. On encountering stress, for example, in an interpersonal situation, one usually uses a relatively habitual and more or less automatic means of coping. If this does not work one seeks other means of dealing with the situation. One tries to define and clarify the problem. Then one tries to modify the situation and, if this fails, either modifies one's own attitudes and expectations or finds a way of getting away from the stress. Failure may lead to the development of an Adjustment Disorder (cf. Chapter 6). However, one may seek professional help before developing symptoms. (Example: A student is warned that he is doing failing work. In the past, when his grades have dropped he has reduced the time spent in some other activities and given more time to study. He tries this but his grades do not improve. He discusses the situation with faculty members. He may employ various techniques in talking with them, perhaps ways of dealing with people that have been effective with other teachers or with his parents, to gain extra help, approval, or sympathy. He asks for and follows advice concerning study habits. He may try getting help from other students or from a tutor. If things still go badly, he may consider the pros and cons of withdrawing from the course. At this point, he may consult a counseling bureau or student health service, though he is still using more or less appropriate coping methods and is asymptomatic. He does this to obtain help with a problem, however, and not to provide himself with the excuse "I'm not doing well because I'm sick.")

CLINICAL IMPLICATIONS
OF THE CONCEPT OF MENTAL HEALTH

The definition of mental health is clinically useful in:

1.   Routine examination of patients
2.   Evaluation of patients who are apparently not mentally ill but who wish professional help with personal problems
3.   Selection of treatment goals for psychiatric patients
4.   Vocational screening
5.   Community mental health activities

The comprehensive medical care for any patient should include such psychiatric attention as is needed. Hence, the examination of a patient is not complete without a psychiatric appraisal. On the basis of the concept of mental health which has been described, this should include more than the search for an identification of symptoms of illness. The examiner must also decide whether the patient is functioning at full physical, intellectual, and emotional capacity. As well as looking for maladaptive character traits, the examiner should also look for those character traits which are congruent with mental health. The patient's insight into his or her own personality, and the amount of repressive mechanisms needed for effective functioning are also evaluated. Some idea is obtained as to the patient's self-esteem and the qualities on which it is based. From the patient's history one gains some knowledge of his or her skills in interpersonal relationships, decision making, and ways of dealing with stress.

The purpose of an evaluation of mental health, along with that of mental illness, is not only to identify the well and the sick. It helps identify those people who are not clinically sick but who still are not completely mentally well or who have limited ego strength. These are persons who are psychiatrically at risk. Their mental health requires some ongoing observation. They may actually need some counseling or some help in developing healthier patterns of living. Even if this is not indicated they are likely to need professional assistance at times of stress and may need professional help in decision making.

It is important to remember than an unusual personality or life style is not necessarily unhealthy. In such cases one does, however, need to look for possible discomfort or dissatisfaction, maladaptive quality, and potential future health risks.

Even persons who are completely well mentally need periodic reassessment. Mental status examination is supplemented by questions about work performance and work satisfaction, family life and interpersonal relationships, leisure time activities, and life style. One may have the patient describe the activities of a typical working day and a typical nonworking day, and the feelings accompanying them. Among other things, one looks for possible needs for recreational activities or for changes in life style. Even the healthy person may need a better balance of activities or may need to develop greater assertiveness or better communication skills.

A definition of mental health is also important in setting treatment goals in working with psychiatric patients. Of course, there are times in therapy when the goal is simply the relief of a symptom or the resolution of a crisis. In long-term therapies in which there is some effort to deal with the total personality, one must decide what goals are most appropriate. Is some amelioration of discomfort or symptomatic behavior all that can be expected? Is the goal a reasonable adjustment? Is the goal mental health?

Vocational screening presents a variety of problems in the application of a definition of mental health. While the mentally healthy worker at any job is more likely to be productive and creative than the person with psychiatric problems, and is also likely to have less absenteeism and to be less frequently involved in personality clashes, few jobs require perfect mental health any more than they require perfect general health. One cannot legally reject the mentally handicapped job applicant because of a history or findings of mental illness alone, and even if one could, the prevalence of emotional disturbance is too great to make it practical to screen out all emotionally disturbed job applicants. Also, while emotional problems reduce efficiency, a person of superior ability may be more effective despite this than would be a mentally healthy but less skilled worker at the same job.

Obviously, some vocational situations require a high level of mental health and ego strength (e.g., work in Antarctica where one would be exposed to physical hazards and isolation as well as having to get along with other people in close quarters). In most vocational screening, one is not as much interested in overall mental health, as such, as in the particular symptoms and personality traits which would interfere with the job, and those personality characteristics which would contribute most to effectiveness. Past work records and work attitudes are particularly important in vocational screening.

The capacity for work is an attribute of mental health. Work history is a good predictor of mental health. The ability to work consistently and effectively as a child or adolescent, whether demonstrated in gainful occupation or in school work and activities, is among the best predictors for both mental health and vocational adjustment. Work also helps maintain mental health and may be desirable for some who do not need work for its financial rewards. The importance of work must be taken into account in retirement planning.

Occupational medicine involves much more than the screening and selection process. Because of this the concept of mental health has the same significance in the occupational examination as it does in all routine examination of patients.

CONDITIONS NOT ATTRIBUTABLE
TO A MENTAL DISORDER

When a person without symptoms or obvious signs of psychiatric disorder asks for psychiatric consultation for assistance with a personal problem or in making a decision it is important in the differential diagnosis to recognize the mentally healthy elements in the personality. The more evidence there is of overall mental health, the more appropriate it is to deal with the problem at face value. In the absence of positive indications of mental health there is a strong probability that a stressful situation may result from maladaptive character traits, repetitive patterns of behavior, or unconscious factors stemming from neurotic conflict, in which case the correct psychiatric diagnosis is made. However, when no psychiatric diagnosis is appropriate, one may use the classification of the third edition of the *Diagnostic and Statistical Manual of Mental Disorders* (DSM-III) for conditions not attributable to a mental disorder. Some of these are mentioned in other chapters because of their relationship to, or the need to distinguish them from, other diagnostic entities. These include:

1. Malingering — Chapter 8
2. Borderline intellectual functioning — Chapter 16
3. Adult antisocial behavior — Chapter 7
4. Childhood or adolescent antisocial behavior — Chapter 17
5. Parent-child problems — Chapter 17
6. Uncomplicated bereavement — Chapter 10

Other diagnoses which may be used for persons without mental disease are:

1. Marital problems
2. Other specified family circumstances
3. Other interpersonal problems
4. Occupational problems
5. Academic problems
6. Phase of life problems
7. Noncompliance with medical treatment

The quality of one's interpersonal relationships is important to successful and happy living. If one has recurring problems in dealing with people, or a serious problem in dealing with a significant person, one may be wise to seek professional help. In differential diagnosis the person consulted about a problem in interpersonal relationships must rule out the possibility that the problem is secondary to a Personality Disorder or Anxiety Disorder before simply taking the problem at face value and offering advice rather than recommending therapy.

A similar problem in differential diagnosis arises when an apparently healthy person seeks advice about his or her interaction with another person whom the patient believes to be emotionally disturbed.

Likewise, when a patient appears to have an uncomplicated vocational problem, one has to be sure not only that the patient is not involved in the problem as a result of a Personality Disorder, an Anxiety Disorder, or other mental illness, but also one has to be sure that the problem is not creating sufficient stress to give rise to an Adjustment Disorder.

There are problems peculiar to various stages in the life cycle. Patients may seek professional guidance in coping with these problems. The key questions that arise in evaluating these patients and their difficulties are:

1. Is the difficulty secondary to mental disorder?
2. Is the problem producing stress-related symptoms that warrant a diagnosis of an Adjustment Disorder?

If the answers to both of these questions are negative, one regards the condition as not attributable to mental disorder, offers appropriate advice or counseling, or refers the patient for nonmedical counseling. However, since ongoing stress can produce symptoms, persons simply advised about a problem, or referred for nonmedical counseling, should have the opportunity for reevaluation if advice does not lead to amelioration of the difficulty.

MENTAL HEALTH
AND COMMUNITY PSYCHIATRY

The concept of mental health is particularly important in community psychiatry. Preventive and social psychiatry includes public health activities and focuses not only on the prevention of specific diseases and difficulties (e.g., alcohol dependence; Schizophrenic Disorder; delinquency), but also in the development of a mentally healthy community. Any research or pilot projects to determine the effect of educational, welfare, and public health programs on mental health must measure the results not only in terms of the incidence and prevalence of disease and indications of malfunction (e.g., unemployment; crime rates; divorce rates), but also on the definition and measurement of health itself. A healthy society is not one composed merely of tranquil, well-adjusted people, but is progressive, dynamic, and creative.

REVIEW QUESTIONS

1. In what ways is a definition of mental health useful?
2. What are the applications of a concept of mental health to selecting control subjects in research? To what extent should normal controls be mentally healthy?
3. What is the concept of ego strength employed in this chapter? Look up definitions of ego strength from at least two other sources. How much do they differ from the definition here?
4. Name three or more important historical figures whose biographies indicate the presence of major emotional problems but who made useful or desirable contributions to society. Speculate on whether their achievements were made because of or in spite of emotional disturbance.
5. Define mental health. How could Systems Theory be used in defining it?
6. From what stage of psychosexual development is optimism chiefly derived? How might you account for an excessive or maladaptive degree of optimism? What is the relationship of optimism and pessimism to mental health?
7. A woman reports that she gets along very well with men but has never liked women. She feels that they are petty, selfish, and uninteresting. What does this suggest concerning her own self-image? Her self-esteem? Her sexual identification? Her ego strength? Her mental health?
8. A woman hospitalized after reporting symptoms of schizophrenia is not sick, but rather she is a student participating in a research project. Would you recognize that she is mentally healthy? How?
9. A young man has a tendency to idealize his girlfriend, though he sees some potential obstacles to a happy marriage. He becomes engaged to her. Immediately after the engagement, will the tendency toward idealization become greater or less, in all probability? Why? How will this be influenced by the level of the young man's mental health?
10. Define empathy. Discuss relationships between empathy and projection. Discuss the role of empathy in decision making by the healthy adult.

SELECTED REFERENCES

1. Berne, Eric: *Games People Play.* New York, Grove Press, 1964.

2. De-Nour, A. Kaplan, and J. W. Czaczkes: The influence of patient's personality on adjustment to chronic dialysis. *J Nerv Men Dis* 162(5):323-333, 1976.

3. Eisenstein, Victor W.: *Neurotic Interaction in Marriage.* New York, Basic Books, pp. 3-100, 1956.

4. Grinker, Roy R., and Beatrice Werble: Mentally healthy young men (homoclites) 14 years later. *Arch Gen Psychiatry* 30(5):701-704, 1974.

5. Grinker, Roy R., Sr.: Normality viewed as a system. *Arch Gen Psychiatry* 17(3):320-324, 1967.

6. Koranyi, Erwin K.: The normal and its deviations. *Psychiatr J Univ Ottawa* 3(2):103-109, 1978.

7. Offer, Daniel, David Marcus, and Judith L. Offer: A longitudinal study of normal adolescent boys. *Am J Psychiatry* 126(7):41-48, 1970.

8. Offer, Daniel, and Melvin Sabshin: *Normality.* 2nd ed. New York, Basic Books, 1974.

9. Rothenberg, Albert: Janusian thinking and Nobel prize laureates. *Am J Psychiatry* 139(1):122-124, 1982.

10. Stein, Stefan P., Stephen Holzman, T. Byram Karasu, and Edward S. Charles: Mid-adult development and psychopathology. *Am J Psychiatry* 135(6):676-681, 1978.

11. Vaillant, George E.: Natural history of male psychological health: VI. Correlates of successful marriage and fatherhood. *Am J Psychiatry* 135(6):653-659, 1978.

12. Vaillant, George E., and Caroline O. Vaillant: Natural history of male psychological health: X. Work as a predictor of positive mental health. *Am J Psychiatry* 138(11):1433-1440, 1981.

13. White, Robert W. (Ed.): *The Study of Lives.* New York, Atherton Press, 1964.

14. White, Theodore C.: The coping functions of the ego mechanisms. In: *The Study of Lives.* Robert W. White (Ed.). New York, Atherton Press, 1964, pp. 179-198.

Chapter 6

REACTIVE AND ADJUSTMENT DISORDERS

THE EFFECTS OF STRESS

A stress situation exists when something in the environment causes a threat to life; a risk of injury; or an actual or potential loss of security, self-esteem, or important sources of satisfaction.

Life is never without stresses. The healthy person has a variety of conscious techniques and unconscious mechanisms for coping with them. When a person is unable to cope adequately with external pressures, stress may:

1. Be a contributing factor in the development of various mental illnesses
2. Precipitate an episode of mental illness
3. Cause an increase in symptoms of an on-going illness
4. Result in an Adjustment or Reactive Disorder

If the effects of stress are sufficient to produce transitory psychotic symptoms such as incoherence, delusions, hallucinations, or grossly disorganized behavior, the diagnosis of *Brief Reactive Psychosis* can be made. A Brief Reactive Psychosis lasts from a few hours up to 2 weeks. In making the diagnosis, one indicates an expectation of rapid remission; if the symptoms persist over 2 weeks, the diagnosis is revised. One makes this diagnosis only when there is a clearly identified major stress that would be upsetting to almost anyone. Though the diagnosis is usually used for people who are otherwise mentally healthy, a person with another psychiatric disorder can have a Brief Reactive Psychosis superimposed upon it, but one does not make that diagnosis when stress merely increases the severity of an already existing disorder.

When stress produces less serious symptoms or interferes with adequate social or vocational functioning, a diagnosis of one of the *Adjustment Disorders* may be considered. The Adjustment Disorders are subclassified on the basis of the presenting, or most prominent, symptom. Adjustment Disorders include those with:

1. Depressed mood
2. Anxious mood
3. Mixed emotional features
4. Work (or academic) inhibition
5. Disturbance of conduct
6. Mixed disturbance of emotions and conduct
7. Withdrawal
8. Atypical features

One of the criteria for the diagnosis of an Adjustment Disorder is that it occurs within 3 months of the onset of a stressor. However, if symptoms clearly attributable to a stressful situation arise later, the diagnosis of Adjustment Disorder with Atypical Features may be used.

REACTIONS TO GROSS STRESS

Disasters such as tornadoes, floods, earthquakes, riots, fires, and explosions that destroy large areas together with certain military situations represent a special kind of stress. In ordinary life one encounters grave threats to survival, e.g., illnesses, accidents, and other dangers. Catastrophes make no greater threat to survival, but they are more disorganizing to the personality, since to danger is added several, sometimes all, of the following features:

1. Unexpectedness
2. Unfamiliarity
3. Prolonged duration
4. Lack of opportunity for effective action
5. Lack of opportunity for escape
6. Unavailability of others on whom to depend

Symptoms and Course

The normal reaction to a threat to survival is fear. Fear mobilizes a person's capacity for fight or flight. In a catastrophe, when neither fight nor flight is possible, fear increases. If it becomes overwhelming, a normal urge to get away can be represented by aimless, useless running, possibly even running in the wrong direction. The urge to attack the source of danger may be displaced in what appears to be a purposeless destructive attack on something else in the vicinity. Overwhelming fear can be paralyzing; the person may be frozen, mute, unable to act in any way. Any of the person's prevailing defense mechanisms, however inappropriate, can be called into play, and the resulting behavior may simulate that of any of the psychoses or neuroses.

The particular effort at adaptation sometimes represented by peculiar behavior at the time of a disaster is often difficult to identify. Since the motivation is largely unconscious, subsequent inquiry yields little information. For example, during a catastrophe, women sometimes disrobe. Does this come from some feeling that escape might be easier if one is not hampered by clothing? Is it a regression to childhood? Is it an effort to shock people so that they will do something about the situation? Is it a symbolic offer of sexuality in exchange for protection?

If the patient is removed from the stress situation, symptoms are likely to subside promptly. However, if the stress has been of relatively long duration, residual anxiety manifested by tremor, restlessness, startle reaction, insomnia, and nightmares can persist for weeks or months. Other residuals include specific fears, sometimes at the phobic level. Secondary symptoms can arise from guilt, shame, or loss of self-esteem over one's behavior during the crisis. Examples: (1) A soldier evacuated from combat feels that he has let his buddies down, blames himself for other casualties, and becomes depressed. (2) During a flood, a woman fled from her home without looking for her children; they are rescued unharmed, but she develops an obsessive rumination about abandoning them.

Though most Brief Reactive Psychoses and Adjustment Disorders produced by gross stress resolve spontaneously after the stress is over, some patients may, in the absence of adequate treatment, develop other psychiatric disorders, including neuroses (including Post-traumatic Stress Disorder, which is discussed in Chapter 8), psychoses, or addictions (especially alcoholism). These disorders often represent the patient's failure to overcome the primary or secondary residual symptoms described. In other instances the stress serves as the precipitating event for another illness in a predisposed individual.

Differential Diagnosis

Theoretically, exposure to gross stress, appearance of major mental symptoms, and a history of a normal premorbid personality should make accurate diagnosis easy. Practically, a history usually cannot be obtained during a catastrophe. In the absence of a history, this condition often is indistinguishable from some of the Anxiety and Dissociative Disorders. Findings identical to any of several other major psychiatric syndromes may likewise make immediate differential diagnosis impossible.

Fortunately, treatment can be started before a positive diagnosis is made. However, if amnesia or confusion are among the presenting symptoms, head injury must be ruled out before sedation is administered.

Within a few days after the patient has been evacuated from the disaster area, progress and additional available history should be sufficient to confirm the diagnosis.

Prevention

Catastrophes cannot usually be prevented. At least their prevention is, with the exception of epidemics (cf. Defoe's *Journal of the Plague Year*), outside the realm of the physician. However, a number of reactions to gross stress can be prevented.

Disaster planning should take into account prevention of these disorders. Military planning must consider it also. Shelters, evacuation routes, food, water, and first aid supplies are only a part of disaster planning. Preparation of the population for possible disasters eliminates much of the unexpectedness and unfamiliarity which compound the stress. An opportunity to do something constructive in the nature of fight or flight is excellent prophylaxis. Advance planning facilitates this. Even at the time of crisis, putting the frightened person to work, providing something to do, may avert serious symptoms.

Leadership at times of crisis is essential. People should know who is in charge and who will take charge if leaders become casualties. Leaders must be recognizable. Whether the leader is in a position to do anything about the catastrophe or not, his or her presence meets dependency needs.

Selection of suitable leaders is not easy. It is difficult to test how they will tolerate a major stress because gross stress is not easily simulated. General measures of mental health and ego strength are of some value. Ability to tolerate the stresses of everyday life as evidenced, for example, by a good work record, is of some predictive value.

The presence or absence of free-floating anxiety, within certain limits, is of less prognostic value. Some people who externalize their anxiety, who show nervousness, rise to the occasion at times of crisis. The natural leaders who sometimes emerge during a catastrophe are not always people who would be selected as examples of emotional stability and complete mental health on the basis of usual examination criteria.

The behavior of a frightened and disorganized person contributes to panic in others. There is a contagious quality to gross stress reactions. In order to reduce the number of additional cases, psychiatric casualties should be evacuated promptly.

Treatment

In early or mild cases, meeting the patient's needs for dependency, direction, and constructive activity by reassurance, encouragement, and assignment of an appropriate duty may be effective. Mild sedation, or even a placebo, accompanied by positive suggestion that the patient will soon feel better and function effectively is helpful. If fatigue or loss of sleep contributes to the stress, a stimulant rather than a sedative may be indicated.

More severe cases must be evacuated from the disaster area. For the extremely disorganized patient a sufficient dose of a hypnotic to produce sleep may be necessary prior to evacuation. Ideally, it is better to defer sedation until thorough examination can be accomplished (the patient may have injuries in addition to the psychiatric disorder, and after evacuation might be able to report pain and otherwise cooperate in examination). Often, it is impossible to do more than check for obvious signs of head injury before deciding between sedation or restraint if the patient is not in sufficient control to cooperate during the evacuation procedure. Sedation saves the patient considerable suffering, removes some danger of being injured while struggling against restraint, and makes the person less disturbing to others.

Upon arriving at a hospital, after additional examination the patient should be put to sleep for several hours; after awakening, the condition should be assessed to determine the need for additional or lighter sedation or tranquilizing medication. A patient able to communicate should be given an opportunity to talk about the experience and the feelings it has produced. Fears and guilt feelings can be brought into the open, and discussion of them leads to some desensitization. Reassurance of present safety and explanation of the situation is indicated. The patient may not have a clear recollection of what has happened, and information helps one reorganize one's thoughts. Genuine reassurance about the safety of family, friends, or property can be helpful; false information should not be given because the long-range harm outweighs the short-term benefit. When answers to some questions are unknown, it is preferable to say so and let the patient talk about the fears rather than covering them up with meaningless encouragement that everything will be all right. If symptoms clear rapidly, a prompt return to duty for the military casualty, or for the civilian a prompt discharge from the hospital with resumption of work and responsibilities is preferable to prolonged hospitalization for convalescence. The damage to self-esteem from having "cracked up," the feeling that one is weak or cowardly, flourishes in idleness.

Residual symptoms which preclude a return to duty or usual activities require additional psychotherapy which should be started without delay. Symptomatic medication can be used. The psychotherapeutic methods are essentially the same as those used for the neuroses. The probability that guilt feelings play a part in residual symptoms should be kept in mind. Diagnosis must be reevaluated in all cases in which the patient does not recover in a few days.

For persons experiencing it for the first time, being in prison is a highly stressful life event that has some features in common with gross stress situations. Though the Ganser Syndrome seen in newly incarcerated prisoners is currently classified as a Factitious Disorder, some clinicians believe it is stress related. It is also called the syndrome of approximate answers or the nonsense syndrome. A patient asked to multiply 3 by 5 may answer, "14" or, if asked to touch the left ear, may touch the left temple. Differential diagnosis must include the possibility of organic brain disease. A high incidence of this syndrome in a prison may suggest deficiencies in the admission program. A suggestible patient is made worse by repeated questioning, especially if questions are asked that the inmate perceives as foolish or as patronizingly simple. The nature of a question determines the nature of the answer, and foolish questions beget foolish replies. Treatment is supportive and expectant.

ADJUSTMENT DISORDERS
CAUSED BY OTHER LIFE STRESSES

The three primary components of an Adjustment Disorder are:

1. A difficult situation
2. A normal personality (usually)
3. The failure of coping mechanisms

The diagnosis implies that the stressful situation involved is one which would be upsetting to most healthy people. A wide range of problems which occur at school, at work, in the home, or in relationships with significant people threaten some loss of security or interfere with sources of satisfaction. The period of adjustment to a change in environment (e.g., moving to a new community, changing jobs, a promotion involving new duties and responsibilities) is one in which various sources of insecurity arise.

Though this diagnosis is usually used for the stress reactions of otherwise healthy adults, one can make the diagnosis appropriately for a person who has another psychiatric illness, if the stress reaction is clearly a separate phenomenon.

The effect of a stress upon the healthy person depends on a number of factors, which include the following.

1. The actual magnitude of the stress. Some situations would be disturbing to *any* healthy adult.
2. The particular effects of the stress on the patient's life situation. The loss of a job could range from being a minor inconvenience to being a major personal tragedy.
3. The relation of the stress to the psychic structure of the individual. Healthy people are not free from intrapsychic conflict; their conflicts are usually controlled by effective ego defense mechanisms. A stress that impinges upon a conflict area is more difficult to manage than one that does not. For example, having a handicapped child creates a problem for anyone. It is a greater problem for a mother who doubts her own adequacy as a woman even though her doubts were adequately repressed until the child's disability became apparent.
4. Past experiences which prepare the person to meet the situation. A youngster who was away from home for short visits to relatives and who attended summer camps is better prepared for going away to school than if he or she had not had those experiences. A woman who has helped care for younger siblings

and did babysitting as an adolescent is better prepared to care for her first infant than a woman who has literally never held a small baby. In other situations or impending situations, past successes or failures in similar circumstances lead to relative optimism or pessimism and make the stress less or more disturbing.

5.   Available practical solutions to the problem. The effect of losing a source of satisfaction is somewhat dependent upon the number of other available ways of obtaining gratification. Some difficult situations could be handled in any of several more or less effective ways; others are traps in which any action is fraught with undesirable consequences, and in some there is actually nothing than can be done.

6.   The number of other stresses occurring at the same time.

The healthy adult encountering a stress is usually aware of some discomfort and experiences some concern or worry. In some situations there is fear, anxiety, grief, annoyance, or anger. Then one begins to do something about the situation. One may already have established a way of dealing with similar situations. If this does not work, one tries something else. Appropriate ego defenses give unconscious support to voluntary coping mechanisms.

For example, a man becomes aware that his girlfriend is becoming interested in a rival and he feels that he is about to lose her. He is worried by this threat to satisfaction (and perhaps security). His first effort at coping with this situation may be to talk to her about it. In the healthy individual this is more likely to begin by asking some questions, in hopes perhaps of obtaining some reassurance concerning her feelings about him and the rival. Possibly he seeks to identify and resolve misunderstandings. If this fails, he may, depending on his personality structure, plead with her or express strong disapproval of her seeing the other man. Still unsuccessful, he may try to win her back by being more attentive and doing more of the things he knows she likes. He may increase his commitment to her by a definite proposal of marriage or he may become more ardent in his sexual advances. To minimize his discomfort during these efforts to solve his problem he may talk it over with close friends, partly for advice, partly for emotional support. He probably consciously seeks other things which he knows take his mind off worries: recreation, hard work, or a few beers. His ego defense mechanisms prevent the situation from posing too much threat to narcissism, his masculine self-concept and concern over male adequacy, and residual childhood fears of rejection or abandonment. Sublimation, denial (refusal to recognize some of the signs of failure in the courtship), and isolation (contemplating possible loss without a feeling of loneliness) are utilized effectively, that is, enough to protect him from too much discomfort, but not so much as to prevent appropriate action.

If it becomes apparent that his efforts to salvage the relationship are doomed to failure, he begins to make new plans. He decides to give up the thought of marriage for a time and concentrate on his career. He finds other sources of satisfaction. Perhaps he spends money he was saving for an engagement ring for a luxury he has wanted for himself. He has a few dates with other girls. New mechanisms come into action. Rationalization helps him convince himself that marriage to the girl would not have worked well after all. The blow to his ego sustained in losing to a rival is softened by a conviction that the rival is not truly a better man but has only a convincing line and that, after all, the young woman is not a good judge of character. Displacement occurs, and though he had intended to give up romance for a time, he suddenly finds himself feeling about a new girl much as he did about the last.

At any point in this sequence, however, if his normal coping mechanisms are manifestly unsuccessful and his conscious search for support and substitute gratifications, together with the unconscious defenses, fail to minimize discomfort enough, he begins to show the symptoms of an Adjustment Disorder.

Symptoms and Course

The symptoms of an Adjustment Disorder vary in number and severity, but they often include:

1.   Anxiety and its derivatives
2.   Psychophysiological disturbances
3.   Behavioral disturbances
4.   Inefficiency and poor morale

The patient's discomfort most often takes the form of anxiety manifested by tremor, tension, sweating, restlessness, irritability, and difficulty in concentration. Mild depression with feelings of inferiority, guilt, and hopelessness may be present. Occasionally there may be an obsessive preoccupation with the situation or, as a result of displacement, with something else.

Somatic complaints may be more apparent than overt anxiety in some cases. These usually are limited to insomnia, anorexia, asthenia, fatigue, and/or tachycardia, but more serious psychophysiological disturbances sometimes appear (e.g., a coronary attack or perforation of a peptic ulcer). Stress affects body chemistry (e.g., students' cholesterol levels tend to go up before examinations). Production of some hormones is increased under stress, while other endocrine activity is suppressed. These changes may contribute to symptom formation.

Behavioral disturbances stem from:

1.   Maladaptive efforts to cope with the situation. Becoming abusive or assaultive does not normally obtain affection from a person who is denying it, salvage the job of a person who is in danger of being fired, or resolve a difference with a neighbor over property boundaries.
2.   Efforts to reduce anxiety or seek alternate satisfactions. Sometimes socially undesirable activities (e.g., drinking, gambling, promiscuity) are chosen, though they would normally be rejected, since the patient feels hopeless and no longer cares much about consequences.

Even in mild cases an Adjustment Disorder interferes with efficiency at work. The patient's discomfort and preoccupation with problems take attention away from duties. Displacement can lead to complaints about work or to personality clashes which are unrelated to the actual stress situation. Work attitudes deteriorate.

Symptoms are often mild and may be limited to one or two minor ones or may be so numerous and severe as to resemble a personality disorder or an acute neurosis.

Many of the stresses of living are self-limited (e.g., an examination; a court trial; an acute illness of a family member). When the stress is over, symptoms disappear promptly. Example: A student experiences anxiety, difficulty in concentration, insomnia, and has mild gastrointestinal symptoms prior to an examination. After the examination he feels tired and mildly depressed; he drinks more than he usually would that night. The next day he learns that he passed the test. He may still feel let down and tired for a day or two, but within a week at the most, all symptoms are gone.

Ongoing stress (e.g., protracted job insecurity; a difficult parent-in-law in the home) may lead to a gradual increase in symptoms. On the other hand, after a brief period of showing symptoms, some patients find effective coping devices, or ego defenses reorganize and symptoms abate or vanish.

Prolonged symptoms accompanying a long period of stress do not abate as promptly after the stress is removed as do those of short duration. Anxiety and related symptoms sometimes persist for weeks or months after the problem that produced them is resolved. Maladaptive behavior patterns can become habitual and remain as permanent residuals. Though one usually thinks of an Adjustment Disorder as resolving completely after the stress is removed, one seldom passes through a long and very difficult stress situation without having some scars remain in the personality. Cheerfulness and optimism may return after long grief and suffering, but unpleasant memories are not fully obliterated; life is not quite the same. The consequences of some situations, or one's feelings about behavior during them, can do almost irreparable damage to self-esteem.

When a stress situation fails to be resolved, a patient may, in the absence of successful treatment, go on to develop other psychiatric disorders.

Disability

The minor subjective discomfort accompanying some Adjustment Disorders is not appreciably disabling. Other symptoms are totally incapacitating. In some cases the true degree of disability is not immediately apparent. A patient's reduced attention to work may impair productivity and creativity. Personality clashes resulting from fatigue and irritability, from displacement, or from ineffectual efforts to cope with a situation at work can hamper organizational efficiency and jeopardize individual careers. Various manifestations of a patient's stress-induced behavior are in themselves stressful to coworkers. If the patient has a relatively important position, the disturbed behavior (e.g., an impulsive decision) may set off a chain reaction that creates stresses for numerous others. One executive's personal headache can have an entire organization taking aspirin.

Differential Diagnosis

The Adjustment Disorders are to psychiatry what the common cold is to internal medicine. Though, because of chronicity, some other disorders, notably the Passive-Aggressive Personality, have a higher prevalence, the incidence of situational disturbances is the greatest of any psychiatric syndrome. Almost everyone has experienced stress situations which have given rise to symptoms or symptomatic behavior. Most people have had several such experiences.

The high incidence of stress in daily living complicates differential diagnosis. Almost any psychiatric history will reveal stresses; many contain stresses sufficient to produce symptoms in some healthy adults.

The time relationship between the onset of the supposedly causative stress and the emergence of symptoms must be determined. Obviously, if the stress is etiological, it must antedate symptoms.

One must distinguish between stress situations that arise spontaneously in the patient's life and those that result from the recurring or prevailing behavior patterns associated with a Personality Disorder or a chronic neurosis. This distinction is essential for prognosis and treatment planning. Examples: (1) A man reports anxiety, irritability, and job dissatisfaction. It is apparent that a disturbed relationship with his supervisor immediately antedated and has accompanied these symptoms. If the condition is an Adjustment Disorder, a change of jobs or transfer to another department would be one effective solution to his difficulties; however, if his difficulties with the supervisor stem from a rebellious attitude toward father surrogates, a transfer would provide, at best, only temporary relief. (2) A woman complains of insomnia, anorexia, and weight loss. The symptoms appeared shortly after her marriage to an alcoholic. History reveals three previous marriages, all to men who had alcohol problems; one of them ended in divorce after the husband had been treated for alcoholism and had remained sober for over a year. It is possible that an alcoholic spouse meets one of her significant emotional needs and that treatment directed at the immediate situation (e.g., helping her to get the husband to stop drinking) would fail to help her materially. (3) A woman complains of being generally unhappy. She is becoming inefficient in her housework. She attributes this to her husband's frequent absences from home and his presumed involvement with other women. Assuming a previously normal personality, this could be regarded as an Adjustment Disorder. However, if the difficulties at home resulted from the patient's inhibited sexual desire and neurotic conflicts over sex, treatment planning would have to take this into account.

A stress may be the precipitating event for almost any acute psychiatric illness. The specific symptoms, and their persistence after the removal of the stress, usually make differential diagnosis possible. If the stress is continuing, the distinction is more difficult.

Since the diagnosis usually implies a healthy premorbid personality, previous history is helpful in diagnosis. The past history may be deceptive if the patient tends to minimize or rationalize previous difficulties. In some cases, psychological testing will reveal the presence of a chronic disorder.

The diagnosis may be missed if the patient fails to report the situation. A man may be aware of a difficulty in his life but not aware that it contributes to symptoms. If his concept of being an adequate man includes guts, being able to take it, or something of the sort, he is unwilling to recognize, and even more unwilling to tell someone, how much some situations bother him. The situation itself may be embarrassing; it can be something that the patient has been unable to discuss with family and friends (e.g., the break-up of an extramarital affair).

Prevention

Life is never easy, simple, and free of stress. However, as civilization progresses, some stresses can be eliminated or ameliorated through development of social institutions (e.g., unemployment compensation; rehabilitation programs). Stress can be reduced in vocational settings. The industrial physician and the employer should recognize that vocational stresses reduce productivity. Personnel policies that enhance job security are not incompatible with those that promote healthy competition, incentive, and challenge. Assigning employees tasks that are within the range of their capacities is both good business and good mental hygiene. An assignment that leads to frustration and failure hurts the organization as well as the employee. Clear job descriptions, channels of communication, and lines of authority lessen occupational stress. Policies in regard to transfers should take into account the adjustments required in relocation.

Preparation for the common stresses of living reduces their impact. The family physician should know whether a youth is prepared to go away from home to school; whether a young patient is prepared to make reasonable vocational plans in keeping with capacities and interests, and unlikely to lead to failure and disappointments; whether patients know the responsibilities and adjustments that go with marriage and having a family and are prepared to cope with them; whether patients are prepared to deal with other usual stresses and adjustments of adult life.

Worrying about some misfortunes that may never occur can be symptomatic of the Compulsive Personality. Constructive worrying, planning what to do if things go wrong, reduces the danger of an Adjustment Disorder.

Having an adequate number of sources of security, satisfaction, and self-esteem lessen the consequences of losing any one. Another thing important in prevention of Adjustment Disorders is the availability of counseling, of help with problems before they become overwhelming, of emotional first aid. To a certain extent the physician can be available for this purpose. Support of social agencies in the community contributes to this; appropriate referrals to these agencies can prevent Adjustment Disorders. In industry, since these disorders, like other illnesses, impair productivity, the employer has a practical, not merely an altruistic interest in seeing that stress situations, vocational and otherwise, which affect employees, are recognized. If help with personal problems cannot be given by the supervisor, the personnel department, or the medical department, at least someone should know the community resources for help with various personal problems well enough to direct the employee to them.

Treatment

If the stress situation is likely to be self-limited and of relatively short duration, treatment is primarily supportive. The patient needs an opportunity to discuss feelings about the problem. It may be possible to offer some helpful information or advice. Encouragement and reassurance are often possible. Symptomatic medication can be used.

A continuing stress situation requires a more comprehensive psychotherapeutic approach. In those instances in which the patient does not recognize that a situation is stressful, minimizes it, or fails to see its relation to symptoms or behavior, helping to clarify this is a first step in treatment.

Symptomatic medication is often useful but is never adequate as the sole treatment, as it might be in some self-limited stress situations.

A recognition that some ineffectual efforts at coping are doing more harm than good, or that symptomatic behavior is making the total situation worse instead of better, can be helpful. This can often be brought out through questioning in an accepting, noncritical manner compatible with usual psychotherapeutic procedure. If the patient does not readily recognize maladaptive behavior once it is discussed openly, and makes no effort to modify it, work with this aspect of the disorder is best deferred until the stress situation itself is relieved.

The main focus of therapy is upon exploration of all aspects of the situation and the patient's feelings about it. The possible courses of action are all explored in detail. There are three basic options in any stress situation:

1.   The patient can do something to change the situation.
2.   One can get out of it.
3.   One can change oneself so as to live more comfortably with it.

The last could involve the acceptance of an unpleasant reality, a change in attitudes and expectations, or methods of gaining satisfaction and security in other areas of living so as to make an otherwise unbearable situation tolerable.

In a given situation there may be several different possible ways of achieving each of the basic solutions, or there may be few practical alternatives.

The patient's own failure to find a workable solution may come from failure to think of a possibility or arbitrarily dismissing it as impractical or unacceptable without full consideration. Examples: Though obtaining help from a public agency is clearly possible, a patient may have failed to investigate it because of the mistaken belief that the agency serves only indigents, or because of an emotional reaction to what is seen as taking charity. (2) Because of something she has read, a woman assumes she could not obtain legal redress, and has never actually consulted a lawyer.

A person may persist in coping methods that are not working without really giving much thought to defining the actual problem and seeking the best possible solution. Instead of thinking through all possibilities, one may go over and over a limited number of obviously unsatisfactory ones.

The therapist draws from the patient all of the possible courses of action and their probable consequences, advantages, and disadvantages. It is the patient who selects the solution. Sometimes the patient feels that a situation is a trap. It is painful and has numerous adverse effects. Yet each way out seems blocked by consequences that are equally damaging. The therapist may or may not be able to help the patient find a good way out of the trap or a way to live in it asymptomatically. If neither can be done, perhaps the patient can be supported in taking the alternative that involves the least detrimental consequences. Sometimes the consequences can be seen as worth taking, either because of long-range advantages or because of the ultimate consequences of *not* doing anything about the situation. Examples: (1) A man realizes that his job is responsible for symptomatic behavior. His therapist realizes that the stresses are genuine and that a successful adjustment to them is unlikely. The patient has rejected changes of occupation open to him because of income reduction and its effect on his family. However, he is helped to recognize that his behavior in the situation will ultimately lead to his losing the job anyway, and chooses the most acceptable of available alternatives. (2) A woman in an intolerable domestic situation has failed to consider terminating her marriage because of the anticipated effect of separation on the children. She recognizes that the children are being harmed more by the domestic strife in the home than they would be by the breakup of the marriage and decides on separation. She is not advised to do this; she reaches the decision after considering all of the factors, some of which she had previously omitted from her thinking.

Sometimes help with a situational problem can be obtained from a nonmedical counselor. Help with marital difficulties may be obtained from a clergyman, a lawyer, or a social worker. Likewise, there are other resources available for help with educational and vocational problems. There may be people who would have a better knowledge of possible solutions than the physician. Before the problem situation becomes a situational reaction, before coping mechanisms fail completely, before symptoms appear, there is no doubt that some such referrals are equal or superior to medical management. However, when symptoms appear, the disorder becomes primarily a medical problem because of the potential usefulness of adjunctive medication, the need for ongoing consideration of differential diagnosis, and the risk of a more serious psychiatric disorder if the problems are not resolved. This does not exclude the use of other counseling in addition to that given by the physician.

For example, a college student elects a premedical course, in part at the urging of his parents. After two or three semesters it is obvious that his grades will not qualify him for admission to an accredited medical school. He is worried about his future and undecided what to do. It may be that he lacks the intellectual capacity for the course he has chosen and is almost certain to encounter further frustrations if he persists. It may be that his study habits are at fault, or perhaps his wish to please his parents by becoming a physician is in conflict with a desire to pursue some other career of which they would not approve, and poor motivation accounts for his academic difficulties. An educator might be able to determine the cause and suggest a solution more easily than a physician. However, the case described is not an Adjustment Disorder; the boy is not sick. Suppose the student does nothing about his problem and during the next semester begins to have trouble in concentration, insomnia, headaches that frequently cause him to miss classes, and he comes to the dean's attention for several violations of college rules. His case is diagnosed as an Adjustment Disorder. It is now a medical problem. The physician may wish to have intelligence and vocational preference tests done, and on the basis of findings may want to consult, or have the patient consult, a faculty advisor for help in appraising the reality of the situation and the possible alternatives. She or he may even refer the patient for counseling; however, one remains active in the management of the case. Whether one sees the patient for psychotherapy or refers him for nonmedical counseling, one will probably prescribe medication for the headaches and will periodically reevaluate differential diagnosis and progress.

ADJUSTMENT DISORDERS OCCURRING IN LATE LIFE

There are specific stresses which arise during late life including:

1.   Physical changes
2.   Retirement
3.   Loss of family members and friends

The effect of changes in appearance and physical abilities which accompany normal aging depends not only on how these qualities have contributed directly to obtaining satisfaction and security but also on what their role has been in the self-concept.

Retirement requires new adjustments. Often it means a change in income and standard of living. The newly retired person may move (moving itself is stressful), and if the move is to smaller quarters, one may have to dispose of a number of familiar personal possessions. Retirement requires finding ways of using increased leisure. It interrupts a number of meaningful social contacts. Often a job contributes to self-esteem. Retirement takes away some feelings of status, importance, and usefulness.

A number of significant relationships are disrupted during late life. Children grow up and leave the home. Family members and friends die. Other friends retire and leave the community.

Differential diagnosis is difficult in late life. The patient is almost certain to be experiencing some fairly major stresses and encountering needs for new adjustments. Past history and careful study of the circumstances surrounding the onset of symptoms is helpful.

Some Adjustment Disorders with depressed mood occurring in patients in the late 50s and early 60s must be differentiated from other Affective Disorders. The possibility of brain syndromes, especially Alzheimer's Disease and Multi-infarct Dementia, has to be considered. The fact that psychological tests reveal minimal "organic signs" does not, however, establish a diagnosis or rule out situational factors. Planning for old age is important in prevention of Adjustment Disorders in late life. Industry and labor groups are taking a growing interest in retirement planning. The physician should encourage this and also accept the responsibility to help patients meet the stresses of late life as well prepared as possible.

If a patient keeps physically and intellectually active, changes resulting from disuse are less likely to occur. New interests, activities, and sources of satisfaction must be planned to take the place of those lost as a result of aging itself, or forced upon the individual by compulsory retirement.

Since significant people are going to be lost at an increasing rate, the aging patient must have ways of meeting new people and establishing new relationships.

Diet, general maintenance of physical health, and correction of visual and hearing disorders are important adjuncts to prevention and treatment.

Treatment is essentially the same as that for Adjustment Disorders occurring earlier in life. The younger therapist may have some difficulties in grasping and empathizing with the problems of the aging patient. One must be alert to the possibility that one's own fears of growing old influence attitudes toward the elderly. One is particularly likely to experience countertransference difficulties.

SITUATIONAL CRISIS
IN CHRONIC PSYCHIATRIC ILLNESS

Patients with personality disorders, chronic neuroses, and chronic mild psychoses often make fairly satisfactory social and vocational adjustments. They are exposed to all of the stresses and adjustment needs that are encountered by other adults (in addition to a few others of their own making). They have less effective coping techniques and ego defense mechanisms and hence will show more marked symptoms in proportion to the severity of a stress than do healthy adults.

While we usually think of Adjustment Disorders as occurring in otherwise healthy adults, an Adjustment Disorder can occur in a person with other mental illness. Many chronic patients seek medical help only when situational anxiety is added to their other problems in living. Whenever a patient seeks treatment for a psychiatric disorder of more than a few weeks' duration, one must ask oneself and the patient, "Why now?" Sometimes there are other reasons, but often a situational problem will be discovered. Then there are two relevant questions: (1) Does the patient want treatment for the underlying condition, or is help being sought only for an increase in discomfort stemming from an immediate problem in living? This distinction may or may not be consciously formulated by the patient. (2) Is the stress situation a recurring type of difficulty produced by the patient's behavior patterns or resulting from symptoms of the underlying disorder?

A patient who is really coming for help with an immediate problem is unlikely to continue to come for an extended evaluation or for treatment focused on the total personality rather than the present difficulty. Initial treatment is for the Adjustment Disorder. If the underlying condition is so disabling as to require treatment on its own merits, the patient can perhaps be helped to see this after adequate attention has been given to the situational difficulty.

Situational problems of a recurring character based upon habitual maladaptive behavior must be treated, however, in the context of the total personality disorder. The patient must be helped to see that the pattern is repetitive and that a quick solution to the present problem will not be adequate treatment.

A major difficulty in differentiating between those chronic patients who come for help with their basic disorder and those who seek first aid for a crisis is the tendency of some patients to use a relatively minor problem in living as an excuse to see the physician. The patient may want to give a reason for coming, but at the same time may hesitate to be completely candid about ongoing difficulties. If the patient spontaneously digresses from a discussion of the presenting problems, or shows any resistance to the therapist's attempt to focus discussion on it, this possibility can be suspected.

Recognition of the patient's actual purpose in seeking help leads to more accurate selection of treatment focus and method. It also reduces "drop-outs" from therapy.

REVIEW QUESTIONS

1. Name several stresses sufficient to cause symptoms in a healthy adult.
2. A patient with a chronic psychiatric disorder seeks help with symptoms which apparently have been produced by situational stress. How do you decide whether or not to make a diagnosis of Adjustment Disorder?
3. What factors contribute to the disorganization of personality in a Brief Psychotic Reaction or an Adjustment Disorder caused by gross stress?
4. What preparations can be made in advance to diminish the impact of a catastrophe in the civilian population? In the military?
5. In an Adjustment Disorder, what are some of the factors which influence the effect that a particular stress situation will have on the person experiencing it?
6. What are some common presenting symptoms in an Adjustment Disorder? What clues might the general physician have that the complaints result from situational factors?
7. How does treatment of a person in a self-limited stress situation differ from the treatment of a person in a continuing stress situation?
8. In exploring the situation with the patient, the physician keeps in mind the three basic options for coping with stress situations. What are they? Give examples in which each method of coping with the situation would be appropriate.
9. What stresses may contribute to an Adjustment Disorder in late life? How can the effect of these stresses be minimized?

SELECTED REFERENCES

1. Andreasen, Nancy C., and Paul R. Hoenk: The predictive value of adjustment disorders: A follow-up study. *Am J Psychiatry* 139(5):584-590, 1982.

2. Andreasen, Nancy C., and Patricia Wasek: Adjustment disorders in adolescents and adults. *Arch Gen Psychiatry* 37(10):1166-1170, 1980.

3. Caplan, Gerald: Mastery of stress: Psychosocial aspects. *Am J Psychiatry* 138(4):413-420, 1981.

4. Eaton, M.T., Jr.: Investigative psychotherapy in general practice. *Med Times* October, pp. 942-947, 1963.

5. Eaton, M. T., Jr.: Situational anxiety: Diagnosis and treatment. *Am Pract* 13(9):598-600, 1962.

6. Eaton, M. T., Jr.: Executive stresses do exist — But they can be controlled. *Personnel* March/April, pp. 8-28, 1963.

7. Hendrie, H. C., D. Lachar, and K. Lennox: Personality trait and symptom correlates of life change in a psychiatric population. *J Psychosom Res* 19:203-208, 1975.

8. Horney, Karen: *The Neurotic Personality of Our Time.* New York, Norton, pp. 90-92, 1937.

9. Horney, Karen: *Self Analysis.* New York, Norton, pp. 252-273, 1942.

10. Kreuz, Leo E., Robert M. Rose, and Richard Jennings: Suppression of plasma testosterone levels and psychological stress. *Arch Gen Psychiatry* 26(5):479–482, 1972.

11. Looney, John G., and E. K. Eric Gunderson: Transient situational disturbances: Course and outcome. *Am J Psychiatry* 135(6):660–663, 1978.

12. Titchener, James L., and Frederic T. Kapp: Family and character change at Buffalo Creek. *Am J Psychiatry* 133(3):295–299, 1976.

Chapter 7

PERSONALITY AND IMPULSE
CONTROL DISORDERS

A DISORDERED WAY OF LIFE

The Personality Disorders are:

1.   Lifelong processes (usually)
2.   Manifested by recurring maladaptive behavior rather than symptoms

The lifelong nature of these disturbances distinguishes them from acute psychiatric syndromes. An increase in severity, often associated with external stress, may bring the patient into treatment, but careful history-taking will identify the pathological behavior during all stages of adult life, adolescence, and usually childhood.

The few cases which do not have a lifelong history of disturbed activity are those in which a personality disturbance remains as a residual of an unresolved Adjustment Disorder.

Manifestations of repeated maladaptive, self-defeating actions are observed in the patient's:

1.   Pursuit of basic instinctual goals
2.   Adjustment to society
3.   Relationships with significant people

Except when there is external stress, either coincidental or in reaction to the patient's behavior, anxiety is absent. Other subjective complaints are rare; when present, they are usually rationalizations or conscious efforts to excuse failures.

Since these patients experience problems in living rather than symptoms, they often fail to seek professional help; when they do, it is likely to be:

1.   For symptoms arising from a superimposed stress situation

2.   Because of a gradual awareness of an unsatisfactory way of life
3.   At the urging of another person (e.g., spouse; employer)

Corollary to the presence of ineffectual ways of dealing with life's problems is an absence of effective ego defenses and coping mechanisms. Hence, stress is poorly tolerated. Minor difficulties and frustrations evoke anxiety; moderate ones which could be tolerated by a healthy personality lead to transient psychotic episodes. Pressures of daily living, unrelated to the personality disturbance, can cause enough discomfort to require treatment. Also, self-defeating activities get the patient into repeated stress situations (e.g., frequent conflict with employers or supervisors).

Failures to achieve goals are easily attributed to circumstances beyond one's control. Difficulties in interpersonal relationships are readily ascribed to the other person. However, after repeated failures, an intelligent person may have enough insight to recognize a need for change. Unfortunately, in modern society a person often fails to get the feedback that would help in reaching a decision.

The vocational setting is an important part of living, and mastering it effectively contributes to many basic goals. Employees whose behavior, rather than lack of technical ability, prevents advancement or leads to dismissal, are rarely told the true reasons or given encouragement to change.

A need for treatment is sometimes recognized by employers who hope to salvage an otherwise desirable employee. Vocational counselors, welfare workers, and others who encounter the consequences of maladaptation make additional referrals. Etiological factors probably include:

1.   Constitutional predisposition
2.   Identification with significant people who have similar personalities
3.   Childhood experiences which encourage aberrant behavior

Constitutional, hereditary, or development factors cannot be excluded as part of the cause of any of these conditions. In some of them (e.g., the Schizotypal Personality) these possibly contribute to the symptomatic behavior patterns. For the others, it is likely that some individuals start life with more adaptive capacity, with more of some quality — call it gumption, libido, or élan vital — than others.

Adaptive mechanisms are acquired early in life through identification with parents and other significant persons; maladaptive ones are similarly incorporated into the self. The child of a pathologically suspicious parent is not likely to be a trusting little soul. The poet may not have been correct in crediting the sons of policemen with the flattest kind of feet, but the daughter of the floozy more likely than not *will* have the wiggle in her seat, and very possibly a maladaptive one.

There are several types of experiences that encourage the development of maladaptive behavior. Among these are:

1.   Situations in which the behavior is rewarded. Examples: (1) A child who is refused something gets it after a temper tantrum, not once but repeatedly. (2) Unduly conscientious and overly conforming behavior wins praise, while initiative and originality are ignored.
2.   Circumstances in which normal behavior is not allowed to develop. Examples: (1) Parents make unreasonable demands and will not listen to a child's reasons for refusal; to avoid punishment he substitutes procrastination or half-hearted compliance. (2) A child from a minority group is rejected by playmates in his neighborhood; he begins to avoid social situations.
3.   Failures in parental guidance. Examples: (1) A youngster gives up easily; he

starts things but does not finish them. He is given no encouragement to complete tasks or tolerate temporary frustrations, nor is his occasional success in doing so rewarded. (2) A little girl rarely thanks adults for presents or favors; she is sometimes rude to visitors. There is no punishment for this, no reward for "good" behavior, and no explanation of what is socially acceptable. Even if she wanted to be polite she would not know how.

In using official nomenclature (of the *Diagnostic and Statistical Manual of Mental Disorders,* DSM-III), the Personality Disorders are coded on Axis II (see Chapter 4). On this Axis one can also record prominent personality traits that are not maladaptive or that are not sufficiently maladaptive to merit a diagnosis of a disorder. The Personality Disorders include: (1) Passive-Aggressive Personality, (2) Dependent Personality, (3) Compulsive Personality, (4) Histrionic Personality, (5) Narcissistic Personality, (6) Schizoid Personality, (7) Schizotypal Personality, (8) Avoidant Personality, (9) Borderline Personality, (10) Paranoid Personality, (11) Antisocial Personality, and (12) Atypical, Mixed, or Other Personality Disorder (a category to permit flexibility).

Each of the Personality Disorders will now be described briefly. In reading these descriptions remember that, as in other psychiatric conditions, there is a continuum between normal and grossly pathological states. The clinical diagnosis implies an appreciable degree of disability. Subclinical variants and borderline cases of all of these syndromes may be found. In fact, any healthy person may occasionally display maladaptive behavior characteristic of one of the Personality Disorders. The difference lies in degree, frequency, and consequences.

Manifestations of Personality Disorder and neurotic conflict coexist. Everyone has some intrapsychic conflict. Some patients with Personality Disorders have no more internal conflict than the average healthy person. That which is present contributes little, if any, to problems in living. Others, while not having enough to produce a neurosis, show some neurotic symptoms, and their conflicts play a significant part in their Personality Disorders. Still others have both a Personality Disorder and a neurosis.

Patients often have signs of more than one Personality Disorder. In some cases a single diagnosis is appropriate, though the additional symptoms must be taken into account in treatment planning. In other cases, more than one Personality Disorder can be diagnosed.

THE PASSIVE-AGGRESSIVE PERSONALITY

The Passive-Aggressive Personality is one of the most common psychiatric disorders. Its exact prevalence is difficult to estimate because of the number of subclinical and borderline cases and the number of cases with definite disability who fail to seek medical attention.

A passive-aggressive person habitually reacts negatively to the expressed wishes of others, but usually demonstrates this resistance covertly rather than openly. The term passive-aggressive implies two assumptions about the cause of this type of recurring negativistic behavior:

1.   A person with this disorder has a pervasive feeling of hostility toward others.
2.   He or she is afraid, unable, or unwilling to express aggression openly.

Pervasive hostility, whatever the cause, tends in itself to be maladaptive. The feeling tone in interpersonal relationships is reciprocal; a basically unfriendly person does not have many friends. Moreover, the affective component of hostility is unpleasant; when one is angry, one is not likely to feel happy.

Psychoanalytic theory attributes a biological basis to aggression as a manifestation of the death instinct, Thanatos. As such, it is destructive unless sublimated or successfully fused with the life instinct so as to facilitate constructive attacks on obstacles (e.g., a pioneer clearing fields of rock and underbrush; a businessman making a success of a new venture despite well-established competitors; a health officer "stamping out" an epidemic). There is, however, some evidence from anthropological studies and from laboratory experiments with other species that hostile, destructive aggression is not instinctual, but arises from frustration, or is learned within the cultural milieu. In any case, it is not aggression itself that is pathological. It is its pervasive character and inappropriate expression.

One can speculate on reasons why a person would not express hostility openly other than in occasional outbursts. Factors may include fears of abandonment, or retaliation, or even of the consequences of one's own angry impulses. It is easy to see how such fears could be acquired through experiences in early life. Society, perhaps because of population growth and the need of people to live together in relative harmony, has increasingly reinforced restrictions on aggressive activity and even some of its sublimation (e.g., competition is discouraged in schools by de-emphasizing grading; humor is edited to avoid giving offense to others). Certainly there are advantages to controlling aggression and times when its open expression is maladaptive. Again, the clinical concern is not that the patient inhibits aggressive activity, but that he or she does it habitually, inappropriately, and maladaptively.

Symptoms and Course

As in other Personality Disorders, symptoms appear early in life. The main symptoms are shown in relationship to authority, the need to conform to society's requirements, and to the needs, requests, and demands of others in close personal relationships. Symptomatic behavior is apparent in any situation calling for competition or compromise.

In response to authority the patient is stubborn and uncooperative. In the vocational setting, for example, she or he does not refuse to carry out an order, but compliance is half-hearted and accompanied by complaints (more often addressed to others than to the person giving the order). There is procrastination, ways are sought to avoid conforming to regulations, part of them are overlooked, loopholes are found, or the letter of the regulation is obeyed but the purpose defeated.

When a passive-aggressive person is in a position of authority or is dealing with persons perceived as being inferiors or unable to retaliate, he or she is often rude, overbearing, or inconsiderate.

In personal relationships the patient contributes less than his or her share, and when others want something, is obstructionistic and frustrating to them. When pressed, he or she does what is wanted but spoils it with complaints, or by the manner in which it is done.

Passive-aggressive behavior is usually self-defeating. In most instances it has the combined disadvantages of both compliance and noncompliance, and the advantages of neither. The alternate possibility of compromise is neglected. Examples: (1) An employee is asked to work overtime at an unpleasant task. If he accepts the assignment willingly and does his best at it, he wins his employer's approval. If he refuses flatly, he avoids the task but loses approval and possibly risks his job. He might try to reach an understanding with the employer and arrange a mutually satisfactory compromise. If he behaves in a passive-aggressive manner, he will stay but will grumble and do the work carelessly. He has the disadvantage of having to do the task; he loses the advantage of winning approval. (2) A married student comes home expecting to study for an examination but his wife wants to go to a movie. If he takes her cheerfully, he succeeds in pleasing her, perhaps enjoys the movie, but he does not get his studying done. If he refuses, he has an angry wife, but may have a better grade on the examination. Compromise is likely to be possible; an offer to go to the movies the next night, perhaps. The passive-aggressive would take her to the movies — he would complain, probably get there late, pout during the show, forget that his wife likes popcorn, blame her for his poor grades, and generally ruin the evening. Result: An angry wife *and* another poor grade.

As passive-aggressive patients grow older, the condition tends to become worse. They are less likely to be employed, are more socially isolated, and have numerous somatic complaints (a feature of this disorder which is sometimes overlooked).

Disability

The self-defeating quality of the passive-aggressive behavior makes it disabling. It is a major factor in educational, vocational, and domestic failures. Careful history-taking is necessary, since patients who have lost jobs or failed to advance because of passive-aggressive traits are often unaware of the reason.

The Passive-Aggressive Personality, and to some extent other Personality Disorders, contributes to disability from other illnesses and injuries. These patients are more likely to become disabled because their personality interferes with participation in treatment and rehabilitation programs, and possibly because there is some secondary gain associated with escape from frustrating life situations provided by a disability. Personality disorders are overrepresented among disability claimants.

Differential Diagnosis

Generalized passive-aggressive behavior sometimes accompanies an Adjustment Disorder. History of an acute onset and identification of stress sufficient to produce symptoms in the healthy personality suggests the possibility. Passive-aggressive behavior beginning in adult life can represent the character change accompanying an Organic Mental Disorder.

Passive-aggressive behavior in a specific situation or relationship may be adaptive rather than maladaptive. Examples: (1) A prisoner-of-war is ordered to work on the enemy's roads. He knows his captors do not abide by agreements concerning prisoners and that he will be shot if he refuses. His choices are among being a dead hero, a live collaborator who loses his own self-respect and that of his fellows, or being covertly noncompliant. He can malinger, slow down, and sabotage. (2) A man gives as his reason for abandoning an otherwise acceptable hobby, "My wife won't let me." One might suspect passive-aggressive pouting. The implication is quite different from that of a remark to the effect that the hobby was given up to please the wife, or so that more time could be spent with her. Normally, a grown man does not need anyone's permission for a hobby. However, before jumping to a conclusion, one should have a clear idea of the consequences of other courses of action to the patient, and his reasons for not risking them. They just could make sense. (3) A department head is ordered by her immediate superior to make extensive changes in her department. She procrastinates. In evaluating the gamesmanship used to defer action, one might want to know whether the superior is about to be replaced. (4) The strategy by which Fabius defeated Hannibal, using a series of strategic retreats rather than engaging in a major battle.

Anxiety is not a symptom of the Passive-Aggressive Personality. However, many patients' first motivation in seeking psychiatric treatment stems from anxiety. The passive-aggressive person's behavior invites stress. Examples: (1) An employee is frequently late for work or absent without adequate reason; his work is careless; he disregards instructions despite frequent reminders; he criticizes his supervisor to other employees; when suggestions are made for improvement in his work he replies sullenly or flippantly. Finally, and predictably, he is fired. He is suddenly aware that he has limited job prospects and inadequate savings. He becomes acutely anxious. (2) A wife nags and pouts. Her husband suddenly shows an active interest in another woman who does not. The wife believes that divorce is imminent. She comes to the doctor complaining of tremor and insomnia, symptoms she has not had before. (3) A man complies with the income tax laws "too little and too late." He realizes that the Internal Revenue agents mean business. He is nervous.

The obvious anxiety in such cases, together with the history of stress, can lead to an incorrect diagnosis of an Adjustment Disorder. Adequate history will reveal that the Personality Disorder antedates the stress, even if the patient's own role in inviting the stress situation is not immediately apparent. There are clues in the patient's interview behavior; a prevailing passive-aggressive way of relating to others will include the examiner. Passive-aggressive tendencies are spotted in the *way* that the patient fails to comply with the interviewer's actual or implied requests for information (the fact of noncompliance has many other possible explanations; the style offers the diagnostic clue).

A more complex diagnostic problem exists when the patient has a significantly disabling Passive-Aggressive Personality, and also has an acute neurosis. Unless the existence of the underlying Personality Disorder is recognized adequate treatment planning and accurate prognosis are impossible.

Treatment

Individual or group psychotherapy may be used in treating the Passive-Aggressive Personality. For most patients with this Disorder, therapy begins with helping the patient see the maladaptive character of the behavior, its consequences, and the need for change. If this can be done, one can then be helped to identify the goals of the behavior and find more workable ways of attaining them.

Of the therapist's problems with Passive-Aggressive Personality, the first and greatest is to keep from being antagonized by the patient's behavior. To maintain an accepting attitude toward the patient, one must recognize that being passive-aggressive is after all a way of life that merits sympathy. The patient does not do well at work and does not have the self-esteem that comes from success. Domestic life is unrewarding and friendships are tenuous. That in a sense these things are of one's own doing is irrelevant. Does the patient know a better way of living?

Secondly, the therapist risks having efforts frustrated by the patient's stubbornness and habitual noncompliance. If the therapist wishes to use an expressive therapy, the patient becomes unable to think aloud; if the therapist asks questions, the patient does not remember the answers. However, in many cases, if the therapist avoids making demands or requests of the patient, relatively satisfactory interviews occur. One does not have to be passive-aggressive to have some resistance to recognizing unpleasant truths about oneself and one's way of life. If one is passive-aggressive, one is likely to react to such suggestions with covertly expressed anger or by pouting. The therapist must not react to the patient's indirect aggression with direct or indirect aggression. On the other hand, he or she must not be diverted from the task of therapy into an effort to please the pouting patient. The habitually negative, obstructionistic behavior is not to be mistaken for a resistance specific to the therapeutic relationship.

Medication is not helpful for the condition itself. Tranquilizing drugs are considered for superimposed anxiety, but they are used with caution, since patients are likely to "misunderstand" instructions and fail to take medication as directed. Dependency problems add to risks of habituation.

THE DEPENDENT PERSONALITY

A person with the Dependent Personality disorder behaves as a clinging vine, helpless, unable to make decisions, unwilling to be alone, always looking to another to give direction and assume responsibility. This disorder was formerly classified as a subtype or variant of the Passive-Aggressive Personality in which the passive component is much more apparent than the aggressive. However, one does see some highly dependent people who do not show any signs of a pervasive underlying hostility. One also sees dependent people who are obviously hostile to those on whom they depend. Also, dependency itself can be controlling and manipulative.

Most people with dependent personalities form some stable relationships and function quite well with direction and support. Disability may be minimal. Though the role of women in modern society is changing, a high degree of dependency in a woman is still usually socially acceptable; however, there are limits. A man may be attracted to a grown woman who acts like a helpless little girl; his masculine self-image is enhanced by her need for him. He will find her less attractive in time if she is unable to have a career of her own and/or fulfill her share of the responsibilities of managing a home and raising a family. In some vocational situations, a moderately dependent person of either sex does well. Most employers will agree that there is a place for a person who asks for direction and follows it. Nothing short of a promotion can harm such an employee.

Treatment, if needed, is similar to that for the passive-aggressive patient and, in addition, focuses on helping the patient develop more self-confidence and self-esteem. The therapist's main problem is to keep the patient from becoming dependent on him or her without making the patient feel rejected.

THE COMPULSIVE PERSONALITY

People with the Compulsive Personality have a preponderance of character traits derived from the anal stage of psychosocial development. They are concerned with neatness, orderliness, and promptness. They are stingy. They are conscientious, hard-working, conforming, and adhere rigidly to social customs and moral codes. Though they may appear to have a number of friends, their interpersonal relationships lack closeness. They do a great deal for others, but the services are rendered out of a sense of duty without spontaneity, enthusiasm, or affection. They have few recreations and get little enjoyment out of living. Their energies are directed toward attaining security, not satisfaction. There is a tendency to resent authority, but the resentment is rarely expressed overtly. Occasionally there is a trace of passive-aggressive behavior, but this is outweighed by the overall pattern of conformity.

Their roles at work and in social organizations are in keeping with the personality structure. A woman with a Compulsive Personality, if active in a group preparing a church party, will be on the clean-up committee, not the entertainment committee. She will do more work than anyone else and get less recognition. In a club, she is likely to be elected secretary or treasurer, not president.

Disability

Though the disorder may markedly impair occupational functioning, disability is sometimes slight. Many jobs are open to the hard-working, meticulous, conscientious person. However, the Compulsive Personality is not likely to achieve positions of leadership because of a lack of imagination and originality and because preoccupation with detail leads to slow work; this is a handicap unless the job actually requires that each "i" be dotted and each "t" be crossed with meticulous accuracy. Preoccupation with minor details leads to neglect of major problems. These are not people who fail to see the forest for the trees; they fail to see the tree while counting its leaves.

Even if disability is minimal, treatment is indicated for two reasons: (1) the patient's lack of satisfaction in living, and (2) the risk of more serious psychiatric illness developing in middle age.

Compulsivity is relative; so is the lack of *joie de vivre* that accompanies it. At worst, one rarely sees suffering or a life of quiet desperation, but more often dull, meaningless, and pleasureless existence relieved only by hope that virtue will someday be rewarded, or that the next life will be better.

The Compulsive Personality lives systematically; when the system fails, when all of the planning, the hard work, the saving, and the virtue fail to protect one from stress, one is likely to develop an Obsessive-Compulsive Disorder, a neurosis.

In addition to being susceptible to the Obsessive-Compulsive Disorder, these patients are likely to develop depressions, most often a Major Depressive Episode in middle life. A recognition that life has passed one by, that it is too late for postponed gratifications, and that the Orphan Annie-Horatio Alger philosophy of life which has guided one has failed to produce its expected rewards are contributing factors. Associated with this is the breakdown of fantasy as an ego defense. While denying oneself satisfaction in the here and now, the patient daydreams of a different life in the future.

Here is no imaginative Walter Mitty, escaping grim reality for a few moments in fantasyland. Here is a hard-working, conscientious person dreaming, half planning a new career, a new home, perhaps more money, and a new and better spouse. It cannot quite be foreseen, but lots of things can happen. And there is time aplenty.

Some time between the ages of 40 and 65 comes the recognition that there is no longer a lot of time. At least not time for a new career or for raising a new family. The hard-working bookkeeper who has dreamed of being president of the firm, or at least treasurer or comptroller, is brought face to face with the fact that younger and better trained persons are receiving the promotions he or she once half expected. The woman who dreamed of Prince Charming as she made drudgery of keeping house and raising children, sees in her mirror that if Prince Charming came along, his eye would scarcely be attracted, and even if by some miracle he invited her to mount his white horse, her joints would be too stiff to climb aboard.

Differential Diagnosis

The absence of true obsessions and compulsions helps distinguish this condition from Obsessive-Compulsive Disorder.

Up to a point, compulsive traits are adaptive rather than symptomatic. The opposite of compulsivity is disorganization. Two questions help establish whether a particular compulsive trait is symptomatic: (1) Is it effective in the patient's life situation? (2) Can it be modified at times when it is not appropriate?

The healthy person whose compulsive tendencies help rather than hinder in the pursuit of satisfaction and security enjoys life (as much of the time as anyone else) and forms close, rewarding relationships.

Treatment

In investigative psychotherapy the patient is helped to inspect the way of life and reevaluate goals in living so as to modify compulsive characteristics without losing their useful components. This enables one to strike a better balance between security and satisfaction so as to lead a more rewarding life.

In supportive psychotherapy and in the contacts the generalist has with such patients, the patient's way of life is modified by the physician's attitude. Since the physician is viewed as a person in authority, and the patient tends to conform, one is likely to do what one thinks the doctor expects. Opposed to the conforming tendency is the patient's covert resentment of external compulsion and the parsimonious unwillingness to "give" anything to another person. When there is pressure to conform, or demands are being made, the patient becomes resistive. If the doctor does not attack the patient's rigidity too bluntly, but gently deemphasizes the importance of some nonconstructive expenditures of effort, and at the same time shows approval of recreation and enjoyment, quite a bit of modification takes place. Definite prescriptions for recreation (get a hobby, go bowling once a week) do not work. The patient does as he or she is told, but works at it rather than enjoying it. If the physician is trying to minimize unduly rigid adherence to social customs and moral codes, there is a slight risk of overcorrecting. It is possible to guide a patient into a way of life as unsatisfactory as the one from which he or she is rescued.

Even without formal psychotherapy the physician can give the patient some opportunity to express dissatisfaction with life and encourage realistic planning for future changes. Help with retirement planning well in advance is important.

THE HISTRIONIC PERSONALITY

The Histrionic Personality, sometimes called the Hysterical Personality, is manifested by personality traits resembling those of patients with Conversion Disorder. However, actual conversion symptoms are not present.

Patients with this Disorder seek attention. They try to appear attractive and they often behave seductively. They seek new friends (or admirers?). Their behavior is dramatic and intense; they appear to overreact emotionally. Despite, or perhaps because of, the self-dramatization, others tend to regard them as shallow and insincere. Sexual promiscuity, with or without sexual satisfaction, occurs in some cases.

The Histrionic Personality makes extensive use of the mechanisms of dissociation and denial and/or their conscious analogs. Problems are treated as if they do not exist. Examples: (1) A branch manager is told that the plant in which he works will be closed in a few months and that it will be impossible to transfer him. He goes ahead making plans for the following year's work, incurs new personal debts, and fails to look for a new job. (2) A single woman becomes pregnant. She does not tell anyone, including the man involved; she makes no plans for obstetrical care. She has no arrangements for placing the child nor does she have a plan for caring for it herself.

Incongruous or contradictory personality traits often coexist (e.g., prudishness and promiscuity). Patients are seemingly unaware of the implications of some of their behavior (e.g., a woman wears revealing dresses, flirts, tells suggestive stories, and goes alone to a man's apartment. She is surprised and shocked when he makes a pass).

Disability

Patients do not do well in positions where they are responsible for planning or where they must deal with unpleasant contingencies; denial interferes too much with judgment. Dissociation may get the patient into awkward interpersonal situations. The desire for attention leading to the maintenance of an attractive appearance and the acquisition of social graces helps these people make good first impressions. Even the dramatic and emotionally excitable characteristics often make others find them interesting. However, in a vocational situation, vanity, histrionics, and inappropriate seductiveness in time tend to antagonize coworkers and employers.

Differential Diagnosis

Only in rare cases is there a problem distinguishing between the dissociation of the Histrionic Personality and that of Schizophrenic Disorders. Hysterical dissociation involves large areas of the personality; groups of related activities and ideas. The dissociation of schizophrenia separates ideas and activities into much smaller component groups (e.g., a woman with a Histrionic Personality chooses an entire wardrobe, any item of which is startling to the observer. She has no idea that she dresses to attract attention. A schizophrenic intends to dress inconspicuously and almost succeeds save that she puts on purple hose).

The presence or absence of the primary symptoms of schizophrenia is useful in differential diagnosis. An almost immediately noted difference is the desire for attention of the Histrionic Personality in contrast to the schizophrenic's withdrawal.

Differences between Histrionic Personality and Conversion Disorder include the lifelong character of the Personality Disorder and the absence of definite conversion symptoms. A person may have a Conversion Disorder or some other form of Somatoform or Dissociative Disorder superimposed upon a Histrionic Personality. Persons with this condition may also have Substance Use Disorders which may mask the underlying personality disorder.

It is particularly important to distinguish the Histrionic Personality from mild affective (manic) disorders. Hypomania may be accompanied by histrionic and attention-getting behavior together with emotional excitability resembling that of the Histrionic Personality. Medication is effective in controlling hypomanic symptoms, but does not relieve hysterical ones.

Treatment

Treatment is similar to that for other personality disturbances. However, intrapsychic conflict is more often present, and if this is a prominent feature, more attention should be given to identification of significant ego defense mechanisms, investigation of childhood experiences leading to conflict, and uncovering of repressed material.

Some patients' histrionic or seductive behavior creates problems for the therapist; these are rarely serious if they are anticipated and dealt with objectively.

THE NARCISSISTIC PERSONALITY

The word narcissism is an example of the flowery language sometimes used in psychiatry. It is derived from a Greek legend about a beautiful youth who pined away for love of his own reflection and was transformed into a blooming plant, the narcissus. In psychiatry, narcissism refers to self-love.

In psychoanalytic theory there are two types of narcissism, primary and secondary. Primary narcissism occurs in early infancy as a phase in object relationship development. It is believed that the child does not differentiate the self from the environment. Sources of pleasure are thought to be perceived by the child as coming from within the self, and accordingly the infant is believed to have a sense of omnipotence. Secondary narcissism arises later in life after libido has been cathected to external objects and represents a redirection of libido toward the self.

Though similar in some manifestations, self-love is quite different from self-esteem. Self-esteem implies an appreciation of one's worth as an individual together with a more or less realistic assessment of one's strengths and abilities. Self-love tends to idealize or overrate the self.

When a person is described as being narcissistic, the term suggests that he or she is enamored with the self, is vain, demands attention and admiration from others, and is likely to be vexed when not occupying the center of attention. Everyone has some degree of narcissism which is manifested by occasional showing off, by sometimes exaggerating one's own importance, enjoying admiration, and being attracted to people like oneself.

When one has an excess of narcissism accompanied by grandiose ideas about his or her attributes, the accompanying behavior (e.g., a medical student on clerkship treats fellow students as if he or she were a senior faculty member; a football player of moderate ability demands to be treated as a superstar) is likely to alienate others. Though annoying, narcissism is generally tolerated in people who do have unusual abilities or attributes. One can act like the popular conception of a prima donna and get by with it, if one can sing like one.

Even if narcissism is not severe enough to merit a diagnosis, if it is a prominent personality trait, it can be entered on Axis II along with another diagnosis. If it is severe enough to interfere materially with interpersonal relationships or create problems in vocational adjustment, a diagnosis of Narcissistic Personality may be warranted. People having this diagnosis as well as overrating themselves and demanding attention are usually preoccupied with grandiose fantasies of achievement, reject criticism, and are insensitive to the needs of others, whom they often exploit.

Persons whose narcissism is sufficient to merit a diagnosis often also meet the criteria for diagnosing other Personality Disorders (e.g., Histrionic Personality), and if so, both diagnoses can be used. One should be cautious that one's use of the diagnosis is indeed based upon objective evidence of impairment and does not simply reflect a negative attitude toward the patient, since the term lends itself to pejorative use.

The self-esteem of narcissistic patients is often low. In a way, narcissism can be viewed as a reaction formation against low self-esteem. This possibility should be considered in planning treatment for the narcissistic patient.

SCHIZOID, SCHIZOTYPAL, AND AVOIDANT PERSONALITIES

These three disorders are similar in that they are all characterized by impairments stemming from social withdrawal.

Schizoid personalities are characterized by:

1. Aloofness and indifference to others
2. Inability to form close relationships
3. Difficulty in expressing emotions, especially anger, appropriately
4. Excessive daydreaming

Patients are shy, aloof, and withdrawn. They avoid social activities and contact with others. Some cannot express anger or behave aggressively at all; others are unable to express anger when it is justified, but they displace it and react angrily to trifles. A few show passive-aggressive tendencies. Fantasy is more frequently utilized by these patients than by healthy persons; the content tends to be stereotyped and lacks the imaginative quality and variety of the fantasies of the healthy person or the neurotic. Daydreams are usually of being rich or powerful. Other signs of autistic thinking are sometimes shown; peculiar meanings may be attached to words or situations. The patient may show a variety of eccentricities.

The Schizotypal Personality has, in addition to the characteristics of the Schizoid Personality, signs of disordered communication and/or thinking (e.g., magical thinking; ideas of reference; illusions; autistic language) without meeting the criteria for diagnosis of Schizophrenia.

The Avoidant Personality has problems in interpersonal relationships that are superficially similar to those of the Schizoid Personality. However, social withdrawal in these cases is attributable to sensitivity and fear of rebuff rather than indifference to others. These persons want to have friends and participate in social activities, but they are afraid.

Disability

Total disability may occur. Many patients are able to work effectively in occupations which do not require close contact with others. Subjective discomfort is present and is usually expressed as a general dissatisfaction with life; a feeling that life is meaningless.

Differentiation from the healthy introvert can be made, since the latter does form some close, lasting relationships, though in social settings he or she may appear shy and withdrawn. The healthy introvert can express anger appropriately, usually does not experience dissatisfaction with life, and makes vocational choices compatible with the personality.

Treatment of Schizoid, Schizotypal, and Avoidant Personalities

If the patient is motivated for change, supportive therapy, encouragement in entering group activities, and guidance in day-to-day activities are useful. A few cases will respond to long-term investigative psychotherapy.

Under stress, these patients, especially those having the Schizotypal Personality, are likely to have acute psychotic episodes. If the stress is reduced or if the patient is removed from it by hospitalization, the acute psychoses are transitory.

Unduly vigorous attempts at psychotherapy sometimes arouse enough anxiety, either directly or indirectly by involving the patient in social situations he or she cannot tolerate, to precipitate a psychotic episode.

Patients often seek therapy because of anxiety stemming from superimposed situational problems. Help with these immediate problems is more often indicated than is an attempt at more definitive treatment.

In treating the Avoidant Personality, one initially reassures the patient through one's attitude, rather than words, of uncritical acceptance. Casual comments by the therapist are likely to be interpreted as implying rejection or ridicule, and one must be alert to this possibility in working with these patients. Nevertheless, of this group of disorders, the Avoidant Personality offers the best prognosis for improvement in individual or group psychotherapy.

THE BORDERLINE PERSONALITY

Though descriptions of borderline (or borderland) personalities have appeared in psychiatric literature for nearly a century, this Personality Disorder has only recently been recognized in official nomenclature. Prior to its present classification as a Personality Disorder, this condition was often described as being intermediate between a neurosis and a psychosis. There were some authors who felt that it was a subtype of Schizophrenia and others who regarded it as a variant of Affective Disorder. However, the Borderline Personality, like other Personality Disorders, is a lifelong condition.

Patients with this condition show behavior patterns that are described as unstable, erratic, or unpredictable. Affect shows marked fluctuations. An important characteristic is a pattern of intense, unstable interpersonal relationships; these patients socialize readily and dislike being alone, but their relationships are stormy. The marked shifts in attitudes in these intense relationships are often a result of the mechanism of splitting and the attendant inability to tolerate ambivalent feelings. If a significant person ceases to be perceived as all good, he or she becomes all bad.

Borderline patients are often sexually promiscuous and are likely, periodically, to misuse drugs or alcohol and may have psychotic symptoms when using drugs. They report feeling empty or unhappy, but are not as a rule deeply depressed, though suicide gestures and physically self-damaging acts occur frequently. In addition to having psychotic episodes when misusing recreational drugs, especially marijuana, they may have transient drug-free paranoid episodes, but they do not have prolonged episodes of clearly psychotic symptoms such as delusions or hallucinations.

Disability

Disability is usually marked. These patients are underachievers. Their impulsivity and disturbed interpersonal relationships tend to create vocational problems and lead to frequent job changes. Part of the disability may stem from identity problems and difficulties with self-image. Not feeling that one really quite knows who or what one is keeps one from making firm career choices and setting long-range goals.

Differential Diagnosis

In addition to distinguishing this condition from other Personality Disorders, one must distinguish it from Schizophrenia and from the neuroses. Though one uses all criteria in differential diagnosis, among the most reliable in distinguishing the Borderline Personality from Schizophrenia is the strong affect of the borderline patient together with the pattern of intense but stormy interpersonal relationships. In distinguishing Borderline Personality from Neuroses, helpful clues include the borderline patient's tendency to misuse drugs and to have psychotic episodes related to drug use, the more frequent and sustained dysphoria and anhedonia of the borderline patients, the tendency toward sexual promiscuity, the intolerance of being alone, the unstable relationships, and the lower school or work achievement.

Treatment

Though these patients often have symptoms that one would expect to be able to relieve with medication, one should use caution in prescribing for them because of the risks of misuse of medication and of suicide attempts or gestures. Any medication used should be carefully evaluated for benefit, bearing in mind the chronicity of the disorder and the possible side effects from long-term drug use. Antipsychotic drugs are sometimes effective (especially if the patient is really a latent schizophrenic?). Antidepressants may be used if the patient has frequent episodes of severe depression or has persistent marked dysphoria and anhedonia. Also, it should be borne in mind that some of the other behavior patterns, including those related to a search for excitement leading to antisocial behavior, may be depressive equivalents. Lithium is sometimes used for patients who have aggressive episodes, and phenytoin (Dilantin) has occasionally been used successfully for patients whose symptoms are episodic. For most patients, milieu therapy is probably the most likely to be successful, and while inpatient treatment is sometimes necessary, day patient care or care in a boarding home where the patient can experience a warm accepting attitude and direct advice about problems in living is preferable for many patients. Though some authors feel that psychotherapy aimed at insight is contraindicated, it can be considered. It is difficult for these patients to engage in a productive therapeutic relationship. The patient is likely to behave seductively toward the therapist and will bring to the therapeutic relationship the same problems in relating to people that are an essential feature of the disorder. Frustration tolerance is low and the patients are likely to be manipulative. Nevertheless, one can work with them. If one recommends psychotherapy, one should make it clear that one is making no promises of improvement. Efforts should be made to minimize transference, and transference interpretations are usually avoided. One supports positive elements in the personality and is cautious and gentle with interpretations.

THE PARANOID PERSONALITY

These patients show the symptoms of Schizoid Personalities, usually in mild form, and in addition are chronically suspicious and jealous. They see the worst in everyone and every situation. They feel slighted and insulted at times when no offense was intended. They are often litigious.

In school, the Paranoid Personality feels that he or she is discriminated against by the teachers and picked on by classmates, and at work feels that the boss is unfair. When another person receives an honor or promotion, it is attributed to favoritism. Friends are suspected of trying to take advantage. A spouse is suspected of infidelity. Quarrels with neighbors and tradesmen are frequent.

Sometimes it is hard to separate the true from the imagined acts of discrimination. The patient's chip on the shoulder attitude antagonizes others and sometimes leads to discriminatory acts. At other times, people who are habitually accused feel that they have nothing to lose by acts which justify the patient's complaints. Examples: (1) An employee habitually complains of discourtesy and poor service in the company cafeteria. This is resented, and in time he is, while treated with studied politeness, regularly given the smallest serving and the toughest meat.

(2) A wife accuses her husband of having an affair with one of her friends. She points out times when she believes the friend is flirting with him. While he knows the former to be untrue, he begins to think that the latter might be possible; this, taken together with some of the discomforts of life at home and the fact that he is being accused anyway, lead him to ask the friend for a date.

Hostility and suspiciousness lead many Paranoid Personalities to enter quasi-political activities. They take great pleasure in joining groups that are against something. With rare and unfortunate exceptions, they do not rise to positions of leadership in such groups. They cannot trust the other members, and the feeling becomes mutual.

Disability

Disability is marked. The tendency to be hurt and offended easily and the expressions of jealousy are not compatible with satisfactory vocational or domestic adjustment. If the patient's abilities are sufficient to enable him or her to hold a job despite the personality pattern, a mild case is often more disruptive to an organization than a severe one. The severely Paranoid Personality is avoided by others; the milder case has more opportunity to engage in gossip and contention.

Differential Diagnosis

Cases are distinguished from Paranoid States on the basis of history and because of the absence of delusions.

Paranoid symptoms and projective mechanisms may be noted in many other psychiatric disorders.

There are life situations in which, to a degree, suspiciousness, skepticism, and cynicism are adaptive rather than maladaptive; in these cases the tendency does not pervade all relationships.

Treatment

The Paranoid Personality is rarely willing to accept any form of treatment. Sometimes, if the behavior leads to stress situations which create enough anxiety to make him or her seek help, a treatment approach similar to that used for the other Personality Disorders is indicated.

THE ANTISOCIAL PERSONALITY

Those who appear to live by the Pleasure Principle alone, who seek to meet instinctual needs as they arise without the modifying influence of superego values, and without regard for the demands of society represent a major problem for the community and for themselves.

The Antisocial Personality is a disorder in which the major manifestations include persistent violations of the laws, mores, and customs of the community. Though there is a tendency to emphasize the harm done to society by a person's repeated violations of rules of conduct, it must be remembered that the sociopath experiences unpleasant consequences of these acts.

The Antisocial Personality, like the other Personality Disorders, is essentially a lifelong process and is manifested chiefly by disordered behavior rather than subjective discomfort. Because of the severity and complexity of this disorder, it is being discussed in more detail than the other Personality Disorders.

Antisocial Behavior as Symptomatic

Even before modern times, it was recognized that there was something wrong with the sociopath. Some violations of society's rules are readily understandable despite the deterring influence of guilt, shame, and fear of consequences. It is easy to see how various motives can impel a person to do something one feels is wrong (e.g., a hungry person stealing food or money to buy food). A rule violation by a person who hopes to avoid detection and/or is willing to accept the consequences is also often readily comprehensible (e.g., a person in a hurry to get home drives through a red light late at night. He knows it is illegal but there is no traffic and he does not feel that it is wrong. His attitude, whether thought out in words or not, is that it is unlikely that he will be caught, and if he is, he will pay the fine). However, it is not so easy to understand a person who breaks laws and rules repeatedly, apparently without having any impelling motives or gaining any particular advantage in doing so, who seems to disregard the risk of getting caught and who repeats the offenses despite punishments and painful consequences.

The Antisocial Personality's failure to follow the rules is not a result of intellectual deficiency, ignorance, thinking disorder, or confusion.

The term Moral Insanity (subsequently Moral Imbecility), introduced by Prichard in 1835 to describe people who behave in this way, implies a lack of or weakness in some quality analogous to intelligence, but relating to a capacity for adhering to ethical standards. This idea is quite compatible with the more modern concept of superego deficiency. In the latter part of the nineteenth century, at a time when constitutional factors in disease generally were emphasized, the term Constitutional Psychopathic Inferior came into use. In this term, too, there is an implicit recognition of a deep-seated weakness or deficiency in the personality.

Failure to establish constitutional etiology led to the substitution of the diagnosis Psychopathic Personality, Sociopathic Personality Disturbance, and now Antisocial Personality for these patients.

Causes

The possibility that there are constitutional factors in the etiology of the Antisocial Personality is suggested by reports of some mothers of children who became antisocial that from earliest infancy these children were different in behavior from others in the family. Also, frequent electroencephalographic abnormalities have been reported, especially 4-6 per second spikes and waves. One group of investigators reported unusual and characteristic autonomic nervous system dysfunction in one type of primary sociopath manifested by exaggerated cardiovascular response to epinephrine and inability to make graded responses to emotionally laden stimuli. Finally, there is some evidence that sociopathic behavior is more common in persons having an extra Y chromosome (XYY males) than in the general population.

Social factors are also implicated. The antisocial person appears to behave in response to id impulses, and to live by the Pleasure Principle. The Reality Principle, which should cause one to defer pleasure and to tolerate frustration is something which, along with the superego, is acquired. This is acquired not only from parents but also from a community, a milieu, in which deferring pleasure, tolerating frustration, and adhering to ethical standards is rewarded. The high incidence of delinquent behavior (much of which is antisocial in diagnostic as well as general sense) in slum areas suggests that poverty plays a role in the etiology of the Antisocial Personality. In fact, it would appear that in some slums, delinquency is more normal than is its absence.

Studies at the University of Pennsylvania showed that in some of the most severely deprived socioeconomic groups, 63 percent of boys would display seriously delinquent behavior before the age of 17. A study of the 37 percent apparently not delinquent showed most of them to be mentally ill in other ways.

Delinquency (which can occur in the absence of a Personality Disorder), though influenced by socioeconomic factors, is not a product of crowding or other features of urban living, but is just as prevalent in rural communities and small towns as it is in large cities.

Another question concerning the biological and sociological basis of psychopathy is: Is man a herd-forming animal? Most evidence suggests that human beings normally live in groups and form societies, and that this grouping together is instinctual. The loner, then, is basically deviant. However, the alternate hypothesis is that man is not naturally a social creature but is forced to form societies for protection from enemies and/or because of population growth. If this is the case, the Antisocial Personality comes closer to being the natural human condition.

Experiential factors contributing to a relative failure in superego development include the following.

1. Lack of opportunity for identification. The child who is repeatedly moved from one foster home to another is exposed to different value systems but does not form a close enough relationship with any parent surrogate to incorporate a set of standards into his or her own personality. A lack of opportunity to learn by identification also affects some children raised in orphanages or other institutional environments, though this may be avoided by staffing patterns that do allow for relationships conducive to identification. The experience of a succession of foster homes is more likely to occur in lower socioeconomic groups, but some well-to-do parents delegate the care of their young to a succession of servants and private schools in a way that makes superego development through stable identifications equally difficult.
2. Parental inconsistency and hypocrisy. The parent who changes rules too often or who gives verbal expression to one set of values and acts according to another may have a child who cannot believe any rules. Examples: (1) A mother punishes a child for a lie, then declines an invitation by claiming a nonexistent prior commitment or a dubious headache. (2) A father preaches honesty and sportsmanship and deplores cheating, but he brags about his evasion of taxes and his success in sharp business practices. (3) A mother is shocked by a four-letter word, but she indiscriminately performs the act it represents.
3. Parents who set an unreasonable standard and make unrealistic demands. If the child acquires a value system that is in constant conflict with many instinctual demands, and is also in conflict with the social environment, adherence may be resolved with the defeat of the superego. When the "preacher's boy" turns delinquent it may not be parental hypocrisy; it may be that daddy is just too good for this world.
4. Some forms of parental and community rejection. If a dog or a boy is given a bad name, he may live up, or down, to it.

Some authors include the acting-out of neurotic conflict, masochism, and guilt among the etiological factors for the Antisocial Personality. While it is clear that acting-out is sometimes antisocial and that a need for punishment can cause a crime, such cases are not properly classed as Antisocial Personality and do not show the characteristic clinical picture. However, if the diagnosis is applied loosely, as it is in some settings, these factors must be considered.

Symptoms and Course

The Antisocial personality is essentially a lifelong process, and grossly symptomatic behavior is generally apparent at or before adolescence. Behavior problems at home, truancy, and delinquency are usual. However, adult patients may withhold history of these difficulties. In the adult the main symptoms and signs include the following.

1. Numerous socially unacceptable activities. Most Antisocial Personalities will have a police record by the time they are in their early 20s. The nature of the offenses varies. However, the Antisocial Personality will show more than one type of antisocial conduct. A single recurring type of illegal activity (e.g., auto theft, prostitution) is more suggestive of a Compulsive Disorder or of the acting-out of a neurotic conflict. The component of aggressivity in the patient's personality has a bearing on the severity of the offenses. A person from the upper socioeconomic classes, if relatively unaggressive, and especially if protected by family members, may not acquire a police record at all. This is especially likely to be true if the patient is a physically attractive woman.

2. Polymorphous perverse sexual behavior. The sexual activity is largely mechanical and is aimed at immediate physical gratification with little emotional involvement. The patient is promiscuous. Heterosexual contacts are preferred if available, but most histories include some homosexual relationships and often relationships with animals. Various unusual sexual practices occur, sometimes as a matter of whim and experimentation, sometimes because of payments or gifts from a deviant partner.

3. Misuse of alcohol and drugs. Daily drinking and prolonged drinking bouts are unusual, but the Antisocial Personality nearly always has a history of episodic drunkenness. Drugs of various types, especially those readily available in the social milieu, are used, usually episodically, but habituation sometimes occurs.

4. Inability to defer pleasure. This is closely related to some of the manifestations already listed. The Antisocial Personality wants instant gratification — he wants what he wants when he wants it. Examples of the relationship of this to antisocial activity: (1) A youth "borrows" a neighbor's car to go joyriding when he could have the use of his family's car the next evening. (2) A man gives a bad check to purchase a new suit, though he has a job that would enable him to save enough to buy it in a few weeks. (3) A girl who has no money with her but does have money at home steals some costume jewelry from a store counter. (4) A housewife seduces a delivery boy between the time her lover leaves in the afternoon and her husband gets home in the evening. The failure to defer pleasure accounts for much of the apparently pointless quality of sociopathic behavior. As a factor in the commission of an offense it suggests sociopathy. Conversely, a history of being able to work, save, plan, and postpone gratifications effectively is incompatible with the diagnosis. The man who puts aside a few dollars each week for a spree in the city and is arrested when the vice squad raids a house of prostitution is behaving in a socially unacceptable way; he may be foolish or even "sick," but he is not an Antisocial Personality.

5. Inability to tolerate frustration. Acquisition of the Reality Principle permits a person to tolerate discomfort, even prolonged discomfort, to obtain satisfaction or to avoid greater discomfort. This ability is lacking in the Antisocial Personality.

6. Failure to modify behavior as a result of punishment. Sometimes the phrase failure to learn from punishment is used. However, this may create some confusion in regard to the definition of learning. The Antisocial Personality does things that are likely to result in punishment in situations in which his or her intelligence, knowledge, and past experience should lead to awareness of the probable consequences. This does not serve as a deterrent. The patient may be repeatedly punished for similar offenses. Time after time, things are done that produce unpleasant consequences. A close study of the behavior pattern shows that the patient does not seem to seek detection and punishment as may some guilt-ridden neurotics, but instead, that the inability to defer pleasure keeps him or her from taking into account the ultimate cost of impulsive action.

7. Lack of lasting close interpersonal relationships. The give and take of a close relationship requires that each person at times defer satisfaction or tolerate frustration in the interest of the other. The Antisocial Personality cannot do this. The patient is rejected by those who might be friends, not so much because of the antisocial acts, though this may be a factor, but because he or she does not contribute to the friendship. The patient takes from others but does not give of himself or herself. One manifestation of this is in the marital history. It is rare for the Antisocial Personality to maintain an even partially satisfactory marriage for very long.

8. Relative absence of anxiety and guilt feelings. Like other patients with Personality Disorders, the Antisocial Personality shows free-floating anxiety only when under external stress. When facing the consequences of behavior she or he expresses feelings of regret, and at times these sound convincing. However, further history-taking will reveal other episodes which would occasion remorse in the average person about which the patient shows no concern or guilt and which, indeed, may be related with apparent pleasure. It may be that the lack of appropriate anxiety and depression is more apparent than real (like the lack of affect of the schizophrenic), but this does not diminish its significance as a diagnostic sign.

9. Defective judgment. This is a factor in several others of the symptoms listed. However, in addition to examples of poor judgment in the history, the patient is likely to answer questions about problem situations (e.g., What would you do if you found a wallet containing money and an identification card? What would you do if you saw a man attempting to drag a woman pedestrian into his car?) in socially unacceptable ways, even if he or she wishes to make a favorable impression on the examiner. The patient often knows, and is certainly capable of learning, the conventional responses, but if they are used, they are often spoiled by a gesture, an inflection, or a cynical comment afterward.

10. Poor school and work history. The tendency to break rules and the inability to tolerate frustration keeps the Antisocial Personality from doing well in school or from holding a job long. Most patients do not complete high school. Some from upper socioeconomic class families who have superior intelligence may complete college and professional courses. Studying is more frustrating to a normal person of average, or moderately superior intelligence than it is for the brilliant sociopath who seeks to get through with minimal effort, and who uses any means of getting a good grade. The latter will likely have been in trouble a number of times, but more often than not talks his or her way out of difficulties, utilizes pressure from an influential relative or acquaintance, or (not infrequently) uses subtle blackmail to avoid punishment. Years ago, it was an axiom that one did not make the diagnosis of psychopathy in any case where the patient had held the same job for as long as 5 years. In the early

1930s, quite a bit of emphasis was placed on vocational histories and there was a considerable increase in the diagnoses of Psychopathic Personality until clinicians realized that it was the Depression, not antisocial character, that was causing many people to lose jobs. Civil service, union policies, and tenure policies, though they offer valuable protection for the average employee, may enable the Antisocial Personality to keep a job despite recognized unacceptable behavior. As in school, the more intelligent upper class sociopath is likely to keep jobs longer even though often in trouble or on the verge of being in trouble. The severe Antisocial Personality does not hold any job long; milder cases do better in some types of work than others. If work permits relatively easy impulse gratification, imposes few rules and restrictions, and gives little opportunity for impulsive cheating or stealing, and if employers are relatively unconcerned about off-duty activities, the mild Antisocial Personality may make a borderline vocational adjustment (e.g., sales work in which the salesman may take time off when he chooses to have a few drinks, go to the races, or pursue a woman, or in which regular hours, detailed reports, and quotas are not enforced, or in which the salesman does not have valuable products in his possession or collect for them himself).

In modern military service, because of the need for discipline, the Antisocial Personality functions poorly. However, if he avoids court martial long enough to get into some types of combat situations in which considerable license prevails, he may perform effectively. The life of a soldier of fortune, a revolutionary, or a guerilla fighter is sometimes compatible with antisocial personality traits. In fact, some heroes of past wars had life histories revealing more than a touch of psychopathy. Despite this, there is ample reason for rejecting the Antisocial Personality from military service, and the judge who offers the antisocial offender the option of enlistment, as is occasionally done in wartime, does no favor to the man or the country.

The antisocial individual is often described as having an outwardly pleasing personality. This is true of the less aggressive sociopaths. The pleasure motive lends itself to attention to personal appearance and to acquiring some skill in social recreations. Added to this is a lack of scruple in using flattery, and in making promises that are not meant to be kept.

The Antisocial Personality, even more than patients with other personality disturbances, is likely to develop transient psychotic episodes under stress (including prison confinement). He or she cannot tolerate frustration and lacks effective coping mechanisms.

Antisocial behavior, having its start in adolescence or before, tends to become more marked in the 20s and early 30s. Sometimes in late middle life there is some gradual improvement; the phrase burned-out psychopath used to be applied to some patients who showed this improvement.

Diagnosis

The tendency to use the term Antisocial Personality, like psychopath, more as an epithet than a diagnosis is deplorable. If the term is applied to all persons who commit antisocial acts, or even to all recidivists, it has little meaning other than disapprobation. The true Antisocial Personality must show all or nearly all of the symptoms and findings listed. Absent signs should be explainable in a way that is consistent with superego deficit.

The antisocial offender is distinguished from the compulsive in that the latter has strong superego values, and in many spheres of activity is able, perhaps too able, to defer satisfaction and tolerate frustration. The compulsive will usually commit only one type of offense, is aware that it is undesirable, and struggles against the impulse.

The patient whose antisocial behavior represents the acting-out of neurotic conflict also usually shows only one or two types of aberrant behavior and does not show the other symptoms of sociopathy. There is a pattern of controlled behavior, but under external stress or because of increasing intrapsychic conflict, the patient experiences mounting tension which culminates in acting-out followed by genuine remorse and guilt feelings. A need for punishment based upon masochism or guilt feelings rather than sociopathy is suggested when the behavior pattern seems to seek detection and punishment actively rather than merely disregarding potential consequences.

Differentiation should also be made from the Borderline Personality, Histrionic Personality, and other Personality Disorders in which antisocial behavior sometimes occurs. Rarely, behavior suggestive of the Antisocial Personality may occur in schizophrenic patients as a result of delusional content or of autistic interpretations of some of society's rules.

Patients with Cyclothymic Disorders or mild Manic Episodes may be mistakenly diagnosed as having Antisocial Personalities. A combination of mood elevation, grandiosity, the desire for excitement, and unrealistic optimism that everything will turn out well may result in antisocial acts.

Now and then one finds a mentally retarded patient who has a pattern of antisocial behavior. Often such a patient commits offenses as a result of persuasion by others in an effort to obtain status in a delinquent group, or to obtain approval and affection from an individual.

Antisocial behavior can accompany the character change occurring with an Organic Mental Disorder. This possibility should be considered when there is an onset of antisocial behavior in adult life.

Prevention

A reduction in the prevalence of Antisocial Personalities might be facilitated by:

1. Steps to eliminate poverty and the unhealthy concomitants of slum living
2. Placing children who cannot live at home in institutions or foster homes that can assure them the possibility of forming stable identifications with adults who have adequate superego structures
3. Early recognition of the possibility of Antisocial Personalities developing in children who show truancy, behavior problems, or delinquency so that environmental problems may be corrected and therapy offered before the disorders become fully established

Treatment

The Antisocial Personality is not usually aware of being sick and rarely seeks help voluntarily. When he or she does, it is sometimes with an ulterior motive (e.g., using "I'm sick" as an excuse for behavior that is getting one into trouble).

Though the prognosis is poor, attempts to treat the Antisocial Personality should be made if he or she appears as an outpatient, whether with a genuine wish to change, with ulterior motives, or under duress. However, if the motive is not a real desire for change, it is helpful if the true motivation can be discussed openly and recognized explicitly from the start. Treatment should also be offered in prisons and other institutional settings.

Individual and group therapy are used. In individual therapy, acquisition of a value system, a superego, by identification with the therapist may occur. The personal characteristics of the therapist are important factors in one's ability to treat these patients effectively. The therapist must be a person who is successful in living. One need not be financially successful, or successful in other material ways, but one must enjoy life. Otherwise, one would scarcely expect a hedonistic sociopath to even begin to form an identification. Further, the therapist must have a comfortable and workable adaptation to society's rules. One cannot have poorly controlled antisocial impulses of one's own; one cannot envy the antisocial personality's tendency to live by the Pleasure Principle; one cannot be a hypocrite. However, while one must have a superego structure, it cannot be too rigid. The Antisocial Personality cannot gain by identification with a similar personality, but he or she cannot hope to identify with a totally opposite one. Otherwise, the therapy of the Antisocial Personality is similar to that of patients with other Personality Disorders.

The therapist working with antisocial patients is often warned against being "conned" (allowing patients to manipulate). This is a sound warning. If the patient feels able to fool the therapist with ease, it leads to a lack of respect for the therapist's ability, values, and advice. On the other hand, the desire to avoid being conned may lead one to refuse perfectly reasonable requests and in so doing to reject the patient in a way that imperils a good working relationship. Sometimes one can point out a manipulative maneuver but at the same time grant the request on its own merit.

Psychotropic drugs are rarely used in the treatment of the Antisocial Personality. Even though they are prescribed for symptomatic relief of anxiety when the patient is under stress, there is considerable possibility that they will be misused. In institutional settings, antisocial patients will try to obtain sedatives or stimulants, sometimes by malingering, in order to sell them to others or to overdose with them as a substitute for alcohol. Patients who show signs of an autonomic nervous system dysfunction may respond to imipramine.

Prefrontal lobotomy has sometimes been recommended for Antisocial Personalities. Generally, since cortical damage reduces impulse control, one would not expect this to work. However, in rare cases in which the antisocial behavior is extremely aggressive and dangerous, it is possible that the procedure might reduce aggression enough to enable the patient to function safely in the community. If one is to consider prefrontal lobotomy or any other neurosurgical procedure, legal counsel is desirable with specific reference to the patient's capacity to give informed consent (or another person's right to give it for him or her). Question has been raised as to whether a prisoner or a committed patient is capable of informed consent, since some element of coercion may be implicit in being confined. Another factor that might bear on the capacity of a person with Antisocial Personality to give informed consent is the defect in judgment which is a feature of this condition.

Dyssocial Behavior

Repeated socially unacceptable behavior is not necessarily symptomatic of Personality Disorder or other mental illness. However, persons who engage in such behavior may want to change or may be referred for diagnostic purposes. The category of Adult Antisocial Behavior which is listed with the Conditions Not Attributable to a Mental Disorder in DSM-III is used to describe these patients.

Like the Antisocial Personality, the dyssocial person violates laws, rules, and customs. There the resemblance ends. The dyssocial person is one who has developed an aberrant superego through identification with a parent and/or a cultural group whose standards are different from those of the society as a whole. He or she may show one or several types of socially unacceptable behavior. However, he or she can defer pleasure, tolerate frustration, form lasting relationships, modify behavior because of its consequences, experience guilt, use good judgment, and unless not working is part of the "code" accumulate a good vocational record.

The dyssocial patient does not feel that the behavior is wrong, but is in disagreement with the mainstream of society. While remaining in a subcultural group with similar standards to one's own, one is unlikely to want to change. If on the other hand, the person is socially mobile, there may be some spontaneous motivation for change if the behavior leads to repeated difficulties. If such a person does enter therapy voluntarily or under duress, he or she is much easier to treat than the antisocial person, since there is a capacity for forming a positive transference to the therapist.

Borderline Antisocial States

There is little uniformity in superego structure. Diogenes would have to look for a long time to find a completely honest man. If a group of subjects are placed in situations in which various types of stealing, lying, or cheating are possible, a few will show a general lack of superego functioning. Others will be honest in most situations but not in all.

Some of the deviations from socially acceptable behavior result from minor dyssocial elements in parent figures. If Mother approved of the white lie, her children probably will too. Sometimes a child identifies with a parent whose neurotic conflict over some type of socially unacceptable behavior is not acted out. The child may carry it into action; sometimes this is done with overt or covert parental approval. Examples: (1) A mother had strong impulses toward premarital sexual behavior but fear and guilt held them in check. She subscribes nominally to the idea that such conduct is undesirable. She shows a great deal of curiosity and interest in her daughter's dates. She encourages her to dress and behave provocatively. She allows her to go out with older boys, to stay out later than most girls her age, and sometimes allows her to have boyfriends in the house unchaperoned. She expresses some surprise when she finds her daughter in a compromising situation, but passes it off with a laughing comment about modern girls. (2) A father who never behaved aggressively as a youngster tells his sons at great length and with enthusiasm of fights and acts of vandalism done by members of his own high school gang. When school authorities complain of the boy's behavior, Father feels that they are being too strict, and "boys will be boys."

Some other gaps in superego function (superego lacunae) result from selective inattention. Children focus attention on those things that produce parental approval or disapproval. Conduct that the parents appear to disregard is unlikely to be important to the child. If a particular type of behavior is apparently neither desirable nor undesirable as far as parents are concerned, the child will approach situations involving it according to the Pleasure Principle.

Relatively minor deviations from socially acceptable behavior are often not diagnosable and may not be of clinical significance. On the other hand, in some instances they may lead to social maladjustment, school or vocational difficulties, or marital problems. If so, treatment, usually individual psychotherapy similar to that used for Personality Disorders, is indicated. Behavior therapies and behavior modification programs may be used to help alter behavior patterns which the patient experiences as undesirable in themselves or because of their consequences.

ATYPICAL, MIXED,
OR OTHER PERSONALITY DISORDERS

This classification provides flexibility. A patient who meets the criteria for more than one Personality Disorder may have multiple diagnoses on Axis II of DMS-III, but if there are features of several disorders that in combination are sufficiently maladaptive as to require professional attention, even though the patient does not meet all of the criteria for any one disorder, the diagnosis of Mixed Personality Disorder can be used.

Some disorders not included specifically in current nomenclature may be classified as Other Personality Disorders. These include:

1. Emotionally Unstable Personality
2. Explosive Personality
3. Asthenic Personality
4. Inadequate Personality

In addition, the condition formerly called Cyclothymic Personality is now classified with the Affective Disorders as Cyclothymic Disorder (cf. Chapter 10).

The Emotionally Unstable Personality

The Emotionally Unstable Personality is characterized by emotional outbursts occurring frequently and with minimum provocation. Usually, all of the emotions are poorly controlled, but in some cases only one type of feeling is displayed with pathological frequency and intensity.

The typical patient is quickly moved to anger or tears. The anger is out of proportion to the situation which evokes it. People are likely to refer to the episodes as temper tantrums. The patient will be regarded as "temperamental," as having a "low boiling point" or "a short fuse," or simply as someone with a nasty disposition.

The patient is as quick to cry as to become angry. He or she sheds tears in church and in the theater. Minor losses or frustrations produce briefly the sort of grief most people would show at a true bereavement. A woman patient may burst into tears on breaking a dish; not a valuable dish, not an heirloom, not part of a set — any dish.

Another easily evoked emotion is fear. Fright occurs not only when there is a risk of bodily harm, but also at the slightest threat to security.

In many cases, amusement, affection, and sexual feeling are likewise quickly aroused, but with the occasional exception of the last, these are less likely to be viewed as symptomatic or to cause difficulties in the patient's living.

The patient does not function well in stress situations. Emotional reactions interfere with successful coping. When emotionality is aroused, impulsive decisions that fail to take consequences into account are made.

If symptoms are at all marked, there will be some interference with vocational adjustment. This depends some on the type of work chosen and the tolerance of superiors. Temperament, including temper, is better tolerated in the star than in the stand-in. Socially, emotional instability is more accepted in women in traditional female employment than in persons in traditional male employment. A female secretary may be able to rush out of the office in tears without hurting her career, but a soldier, male or female, cannot. Instability is often a source of domestic disharmony. It interferes with the establishment and maintenance of close, lasting friendships.

When various types of emotional lability are present, differential diagnosis must include consideration of possible brain disease. An onset in adult life is highly suggestive of this; however, a lifelong history does not exclude it. Careful sensorium examination, psychological testing, EEG, and brain scan may be indicated.

Apparent emotional instability may result from an acute external stress situation, chronic fatigue, or systemic disease. When only one emotion is involved, the emotional displays may be masking anxiety attacks.

Successful therapy usually requires an initial period in which the patient is helped to realize a need for change. The patient must recognize the undesirable consequences of the behavior. Selective inattention, denial, and rationalization prevent this awareness. The patient may make a virtue of the disability by regarding it as an evidence of artistic temperament or sensitivity.

Before the patient can be shown the pattern of behavior and the predictability of its results, the therapist must discover just what these results are. Sometimes the behavior is found to be partially adaptive. Examples: (1) A woman's husband is reluctant to give her money for new clothes; a temper tantrum or a crying spell gets her what she wants. (2) A surgeon is known as a terror in the operating room; only the most experienced nurses and members of the house staff are assigned to assist him. The term secondary gain, though not in precisely correct usage, is often applied to this. When emotional instability works for the patient it usually has indirect consequences that are undesirable; these may be difficult to identify. Also, though an emotional outburst produces results, there are easier ways to achieve them.

The patient needs to realize the effect of the behavior, but abrupt confrontation is rarely helpful. The patient takes it as evidence of the therapist's disapproval, dislike, or rejection. The therapist works patiently, supports self-esteem, indicates approval and acceptance of the patient as a person, but gradually and noncritically brings out the data indicative of the need for change.

Once the patient sees the behavior as symptomatic and can cooperate with the physician in an effort to change it, one can then study the underlying purposes of maladaptive behavior, the circumstances under which it is most likely to occur, and possibly alternate ways of handling the situations. Contributory conflicts are also explored. Conscious efforts at control are occasionally effective. Sometimes one can learn to delay reactions. At times, situations that trigger the outbursts can be avoided; if they are more frequent under certain circumstances (e.g., when the patient is tired), one can recognize this, and time exposures to certain stresses so that they come when one is best able to cope with them. However, substitution of more effective ways of attaining goals is the cornerstone of therapy.

Two cautions : (1) If emotional instability is largely a manifestation of Personality Disorder, it can be removed safely. If it is a symptom of neurotic conflict, its premature removal leads to the substitution of other undesirable symptoms. Accurate diagnosis precedes therapy. (2) Early in therapy the patient may report criticism of his or her behavior by others, or express guilt or shame (with or without conviction) about it. In order to establish rapport, one may be tempted to reassure the patient that the behavior is, after all, fairly normal. The patient is pleased by this, feels that something is being gained from therapy, and, in fact, for a time functions better because of the support given. However, if the behavior is truly maladaptive, the long-term results of this approach are unsatisfactory. It is difficult to help the patient alter it later if the therapist has approved of a behavior pattern at the start.

Tranquilizers, antidepressants, and stimulants are sometimes used in this condition. Tranquilizers and antidepressants are prescribed in the hope of a general reduction of emotional reactivity and stimulants because most patients show more pronounced symptoms when fatigued or mildly depressed. Medication is used with caution and results carefully evaluated. Tranquilizers make some patients worse, as even minimal sedative effects weaken cortical control. Since the conditions are chronic, medications in which long-term use is undesirable because of tolerance, habituation, or cumulative toxicity are to be avoided. The possibility of medication being used in a suicide attempt should be kept in mind when prescribing, since the emotionally unstable patient is impulsive and is often subject to brief, unpredictable periods of severe depression.

The Explosive Personality

The explosive, or epileptoid, person is one whose only major deviation from normally adaptive behavior consists of uncontrolled outbursts of rage. The condition is to be differentiated from Dissociative Disorders. The possibility that the attacks result from cerebral dysrhythmia, that they are epileptic equivalents, must be considered. The EEG is usually helpful, but sometimes when it is negative there may still be enough reason to suspect epilepsy to warrant a trial of anticonvulsant medication. Lithium is also sometimes used in the treatment of aggressive outbursts. Treatment is otherwise the same as for the Emotionally Unstable Personality.

Some patients that would formerly have had this diagnosis are now classified as having a Disorder of Impulse Control, Intermittent Explosive Disorder. However, for the latter diagnosis, according to DSM-III criteria there must have been several discrete episodes resulting in serious assaults or destruction of property. There are Explosive Personalities who are not physically assaultive and do not destroy property (one assumes a golfer breaking his clubs or a teacher hurling chalk at a student is not what the authors of DSM-III had in mind). There are some patients who have not had repeated episodes, or even had one major one, who have a real risk of hurting someone during a temper outburst and need treatment to reduce this risk.

The Asthenic Personality

Throughout life these patients complain of weakness, lack of energy, and fatigue. They are tired all the time and lack interests, enthusiasms, and involvement.

Differential diagnosis includes the Chronic Depressive Disorders, and one must rule out many debilitating diseases of other systems. The condition differs from Inadequate Personality in that the patients make an adequate adjustment in many spheres of activity despite their feelings of fatigue and weakness.

Treatment may include an effort to help the patient acquire new interests and enthusiasms. As the patient becomes more involved in living and has more things to enjoy, symptoms either abate or become less of a source for concern. Attention may be given to sleeping habits and diet. A study of the patient's activities may reveal that such energy as she or he has can be directed in ways to give more satisfaction. In treating these patients psychotherapeutically, one frequently needs to deal with sexual problems, including worries about masturbation. Mild stimulants are occasionally useful, but they are employed with caution, since one is dealing with a lifelong condition and must keep in mind possible risks associated with prolonged use of these medicines.

Inadequate Personality

People with Inadequate Personality are inadequate in all spheres of activity. The diagnosis is not used in cases where physical disease or defective intelligence produces inadequacy. A history of adequate adjustment at any time of life or in any type of activity excludes this diagnosis. If the patient did well in school, was able to hold a job for any length of time, was successful in sports or social activities, or maintained a satisfactory marriage the diagnosis is excluded.

Constitutional factors have been postulated but none have been specifically identified. They are generally believed to play a part in many cases. A poor self-concept arising in childhood from repeated frustrations and failures in attempts to meet parental demands is another possible factor. Likewise, the child who is grossly overprotected may develop this type of personality.

Most patients are permanently and totally disabled for gainful occupation. A few can do some work in a sheltered environment. Subjective discomfort varies. A few patients are obviously distressed by their inadequacy; others, as long as physical needs are met, seem to accept disability as a matter of course and show little interest in attempts to change.

Mental Retardation, chronic physical disease, and chronic mild Schizophrenia should be ruled out. Inadequacy is a relative term. People who make a marginal adjustment in various spheres of activity or who habitually underachieve often represent borderline cases of Inadequate Personality, but for descriptive purposes they are not classified in this group.

The condition is often described as untreatable. True, nothing approaching recovery or normalcy is possible. However, support, encouragement, and practical advice on day-to-day problems results in some amelioration and enables some patients to attain a marginal functioning level. A few cases, especially those in which history reveals a markedly stressful childhood and in which psychogenic factors are of etiological importance, may profit from very long-term investigative psychotherapy. Many patients in this diagnostic group are clients of social agencies; some who would otherwise need institutional care are maintained as outpatients as a result of case work.

DISORDERS OF IMPULSE CONTROL

These disorders are manifested by recurring failures to control detrimental impulses. The patient experiences increasing tension before acting upon the impulse and gains pleasure, or at least a feeling of relief, from the act. The classification is not used for impulse disorders that are otherwise classifiable, such as Substance Use Disorders and Paraphilias. The classification includes:

1.   Pathological gambling
2.   Kleptomania
3.   Pyromania
4.   Intermittent Explosive Disorder
5.   Isolated Explosive Disorder
6.   Atypical Impulse Control Disorder

Formerly, many patients with these conditions would have been viewed as having Personality Disorders, if the maladaptive trait was essentially a lifelong feature of the personality and could not reasonably have been attributed to neurotic conflict. When seen as symptomatic of neurosis, these patterns of behavior were thought of as compulsive. Current nomenclature makes a distinction between an inability to control an impulse to do something and a compulsion to do it. The distinction includes the element of the behavior being enjoyable (egosyntonic), whereas compulsions are unwanted, unenjoyed, and ego-alien. This distinction is easier to state than to verify clinically.

Pathological Gambling

A diagnosis of pathological gambling is made when a person is unable to resist impulses to gamble and experiences recurring domestic and vocational problems as a result of gambling. Often one is struck by the apparent need to lose rather than by expectations of winning displayed by these patients. Pathological Gambling is to be distinguished from social gambling, professional gambling, and the gambling of patients with Antisocial Personalities, Manic Episodes, and Obsessive-Compulsive Disorder. Investigative psychotherapy, behavior therapy, and group therapies, including self-help groups, are used in treatment.

Kleptomania

Kleptomania is characterized by repetitive impulsive stealing. The stealing does not make sense. The things stolen are not necessarily of great intrinsic value; they are not stolen because they are needed or because the patient intends to sell them. In working with these patients, especially ones in the younger age groups, one often finds that the patient feels, with or without reason, unloved and unwanted. The stolen objects in some way make up for intangibles desired from significant others.

Pyromania

The term pyromania implies recurrent failure to resist impulses to set fires. Onset is usually in childhood and patients are often described as frustrated and resentful of authority.

They like to watch fires and are sometimes aroused sexually while watching them. It should be remembered, however, that if the police catch a boy (fire-setting and sexual excitement while watching fires is uncommon among females) masturbating at the scene of a fire, it may suggest that he is sexually excited by watching fires, but it does not prove that he sets them. One distinguishes Pyromania from the normal curiosity of small children about fire, and from purposeful criminal arson. The diagnosis is not made when fire-setting is secondary to another psychiatric disorder.

Intermittent Explosive Disorder

Intermittent Explosive Disorder has the features of the Explosive Personality, but one does not make the diagnosis unless there have been several behavioral episodes of loss of control manifested by serious assault or destruction of property. In differential diagnosis one rules out Schizophrenia, Antisocial Personality, and cerebral dysrhythmia (epileptic equivalents). In regard to the latter, if episodes are frequent, even if the EEG is normal, a trial on anticonvulsant medication may be warranted.

Isolated Explosive Disorder

The term Isolated Explosive Disorder describes the patient who has a single episode of violent activity unwarranted by external circumstance. This presumably represents an acute breakdown resulting from a combination of internal conflicts with mounting tensions and diffuse external stresses. This is the sort of thing sometimes described as going berserk or running amok. The term catathymic crisis has also been used to describe the condition. When this sort of irresistible impulse apparently leads to criminal behavior, one must consider the possibility that the patient is concealing a more logical motive or has some other mental illness (Schizophrenia; Organic Mental Disorder). One must also think of possible drug effects.

Other Impulse Control Disorders

A classification added for flexibility is Other Impulse Control Disorders.

REVIEW QUESTIONS

1. What characteristics distinguish Personality Disorders from other psychiatric syndromes?
2. Discuss the etiology of Personality Disorders.
3. Recall a time that you have behaved in a passive-aggressive manner. Was this behavior maladaptive? Why? What were your other options?
4. How do you account for the fact that patients with Personality Disorders frequently have somatic symptoms and are overrepresented among disability claimants?
5. Why do patients with Personality Disorders tolerate stress so poorly?
6. Describe the affect and the pattern of interpersonal relationship usually found in persons with Borderline Personality.
7. Why is Pathological Gambling classified as a Disorder of Impulse Control? How would you determine that a person who makes daily bets on horse races is *not* a pathological gambler?
8. How do you account for the Antisocial Personality's inability to tolerate frustration?
9. What is the reason that the Antisocial Personality fails to maintain lasting friendships?
10. A young man is seen after he has been expelled from school for cheating. He has had two arrests for shoplifting. He has a history of promiscuous heterosexual behavior and reports some homosexual activity. What is the probable diagnosis? What other data are necessary to confirm it?
11. The patient described in the previous question does not appear depressed, but he says that he is troubled by periods of depression that are relieved by amphetamine. He asks that some be prescribed so that he can have it on hand to use if needed. Would you prescribe it? Why or why not?
12. What are superego lucunae? How do you account for them?

SELECTED REFERENCES

1. Akhtar, Salman, and Jessica Price Byrne: The concept of splitting and its clinical relevance. *Am J Psychiatry* 140(8):1013-1016, 1983.

2. Akhtar, Salman, and J. Anderson Thomson, Jr.: Overview: Narcissistic personality disorder. *Am J Psychiatry* 139(1):12-20, 1982.

3. Angyal, Andras: Evasions of growth. *Am J Psychiatry* 110:358-361, 1953.

4. Cleckley, H. M.: *The Mask of Sanity.* 4th ed. St. Louis, Mosby, 1964.

5. Eaton, M. T., Jr.: *The Diagnosis and Treatment of Personality Disorders.* Behavioral Sciences Tape Library, Ivan K. Goldberg (Ed.). Leonia, New Jersey, Sigma Information, Inc., 1974.

6. Fitzgerald, Michael: Treatment aspects of the hysterical personality. *Ir J Psychother* 2(2):61–64, 1983.

7. Group for the Advancement of Psychiatry. *Urban America and the Planning of Mental Health Services* 5(10):505–509, Discussion — Maurice E. Linden, November, 1964.

8. Johnson, Adelaide M.: Sanctions for superego lacunae of adolescence. In: *Search Lights in Delinquency.* International University Press, 1949, pp. 225–245.

9. Kendler, Kenneth S., and Alan M. Gruenberg: Genetic relationship between paranoid personality disorder and the "schizophrenic spectrum" disorders. *Am J Psychiatry* 139(9):1185–1186, 1982.

10. Lion, John R. (Ed.): *Personality Disorders: Diagnosis and Management.* 2nd ed. Baltimore, Williams & Wilkins, 1981.

11. Millon, Theodore: *Disorders of Personality: DSM-III: Axis II.* New York, Wiley, 1981.

12. Monopolis, Spyros, and John R. Lion: Problems in the diagnosis of intermittent explosive disorder. *Am J Psychiatry* 140(9):1200–1201, 1983.

13. Perry, J. Christopher, and Raymond B. Flannery: Passive-aggressive personality disorder: Treatment implications of a clinical typology. *J Nerv Ment Dis* 170(3):164–173, 1982.

14. Pope, Harrison G., Jeffrey M. Jonas, James I. Hudson, Bruce M. Cohen, and John G. Gunderson: The validity of DSM-III borderline personality disorder. *Arch Gen Psychiatry* 40(1):23–30, 1983.

15. Reid, William H. (Ed.): *The Psychopath: A Comprehensive Study of Antisocial Disorders and Behaviors.* New York, Brunner/Mazel, 1978.

16. Shaffer, John, Kurt Jussbaum, and John Little: MMPI profiles of disability insurance claimants. *Am J Psychiatry* 129(4):403–407, 1972.

Chapter 8

THE NEUROSES: ANXIETY, SOMATOFORM, AND DISSOCIATIVE DISORDERS

MILD EMOTIONAL DISTURBANCE

The neuroses are a group of relatively mild psychiatric disturbances which have the following characteristics.

1. An acute onset. It is usually possible to determine from the history a precise or fairly precise date of onset. Careful study will reveal disturbances of psychosexual development in childhood. During adult life there may be some evidence of maladaptation. Prodromal symptoms may be noted. However, the neuroses are not lifelong overt disturbances as are the Personality Disorders.
2. Relatively mild disability (in most cases). A few patients may be totally disabled for gainful occupation (e.g., a patient confined to home because of a phobia), but the majority are employable. However the neurotic does not function at an optimum level of productivity and creativity.
3. Lack of involvement of the total personality. Many of the patients' interactions with the social environment are unimpaired by these disorders.
4. Maintenance of ego boundaries and of reality testing. The phobic or obsessional patient may not be able to cope with disturbing and unrealistic thoughts, but she or he recognizes them as pathological. There are some exceptions to this, especially in the Dissociative Disorders.
5. Subjective symptoms of anxiety and its derivatives.

THE NATURE OF ANXIETY

Everyone has experienced anxiety. It is an unpleasant affect similar to fear both subjectively and in its concomitant physiological disturbances. Fear has an external object and is proportional to a real or reasonably expected danger to life or well-being. It is an appropriate reaction to an external threat. Anxiety does not have an external object, or is grossly disproportionate to any real external threat (i.e., almost anyone would experience the unpleasant sensation of fear upon encountering a poisonous snake at close range; some people would have a similar sensation, anxiety, even if the snake is at a distance or is known to be nonpoisonous).

When fear occurs, one can overcome it by coping with the source of danger or getting away from it (fight or flight).

Fear warns of an external danger; anxiety of an internal danger. To the extent that each is a warning, though unpleasant, it is useful. The danger warned of by anxiety is an impulse involved in intrapsychic conflict and unacceptable to the ego, a repressed thought nearing consciousness.

The subjective sensation of anxiety at its mildest level is that of an apprehensive expectation, nonspecific and ill-defined; at its most severe level the feeling is that of panic.

Anxiety, like fear, is accompanied by physiological disturbances, including:

1.   Muscular tension
2.   Restlessness
3.   Tremor
4.   Excessive perspiration (hyperhidrosis)
5.   Pupillary dilatation (mydriasis)
6.   Rapid pulse (tachycardia)

Additional symptoms, perhaps secondary to some of the above, include:

1.   Fatigue (this is sometimes attributed to the use of energy, libido, in maintaining repression, but it can be seen as a result of the sustained tension and restlessness)
2.   Insomnia
3.   Irritability
4.   Difficulty in concentrating (e.g., trouble in maintaining attention when reading or listening to a lecture)
5.   Dysfunction of various organs and systems; interference with appetite and with sexual function is common

Pure anxiety, free-floating anxiety as it is sometimes called when it is severe and persistent, approaches being intolerable, and if healthy defense mechanisms cannot control it, the ego uses pathological ones. The combination of pathological defense mechanisms used to control anxiety governs the form of the neuroses, except in Panic Disorders and Generalized Anxiety Disorders, and produces their characteristic symptoms (previously referred to as derivatives of anxiety). The choice of defenses is to some extent a product of the character structure of the patient and hence is determined by the stage(s) of psychosexual development in which fixation occurred or from which the most prominent character traits were derived.

CLASSIFICATION OF THE NEUROSES

The Neuroses, or Neurotic Disorders, are in the current classification system grouped under three headings:

1.   Anxiety Disorders
2.   Somatoform Disorders
3.   Dissociative Disorders

Anxiety Disorders

The Anxiety Disorders are divided into three groups:

1. Anxiety states, including Panic Disorder, Generalized Anxiety Disorder, and Obsessive-Compulsive Disorder
2. Phobic disorders, including Agoraphobia with panic attacks, Agoraphobia without panic attacks, Social Phobia, and Simple Phobia
3. Post-traumatic Stress Disorders

Anxiety States (Anxiety Neuroses)

Generalized Anxiety Disorders and Panic Disorders are the simplest forms of neurosis. The anxiety is experienced subjectively and is accompanied by some or all of the physiological concomitants mentioned (though in very mild cases these may not be obvious during an interview). Anxiety is more or less constant in Generalized Anxiety Disorders, but it occurs periodically in the form of anxiety attacks in Panic Disorders. Panic attacks may occur without apparent external precipitating factors or may appear to be precipitated by mild stresses, including certain social situations. When there are recurring external precipitating factors a distinction must be made from phobia.

These disorders may have spontaneous remissions after periods of weeks or months, may become chronic, or may develop into some other type of neurosis. If there is no remission, chronicity is more likely with mild sustained anxiety or anxiety in the form of attacks; it is unusual for a patient to experience moderate or severe anxiety for a period of more than a year or so at most without developing some defenses which transform the neurosis into one of the other types. The diagnosis of Generalized Anxiety Disorder should not be made unless the condition has been present for at least 1 month. Prior to that one may use the diagnosis of Atypical Anxiety Disorder.

Though grouped with the Anxiety States for purposes of classification, the Obsessive Compulsive Disorder is clinically quite different. It is discussed on pages 121-123.

Phobias

A phobia is a pathological fear. There is a displacement from some object or situation involved in intrapsychic conflict to another type of object or situation which then is feared. The phobic object usually symbolizes the original object or situation. This is, in effect, a neurotic compromise. The patient substitutes fear for anxiety, is still uncomfortable, but on an intellectual level at least knows that the feared object is not really dangerous. Also, the phobic object can be avoided or escaped. Thus, the patient is freed of anxiety and discomfort except on encountering or expecting to encounter the phobic object.

The thing that is feared may be totally harmless. If it is something that is at least potentially dangerous, the fear is greatly out of proportion to the real danger. Some phobias are of things that the average person does not find unpleasant at all (e.g., open spaces); others are of things that most people dislike to some extent (e.g., only entomologists and small boys really like spiders; the average person may feel uncomfortable upon unexpectedly encountering a large spider; a person for whom a spider is a phobic object becomes extremely frightened at the sight of a nonpoisonous spider and is unable to go into an area where there may be spiders).

Though the phobic object usually symbolizes the underlying conflict or something closely related to it, one cannot identify the conflict definitely from knowing the object. Personal experiences, autistic or parataxic associations, and cultural influences govern the meaning of symbols; two patients with identical phobic objects may have totally dissimilar conflicts. For one example, for patients with a morbid fear of dogs, a dog may in some cases symbolize aggressive behavior (fear of aggressive people; fear of one's own aggressive impulses); in other cases the dog is something that bites, hurts, or mutilates (fear of punishment; castration); and in still others, a dog represents freedom from sexual inhibitions (fear of seduction or assault; fear of one's own sexual impulses).

However, some phobic objects have a particular symbolic significance in a high enough percent of cases that when they are encountered, the usual interpretation should at least be considered. Examples: (1) snakes often represent the penis; (2) spiders and sometimes cats may symbolize female genitalia; (3) rats and mice often stand for children (especially younger siblings); (4) high places may represent sexual arousal; (5) fears of being away from home (or familiar surroundings) are often associated with conflicts over voyeuristic impulses (a fear of seeing something; a fear of encountering the primal scene); another common basis of the fear of being away from home is a fear (or really the conflict between an unacceptable wish and the superego) of doing something which is taboo at home; (6) stage fright, which sometimes reaches a phobic level, may be related to conflicts over exhibitionistic impulses, conflicts over an impulse to express hostility toward the audience or toward other people in general, or simply fear of failure and humiliation.

Many of the conflicts of phobic patients are sexual in character and have their inception in the phallic stage of psychosexual development.

Many, perhaps all, people have some irrational fears. Some of these are subclinical phobias, are dynamically identical with neurotic symptoms, and differ only in intensity from clinical cases. The housewife who screams at the sight of a mouse, though she is not necessarily sick or neurotic, is at least subclinically phobic. Clinical phobias vary in degree of disability, general discomfort, and clinical significance from mild to very severe. The variation is partly governed by the choice of phobic object and partly by the degree of discomfort or fear experienced when it is encountered. A patient with a mild claustrophobia (a fear of being in enclosed or narrow spaces) may prefer escalators to elevators and feel mildly to moderately anxious on having to ride an elevator. A person with a more severe claustrophobia simply cannot tolerate the discomfort of an elevator and will walk up many flights of stairs rather than attempt to ride. A person with a phobic dread of tigers needs only to avoid zoos and jungles to stay comfortable; a person who has extreme fear at the proximity of a housecat will be uncomfortable more often. Claustrophobia, agoraphobia (described below), and acrophobia (a fear of high places) each interfere with certain vocational pursuits. The person who cannot leave home because of a phobia is severely handicapped.

The current system of classification divides Phobic Disorders (Phobic Neuroses) into four types:

1. Agoraphobia with panic attacks
2. Agoraphobia without panic attacks
3. Social phobia
4. Simple phobia

The term Agoraphobia is derived from a Greek word meaning marketplace. One would expect it to mean a fear of open spaces or perhaps a fear of crowds and, indeed, the term is sometimes used for such fears. However, by extension it refers to an irrational fear of being away from home or away from familiar surroundings. The diagnosis of Agoraphobia is also used for those whose fear is of being alone or traveling alone. It is among the most common phobias (or at least the most common that are severe enough to require treatment). The diagnosis of

Social Phobia is used when the feared situation involves behavior in public and includes stage fright, fear of blushing, fear of eating in public, and "bashful kidneys." The diagnosis of Simple Phobia is used for persons whose pathological fear and avoidance behavior involves any object or situation which does not meet the criteria for Agoraphobia or Social Phobia.

Some patients with phobic tendencies overcompensate through reaction formation. Counterphobic mechanisms may lead some people to repeated activities that have an element of danger. One should not, of course, jump to the conclusion that a person who chooses mountain climbing or sky-diving as a recreation is overcompensating for a fear of heights, but one should not ignore the possibility.

Obsessive Compulsive Disorder
(Obsessive Compulsive Neuroses)

The Obsessive Compulsive Disorder represents an additional way in which free-floating anxiety is transformed into another symptom. An obsession is a recurring thought which is unwanted and which cannot be voluntarily excluded from consciousness. A compulsion is a recurring irresistible impulse to perform an act or a series of acts. It is, in effect, an obsession in action.

An obsession may be a single thought (e.g., a line of verse that the patient cannot stop repeating; an obscene word that keeps coming to mind, perhaps at any time, or perhaps only when attending church or in social settings in which it would be highly inappropriate). Another type of obsession is obsessive rumination; instead of a single thought, the patient keeps thinking of a subject, a personal problem, or an abstract philosophical topic. The thoughts on the subject are repetitive and stereotyped and no conclusions are reached. A variant of this is obsessive doubting or indecision in which one ruminates over a decision or choice without being able to come to a conclusion; this may involve a relatively important decision (e.g., changing jobs) or a minor one (e.g., selecting a necktie to wear).

Obsessive thoughts and ruminations are to be differentiated from other recurring thoughts and preoccupations. The frequency with which a thought recurs, or the amount of time spent dwelling upon a subject is not the crucial point. An obsessive thought is unwelcome; a young man, or an old one, who spends much of his time thinking about girls, and enjoys thinking about them, may be ruminating, but he is not ruminating obsessively. However, not all unwelcome thoughts are obsessive either; one may be preoccupied with a distressing situation, an impending crisis, or a source of frustration in living. This is not obsessive (even though it may be disproportionate to the situation), if the person can, when the occasion demands, dismiss the subject and concentrate on something else.

If an obsessive thought is foolish, the patient recognizes its absurdity. If it is unreasonable, he or she knows this and will readily acknowledge it. In some instances this may be helpful in distinguishing an obsession from a delusion.

An inhibiting obsession is a recurring thought or fear that one may do something that one does not want to do (the most common is the fear of harming some member of the family). Examples: (1) A housewife is obsessed with the idea that she may accidentally put poison in food that she cooks. She is unwilling to keep ordinary household chemicals in or near the kitchen. She prefers to have someone in the kitchen when she is cooking. (2) A mother is bothered by the recurring thought that she may stab one of her children. When she is alone with the children she prefers that knives and scissors be locked up where she cannot get them. (3) A man has the obsessional thought that he may jump off a high place or out of a moving car. Superficially, his reaction to heights and automobiles is like a phobia, but he is not actually afraid of *them*; he is consciously afraid that he will have the impulse to jump.

The patient with an inhibiting obsession does not actually want to do the thing that is thought about; in fact, the idea is horrifying and repelling. Inhibiting obsessions are not carried into action, but they must be distinguished from other types of fears of harming one's self or others. The person who actually wants to harm someone, with or without a more or less logical reason, and worries that the impulse will be beyond control (e.g., the man, paranoid or otherwise who wants to kill his wife's lover or suspected lover and feels that he may do so if the lover taunts him again, or if he catches them, or if he takes one drink too many) presents an entirely different problem. So does the patient who is aware of periods of confusion or amnesia or outbursts of temper and is afraid of harming someone at such times.

A compulsion may take the form of a single act which the patient feels impelled to repeat (e.g., stepping on cracks in the sidewalk), or a series of acts (e.g., folding clothing in a particular way; facing all of the objects in a room in a certain direction). The series of acts are sometimes spoken of as compulsive rituals. These differ from religious rituals, for example, in that the latter are meaningful, purposeful, culturally determined, and are done voluntarily.

The compulsion may be associated with an obsession. Compulsive handwashing, a relatively common compulsion, is often associated with obsessive thoughts and fears of dirt and germs. Example: A patient is obsessed with a fear of germs, and especially a fear of venereal infection. These thoughts bother him most when he uses a public lavatory (though even at home he may wash his hands so often that they are red and raw). When he uses a rest room away from home he starts thinking about infection. Actually, he knows that venereal disease is not usually acquired in this way. Still, he washes for several minutes, then he starts to turn off the water and wonders if he contaminated his hands on the faucet. He washes again. He gets a paper towel to open the door, but he fears that he may have touched the handle and so washes again. And again.

Compulsivity may take the form of doing things over or rechecking them. Examples: (1) A student is unable to complete a composition. He writes a page or two, feels that it is not neat enough or is not quite accurate in content, and so time after time tears it up and starts over. (2) A woman starts on a trip and, though she has not been cooking, she feels compelled to go home and make sure that she has turned off all the burners on the stove. All is well and she starts again, only to feel once more compelled to return and check the stove.

If one apparently has a compulsion to do something that many people find ego-syntonic (desirable; enjoyable), a distinction must be made from the Impulse Control Disorders described in the previous chapter. For example, overeating, gambling, or sexual promiscuity resulting from a compulsion is not a desired activity. It is something the patient does not want to do and does not enjoy. The same behavior resulting from a difficulty in impulse control is actually desired, though the patient may feel that it ought not to be, and results in enjoyment, or at the very least a feeling of relief. Compulsions, and disorders of impulse control, may contribute to some cases of syndromes classified under other headings (e.g., Substance Use Disorders; Paraphilias).

Though compulsions nearly always involve relatively innocuous activities, a few lead to socially undesirable or criminal acts. These pose difficult problems in evaluation; not all patients who claim that socially unacceptable acts stem from recurring unwanted and irresistible urges are actually compulsive.

The compulsive, whether the compulsion is a single act, a ritual, or a need to recheck things or do them again, does not *want* to act upon the compulsion, but *has* to act. If prevented from the action(s) by force or circumstances, he or she experiences extreme anxiety. The compulsions are not enjoyed and only rarely is there any secondary gain associated with them. They are recognized as inappropriate and maladaptive.

A patient may have only one obsession or compulsion or several. In the transmutation of the patient's basic conflict and anxiety into the obsession or compulsion, the mechanisms of displacement, condensation, and symbolization play an important part. Reaction formation and isolation are often involved.

In some cases in therapy it is found that even before the unconscious displacement became established, the patient consciously substituted the obsessive thought for some other disturbing idea or preoccupation.

The character structure of most patients who develop Obsessive Compulsive Disorders is heavily influenced by the anal stage of psychosexual development. Hence, underlying conflicts often relate to feelings about authority and external control, to hostile or sadistic impulses, and to matters related to neatness, cleanliness, and orderliness. A connection between the symptom and these conflicts is often readily apparent.

In addition to the obsessions and compulsions themselves, most patients show other symptoms, many of which are related to the anal character structure or Compulsive Personality. Within any cultural group one expects to find a fairly wide range of normal behavior in regard to cleanliness and grooming. The obsessive is likely to be outside this range. His or her appearance will be overly neat or markedly untidy, or may show an inconsistency (e.g., outer garments very clean and neat; underwear surprisingly dirty — or the reverse).

In the same way, there will be departures from normal in orderliness and promptness. There are usually problems related to generosity and stinginess. There are problems in the handling of money. Difficulties with authority are frequent. There is likely to be concern over bowel habits and there may be complaints of constipation or diarrhea.

Obsessional patients tend to show a passive resistance during interviews even when they seek help voluntarily (as is usually the case). They seem to resent being questioned. Part of this is a general resentment of authority (the physician is culturally viewed as an authoritarian person); part of it is the feeling that thoughts and experiences are personal possessions which the patient is parsimoniously unwilling to share with another. The patient who has been hostile during the interview is likely to show some undoing near the end and at that point becomes ingratiating.

Most obsessionals have a narrow range of interests. Their emotional range also appears limited, sometimes to a degree approaching the apparent flatness of affect of the schizophrenic.

Isolation may be noted during interviews. The patient may consciously recall early childhood experiences of a traumatic nature that most persons would repress, but he or she recalls and expresses these without much feeling.

There is a wide range of severity and disability associated with Obsessive Compulsive Disorders. Patients with severe cases may be totally disabled. On the other hand, one finds mild subclinical cases, the manifestations of which differ only slightly from those of the minor obsessive tendencies which occur in many, if not all, healthy people at times. Almost anyone can recall times when he or she could not exclude some extraneous thought from consciousness while trying to work (e.g., a song; an advertising slogan) and almost anyone can remember going back to check a door that one clearly remembered locking, or getting out of bed to check an alarm clock that one certainly recalled setting.

At the clinical level, the Obsessive Compulsive Disorder is often among the most severe of the neuroses. It offers the poorest prognosis. Though some cases, especially relatively mild cases in adolescents, have spontaneous remissions, the majority become chronic, and tend to become worse as the patient grows older. During middle age there may be a failure of the obsessive defenses to control anxiety and patients may become psychotic. Some of these cases develop depression with suicidal tendencies; others become schizophrenic.

Post-traumatic Stress Disorders

Post-traumatic Stress Disorders are neuroses that follow a highly stressful experience in military combat, as a prisoner-of-war, or in civilian life (e.g., natural disasters; rape; torture). Symptoms of Adjustment Disorder may or may not have been present at the time of or immediately following the stress period.

Characteristic symptoms include frequently recurring, vivid recollections of the traumatic event, nightmares about it, and symptoms of generalized anxiety. Along with these symptoms there is a tendency toward social withdrawal and loss of interest in activities that were previously enjoyed.

A Post-traumatic Stress Disorder is described as Acute if the onset of symptoms is within 6 months after the stress and symptoms have been present for less than 6 months at the time of the examination. Chronic Post-traumatic Stress Disorder is diagnosed when symptoms have been present for 6 months or more. Delayed Post-traumatic Stress Disorders have an onset more than 6 months after the traumatic experience.

Though diagnosis is usually not difficult, there are three things that should be kept in mind in evaluating possible cases. First, the person who has a highly traumatic experience and subsequently develops psychiatric symptoms of any sort may attribute them to the trauma. A traumatic experience may play a part in the etiology of a disorder other than Post-traumatic Stress Disorder. A person who has been exposed to a grossly stressful experience can also develop a psychiatric disorder totally unrelated to it. Second, many patients with Post-traumatic Stress Disorder have one or more other diagnosable psychiatric conditions. Finally, there are Factitious Post-traumatic Stress Disorders and malingering is also a possibility when, for example, claims for compensation based upon an allegedly stressful event are involved.

One should verify that the history of a major traumatic experience is valid, should look for the characteristic symptoms of Post-traumatic Stress Disorder, and should consider the possibility of additional or alternative diagnoses to account for other findings.

Depressive Neuroses

Neurotic depressions are classified among the Neuroses in the ninth edition of the *International Classification of Diseases: Clinical Modifications* (ICD-9-CM, but in the third edition of the *Diagnostic and Statistical Manual of Mental Disorders* (DSM-III) they are classified with the Affective Disorders as Dysthymic Disorder (Depressive Neuroses). Neurotic Depressions will be discussed along with other Affective Disorders in Chapter 10 of this book.

Somatoform Disorders

The Somatoform Disorders include:

1.   Conversion Disorder (Hysterical Neurosis, Conversion Type)
2.   Psychogenic Pain Disorder
3.   Somatization Disorder
4.   Hypochondriasis (Hypochondriacal Neurosis)
5.   Atypical Somatoform Disorder

All of these, with the exception of Hypochondriasis, were formerly regarded as types of hysteria.

Conversion Disorder

The mechanism of conversion allows conflicts to be represented as physical symptoms involving portions of the body innervated by sensory or motor nerves. This leads to reduction or elimination of free-floating anxiety. The symptom usually symbolizes the conflict or the unacceptable impulse (e.g., a paralyzed hand may be the hand with which the patient might have had an impulse to masturbate or strike someone). The *primary gain* from the symptom is related to the way in which it prevents or inhibits the carrying out of an impulse or creates some compromise of an internal conflict (e.g., aphonia prevents saying something; dysphonia prevents saying it loudly and clearly). Conversion symptoms may include:

1. Sensory symptoms
    a. Areas of anesthesia. These will not follow nerve distribution unless the patient has at some time studied the nervous system or observed a patient with a sensory nerve lesion and (unconsciously) copies that patient. Glove or stocking anesthesias are often conversion symptoms.
    b. Blindness.
    c. Deafness.
2. Paralyses
    a. Aphonia or dysphonia.
    b. Hemiplegia or hemiparesis.
    c. Paralysis or paresis of any muscle group (e.g., the muscles of one hand; a group of facial muscles leading to a slight disfiguration). Paralyses also may fail to follow nerve distribution. In chronic cases atrophy from disuse occurs in the involved muscles.
3. Dyskinesias
    a. Tics (muscular twitches).
    b. Convulsions.
    c. Recurring peculiar movements or postures.

In addition to the conversion symptom itself, patients with Conversion Disorder often show other symptoms and findings, including:

1. Relatively marked sexual problems. Patients with any conversion symptom rarely, if ever, report a normal, satisfactory sexual adjustment. Conflicts over sexuality are revealed in interviews and on psychological testing. (The mechanism of conversion may be directly responsible for some forms of impaired sexual function, but when a disturbance of sexual function is the *only* conversion symptom the case is classified with the Psychosexual Disorders rather than with the Conversion Disorders.)
2. A bland attitude toward the conversion symptoms and the disability produced by it. The patient is likely to discuss the disability with a smile and to seem rather indifferent toward it. This is sometimes called la belle indifference.
3. A tendency to utilize dissociative mechanisms. The commonest manifestation is a tendency to behave seductively without being aware of the implications of the behavior.
4. A tendency to seek attention. This is pervasive and is not limited to attention gained through having the symptom.
5. Suggestibility.

Another feature of Conversion Disorder, and one which sometimes complicates understanding of a case, is *secondary gain*. *Primary gain* has already been described.

Secondary gain refers to other advantages gained by the patient through being sick. Secondary gains may include attention, ability to control or manipulate relatives and other significant people, freedom from certain tasks and responsibilities, and in some instances compensation. Secondary gain is not part of the cause of illness. It arises after the illness is already established. It may appear to be a reason for being, or staying, sick, and in some instances leads to more or less conscious use of the symptoms in a way suggestive of malingering. Secondary gain may complicate treatment but removal of secondary gain does not lead to remission.

Conversion Disorder is more common in women than men. Since the underlying conflicts are often sexual, this may be related to the double standard. Conversion symptoms are apparently much less common now than they were a century ago. There are two possible explanations:

1. Modern society creates fewer conflicts over sexuality. There is less need to repress sexual impulses; one may think about them without undue fear.
2. The population is more sophisticated concerning medical matters. The conversion symptom, to work, has to be so convincing that the patient can logically believe the disability to be from some cause other than emotional conflict.

When conversion symptoms are seen, they are often associated with intellectual limitations, naivete, a history of an unusually sheltered background, or a childhood and adolescence in which more than the usual inhibition and suppression of sexual thoughts and feelings were required.

As has been noted, the mechanism of conversion itself utilizes sensory or motor nerves, but the criteria for the *diagnosis* of Conversion Disorder are broad enough to include some symptoms mediated through the autonomic or endocrine system (e.g., psychogenic vomiting; pseudocyesis). When pain is the only conversion symptom, the diagnosis of *Psychogenic Pain Disorder* is used and the criteria for that diagnosis are likewise broad enough to include other types of psychogenic pain.

Somatization Disorder

This condition, sometimes called Briquet's syndrome, is said to occur primarily in women and to have an onset before the age of 30. It is characterized by multiple physical complaints, frequent hospitalizations, and sometimes polysurgery. Conversion symptoms may be present but are not necessary for the diagnosis. Patients describe themselves as having generally poor health, often report gastrointestinal symptoms, and complain of various aches and pains. Women with this condition report frequent menstrual difficulties.

Hypochondriasis (Hypochondriacal Neurosis)

The hypochondriac is preoccupied with worries about health, is likely to have multiple somatic complaints, and believes that these are symptoms of various diseases. He or she is not reassured by negative examination findings and may feel that something has been overlooked or remains undiscovered. The ideas do not reach a delusional level but may have an obsessive quality. Some patients are at least partly aware that their concern is irrational, and in expressing their complaints they are not actually seeking additional diagnostic studies or treatments, but instead wish help in ridding themselves of disturbing thoughts.

Dissociative Disorders

Dissociation has been mentioned as one of the mechanisms found in patients with Conversion Disorder. In the Dissociative Disorders it is the main mental mechanism and is used to control what would otherwise be overwhelming anxiety. Portions of the ego are split off from the mainstream of consciousness. Classified under the heading of Dissociative Disorders are:

1. Psychogenic Amnesia
2. Psychogenic Fugue
3. Multiple Personality
4. Depersonalization Disorder (Depersonalization Neurosis)
5. Atypical Dissociative Disorder

Amnesia refers to a loss of memory which may be complete or partial. One may have amnesia for a specific period of time or for all past events. The word *fugue* is derived from the Latin fuga, meaning flight. As a manifestation of dissociation one may see a running away, an unplanned and apparently aimless flight. However, the diagnosis of *Psychogenic Fugue* is applied in cases in which there is both fugue and amnesia. A person may suddenly travel away from home, assume a new identity, and be unable to recall his or her past. An unusual dissociative manifestation is the presence of *Multiple Personality* (e.g., the *Three Faces of Eve; Sybil;* Morton Prince's case of Sally Beauchamps). *Depersonalization Disorder* is a less severe manifestation of dissociation. It is manifested by feeling unreal or feeling that one is not oneself. The feeling is uncanny, as if one were looking into a mirror and seeing a stranger. An isolated episode of feelings of depersonalization is not unusual for an otherwise healthy person, and a diagnosis is made only if there are multiple episodes, or if a single episode is unusually distressing or disabling. Another mild dissociative manifestation is sleepwalking (somnambulism).

Major Dissociative Disorders are relatively rare. In the absence of history, some of them may be clinically indistinguishable from Adjustment Disorders resulting from gross stress or, less frequently, schizophrenia.

Factitious Disorders

The word factitious means artificial. A person with a Factitious Disorder, then, is one who claims to have symptoms that are not really present or who does something to produce symptoms or findings (e.g., touches the clinical thermometer to a warm object so as to appear to have a fever; scratches oneself here and there so as to appear to have a skin disease).

There is a distinction between malingering and Factitious Disorder. Malingering is pretending to be ill or incapacitated so as to avoid work or to achieve some other more or less reasonable objective (e.g., avoiding military service; collecting insurance benefits). A person with a Factitious Disorder has no conscious goal other than that of convincing others that he or she is sick, perhaps obtaining the extra attention accorded to persons who are ill, and being a difficult, hence, interesting case. Creating painful lesions, or even claiming unusual symptoms and subjecting oneself to diagnostic procedures that are often uncomfortable and sometimes dangerous is certainly getting attention the hard way and it is obviously not the behavior of a mentally healthy person.

The types of Factitious Disorders classified include:
1. Factitious Disorder with Psychological Symptoms
2. Chronic Factitious Illness with Physical Symptoms

3. Atypical Factitious Illness with Physical Symptoms

Chronic Factitious Illness with Physical Symptoms is sometimes referred to as the Münchausen Syndrome. Patients with Münchausen Syndrome accumulate a history of multiple hospitalizations and, in addition to faking illness, usually make up a variety of other stories about themselves. Their behavior is often histrionic.

THE CAUSE OF THE NEUROSES

Many of the apparent contradictions in the literature about the cause of the neuroses are based upon failure in most studies prior to the last decade or two, and in some contemporary work, to distinguish among the Neuroses, the Personality Disorders, and the Adjustment Disorders.

Identification with an aberrant parent, learning of maladaptive behavior patterns by trial and accidental success, and conditioning are more likely to be important factors in the development of Personality Disorders than in the etiology of the neuroses. Environmental stress is more important in the Adjustment Disorders.

Though there are some opinions to the contrary, many psychiatrists beieve that the important causative factors in the Neuroses are experiential, psychogenic, and related to intrapsychic conflict. This does not exclude other contributing factors, including constitutional predisposition. In evaluating biochemical factors, one must differentiate causative elements, mechanisms, and imbalances produced by illness.

As was described in Chapter 1, an instinctual impulse arising from the id may be in conflict with another instinctual impulse, with the superego, with the ego, or with the external environment. Conflict itself is only a partial explanation of symptom formation. One must seek further for biological explanations of those factors which govern the intensity of basic drives and impulses, for explanations of superego development, and for sociological explanations of the role of culture in producing conflict.

Society requires, both directly and indirectly by way of the superego, the inhibition or repression of certain impulses related to sexuality, hostility and aggression, and dependency. Hence, conflicts arising from these impulses and related needs are often involved in the formation of neuroses.

Conflict is a cause of neuroses. Other factors govern its form. Some of these are related to the stage of psychosexual development in which the conflicts first arose (e.g., conflicts resulting in Conversion Disorders and Phobic Disorders usually arise in the phallic stage of development; conflicts productive of Obsessive Compulsive Disorder derive from the anal stage). Specific events in childhood coupled with a particular precipitating stress may influence the form of some neuroses (e.g., the occasional relationship between a traumatic sexual experience in childhood, the awakening of sexual feelings in adult life, and the onset of a Conversion or Phobic Disorder; the relationship between a childhood experience with a phobic object and the development of a phobia).

Many other factors may play a part in the form of the neuroses. These include, but are not limited to, the following:

1. Identification with a significant person, often a parent, who handled anxiety symptomatically.
2. Parental attitudes. Concern over a child's health may contribute to hypochondriasis, conversion symptoms, or factitious illness. There may be a specific concern such as that manifested by frequent warnings about things which might

impair vision. Repeated warnings about various sources of danger may contribute to phobic symptoms. Undue insistence on neatness and accuracy may lay some groundwork for the development of obsessional problems. Frequent criticism may predispose to feelings of low self-esteem, apprehension, and anxiety. Concern over sexual interests and activities leads to a fear of sexuality, even in its socially permitted forms, which influences symptom formation.

3. Coping devices and defense mechanisms which are adaptive in other situations. A tendency to be highly accurate in one's work, to pay attention to details and to recheck is often adaptive and is rewarded. The person who has found this useful in coping with life situations is likely, unconsciously, to invoke similar patterns of behavior when coping with anxiety. Expressions of sorrow and guilt are also rewarded at times in childhood and adult life by sympathy and by forgiveness. A child, or an executive, who takes the blame when things go wrong may be praised. Such experiences set the stage for the unconscious selection of symptomatic means of coping with anxiety.

SYMPTOMS AND COURSE

The neuroses begin abruptly. The onset is usually early in adult life. Patients who have recovered from a neurosis may have recurrences in middle and late life, but a first attack after the age of 35 is unusual. Neuroses similar to those seen in adults are sometimes found in children and adolescents.

Though the clinical onset is in adult life, the psychopathological process usually begins within the first 6 years of life. Histories of most neurotic patients reveal outward manifestations of adjustment difficulties in one or more of the stages of psychosexual development. Some common findings in the early histories of neurotics include:

1. Feeding problems in early infancy
2. Difficulties in toilet training
3. Nightmares or night terrors
4. Temper tantrums
5. Enuresis (bed-wetting) persisting until age 8 or beyond
6. Thumbsucking or nailbiting persisting throughout childhood and into adolescence

Histories of childhood may also include evidence of a disturbed relationship with one or both parents, marked sibling rivalry, periods of overly aggressive behavior, or symptoms similar to those seen in adult neuroses. There may be a history of some unusual event or situation which one would expect to be stressful, emotionally disturbing, or traumatic, occurring during early childhood.

During the latency period, the outward manifestations of emotional disturbance subside. Symptoms, if any, are subclinical. Careful history-taking will usually elicit some evidences of ongoing conflicts during late childhood, throughout adolescence, and up to the onset of the neurosis. Shyness, sensitivity, and difficulties in interpersonal relationships are not unusual. Situations touching upon a conflict area may evoke transitory periods of anxiety. Conflicts may be revealed in various other ways. Examples: (1) A patient whose major early conflicts were over aggressive impulses, including fears of competing with his father and brother, avoided competitive activities, sports, and games when in high school. He went to a small school and because of height and muscular coordination was needed by the basketball team. He encountered considerable social disapproval when he refused to play, but though he wanted to please the coach and fellow students and was deeply hurt by criticism, the idea of playing repelled him. (2) A young woman patient whose early conflicts were primarily sexual recalled that she did not begin to date until 2 years after most of her girlfriends had started dating. For nearly a year after she began to go out with boys she experienced feelings of tension accompanied by nausea before each date.

These examples illustrate evidences of premorbid conflict in patients who subsequently developed neuroses. Though such evidences of conflict are symptomatic, they often occur in persons who do not regard themselves as ill, are not regarded by others as ill (or abnormal), and who would probably not be diagnosed as neurotic at the time if seen for a psychiatric examination as part of a general clinical evaluation.

There is usually some precipitating event, a stress, or at least an environmental change shortly before the onset of the neurosis. The stress is usually of less magnitude than that which would be sufficient to account for an Adjustment Disorder. Sometimes a precipitating event which is not discovered on initial interview is reported after the patient has started treatment. Its significance is recognized only after some insight has been attained.

In the absence of an external stress, sometimes there is an internal one, a decision to make some change in one's way of life, a feeling that a habit should be given up or a new responsibility undertaken, or a growing urge or impulse to do something about which there are some fears or misgivings.

Clinical manifestations initially are usually those of anxiety (or occasionally depression). Other symptoms are usually preceded by a period in which anxiety itself is the main symptom, though patients who have been ill for some time may not recall this early stage of the disorder.

Many cases (probably the majority, though the number cannot be known until long-range studies in public health and social psychiatry provide new information) have a spontaneous remission in a period of days, weeks, or months. Since the diagnosis of Generalized Anxiety Disorder is reserved for patients who have been symptomatic for at least a month, patients who have an early remission, if diagnosed, are classified as Atypical Anxiety Disorders. A few of these cases do become chronic; the remainder of those who do not have spontaneous remission go on to develop characteristic symptoms of one of the other types of neuroses.

DIAGNOSIS

The diagnosis can usually be made from symptoms, history, and mental status examination. Psychological testing is occasionally helpful.

In general, the neuroses differ from psychoses in that the neuroses are:

1.   Less severe
2.   Less disabling
3.   Do not involve the total personality
4.   Do not interfere with the patient's ability to test reality

Distinction from Personality Disorders is based on the fact that the neuroses have an identifiable onset whereas the Personality Disorders are lifelong processes. Also, the neuroses are manifested primarily by symptoms, subjective discomfort, whereas the Personality Disorders are manifested by habitual or recurring patterns of maladaptive behavior. However, maladaptive behavior sometimes occurs in the neuroses in the form of *acting-out* of neurotic conflict. The term acting-out is often misused, or at least used loosely. It should not be applied, as it sometimes is, to any socially more or less undesirable activity (often when acting-up would be a better phrase). Actually, acting-out need not be socially undesirable. Conflict usually impedes action; even the simplest conflict in conscious thought (e.g., would you rather have pie or ice cream?) causes a moment's hesitation until the conflict is solved by decision one way or the other, or compromise (pie à la mode, thank you). However, one sometimes acts on an impulse without having solved or compromised the conflict. Even after action the conflict may not be resolved. Relatively healthy mechanisms, including rationalization, convince the patient that a wise, or at least a necessary choice was made in deciding to act. Reconsideration of alternative possibilities is suppressed. These protective mechanisms fail when acting-out occurs. The steps in acting-out are:

1. Mounting tension as the strength of a conflicted impulse grows
2. Discharge of the impulse; impulsive action
3. A shift in the balance of the conflicting forces after the impulse has been discharged
4. Guilt feelings

Since guilt feelings are not a prominent feature of most Personality Disorders, their presence is useful diagnostically.

Differentiation from Adjustment Disorders is based on the intensity of the stress involved in producing the Adjustment Disorders and the relative lack of evidence of neurotic conflict in the premorbid personality of patients with Adjustment Disorders.

Differential diagnosis is complicated in cases who present or appear to present a mixture of disorders.

Generalized Anxiety Disorders, though characteristic symptoms are readily elicited and objective signs easily observed, often present problems in differential diagnosis. There are many causes of nervousness. Outward signs of tension similar to those of anxiety are sometimes seen in routine examinations in the absence of any complaint. Such tension differs from anxiety in that:

1. It is more or less appropriate to the patient's situation (one which requires some hyperalertness, readiness for action).
2. It is not in itself a source of gross subjective discomfort. The situation which evokes it may or may not be productive of discomfort. The sensation may even be pleasurable (e.g., the hyperalertness associated with some sports and recreational activities).
3. It is not disabling and does not interfere with effective handling of the situation.

Differential diagnosis may be difficult if the patient has some reason to conceal discomfort or disability. For example, many job applicants are nervous. This is especially true if the applicant is eager to get the job and is "keyed-up." However, if the signs are in excess of what is usually observed and the patient is questioned about anxiety, he or she may deny or minimize symptoms which actually interfere with day-to-day activities.

There are many somatic disorders which produce symptoms suggestive of generalized anxiety or panic (e.g., thyrotoxicosis, hypoglycemia, pheochromocytoma, amphetamine intoxication).

Patients with psychiatric conditions other than the neuroses often show anxiety, either throughout the illness (e.g., some schizophrenics) or when there is a superimposed external stress (e.g., patients with Personality Disorders). Adjustment Disorders are almost always accompanied by signs of anxiety.

The Dissociative Disorders are distinguished from Adjustment Disorders produced by gross stress largely on the basis of history. Differentiation from Schizophrenic Disorders is based on history, identification of neurotic conflict in the neuroses, and the absence of the primary symptoms of schizophrenia. Sometimes malingering must be considered. The fact that a patient is in trouble and that it is convenient to "forget" one's identity or to have a period of amnesia for one's actions does not establish malingering. A complete psychiatric evaluation and a period of observations are necessary.

Conversion Disorders must be distinguished from a number of neurological diseases. Diffuse neurological disorders such as multiple sclerosis can present bizarre neurological findings which do not appear to conform to nerve distribution. Malingering may also need to be considered in some cases. This is not an either-or situation. Exploitation of secondary gain does not mean that the basic illness is simulated. A person with *any* disease or injury may more or less consciously exaggerate symptoms to gain sympathy and attention, to avoid responsibilities, to manipulate people, or even to gain (increased) compensation. Also, a conversion headache, for example, can be intermittent, so that the patient claiming disability for gainful occupation may be symptom-free at some times; the symptom may even interfere with work and not with recreation. To make the diagnosis one must study the history, look for signs of neurotic conflict, and evaluate the presence or absence of the other signs of hysteria. On the other hand, one looks for evidences of sociopathy, and evaluates the extent to which malingering, if present, would be (setting aside moral values) a workable and adaptive way of dealing with a situation, taking into account both the disadvantages of maintaining the symptom and the possible gains from doing so. Even definite malingering does not mean the absence of psychiatric disease; it may be an unsatisfactory coping mechanism chosen by a person with Mental Retardation, Personality Disorder, or Schizophrenia.

Sometimes establishing the element of malingering is more a task for a detective than a physician; however, whether there is malingering or not, the physician is the one to evaluate the degree of mental illness. For legal reasons it is often better not to record a formal diagnosis of Malingering (a term found in DSM-III under the heading Conditions Not Attributable to a Mental Disorder). It is usually enough to present one's findings and indicate that one cannot make a psychiatric, or other, diagnosis.

Phobic Disorders rarely present a problem in differential diagnosis. Of course, a patient with some other psychiatric disorder can have a phobia as one of the symptoms, and some relatively healthy people have disproportionate fears.

Mild obsessions should be distinguished from other types of preoccupation. Patients with Compulsive Personalities differ from those with Obsessive Compulsive Disorders in that the former usually do not have clearcut obsessions or compulsions and present only a lifelong pattern of behavior heavily influenced by character traits derived from the anal stage of development. Their obsessional defenses work — after a fashion. Some patients with Compulsive Personalities develop true obsessions or compulsions under stress; these tend to be transitory and show remission when the specific stress is relieved or when the total stress in the environment is reduced. Problems in evaluating inhibiting obsessions have already been discussed. Severe obsessionals are sometimes hard to distinguish from schizophrenic patients. The latter diagnosis is made if the primary symptoms of schizophrenia are present. In regard to treatment and prognosis in doubtful cases, this differential diagnosis is usually a distinction without a difference.

PREVENTION

Though adequate statistics are lacking, there is little doubt that the prevalence of severe neuroses is less in modern times than in the past. It is indeed difficult nowadays for even a large clinic to assemble a sufficient number of typical severe neurotics for research. This is not altogether a result of more sophisticated diagnoses. Improved child care has done much to prevent neuroses, and in time can do more. Children who are having difficulties negotiating the early stages of psychosocial development can be identified and helped before fixations or major conflicts develop.

Modern attitudes toward sexuality have done much to reduce the occurrence of major sexual conflicts. Almost everyone has minor ones. Society and the individual must regulate behavior stemming from the sex instinct, just as other instinctual behavior must be regulated, but this can be done by conscious intent based on the consequences of behavior, without the need for unreasonable fears, guilts, and repressions.

Conflicts over dependency and aggression are still handled with difficulty within our social framework. Constructive, or at least innocuous, ways of meeting needs underlying these conflicts must be found. The physician, in direct discussion, or indirectly by his or her attitudes, can be helpful to patients who are potentially neurotic because of conflicts related to these needs. Patients can be helped to recognize and accept emotional needs so that these needs may be met in socially desirable ways without anxiety-producing conflict.

Early treatment of neuroses before the more severe and chronic manifestations appear can reduce the incidence of neurotic disability.

Treatment

Acute mild anxiety neuroses often have spontaneous remissions. Many of these do not come to medical attention at all. If they do, while expectant and symptomatic therapy is appropriate, close medical observation is also indicated so that any tendency toward chronicity or toward the development of more serious symptoms can be recognized and more definitive treatment instituted.

Symptomatic treatment is also indicated in some cases of Generalized Anxiety Disorders if disability is not too great. Sometimes disability is difficult to evaluate. The effect of fatigue caused by insomnia and muscular tension (or the use of energy, libido, in maintaining repression?) on vocational performance, the effect of impaired concentration on learning and creative work, and the effect of irritability on vocational and social relationships is hard to measure.

Medication should be aimed at target symptoms, and its effect not only on these but on other symptoms as well must be carefully observed. Suppose a patient has tremor, restlessness, insomnia, difficulty in concentration, irritability, and chronic fatigue. A sedative or tranquilizer will almost certainly reduce the first three symptoms. It may help the others or, almost as frequently, may make them worse. If the fatigue is the most disabling symptom, the patient may feel better and function better with a stimulant. This is also true of irritability in some cases. On the other hand, a stimulant will increase the restlessness and insomnia (though patients worry about this less if it is termed lowered sleep requirement). Tricyclic antidepressants occasionally relieve ongoing anxiety (secondary to depression?), but they are more often effective in the treatment of Panic Disorders. Beta-adrenergic blocking drugs are occasionally effective in the treatment of Panic Disorders or other cases of episodic anxiety (including the anxiety accompanying some Social Phobias). Other drugs which are sometimes useful in treating patients who have panic attacks include alprazolam, a benzodiazepine, and phenelzine, a monoamine oxidase (MAO) inhibitor.

Anxiolytics (minor tranquilizers) are most likely to be effective in relieving observed symptoms. The patient who complains of anxiety but does not show outward signs of it is unlikely to be benefited. Use of tranquilizers in Conversion Disorders and Obsessive Compulsive Disorders is indicated only if there is appreciable free-floating anxiety.

When medication is used in acute cases one does not expect to continue it indefinitely. One also expects to discontinue, eventually, medication that is used in a chronic case as an adjunct to psychotherapy. However, when medication alone is used in a chronic case one must consider possible long-range consequences and should avoid relatively new drugs when the effects of years of use are not fully known. Symptomatic medication usually should not be used in women who may be or may become pregnant unless the safety of the medication during pregnancy has been established.

Anxiolytics may be given in regularly scheduled doses or for use as needed (up to a maximum daily amount). Before prescribing medication to be used as needed one is careful to evaluate risks of drug misuse, habituation, and suicide attempt. Using medication only when needed helps prevent the development of drug tolerance. The competent physician is never casual about prescribing anxiolytics as they are dangerous drugs when misused, but the fact that some patients misuse a drug should not deprive others of its benefits.

If depression is among the symptoms of neurosis, antidepressant medications may be used, though they are not as effective as they are in other types of depression. The tranquilizers may increase depression (and irritability), and they are used with caution, even if anxiety is also present. Rauwolfia derivatives are contraindicated, since they deplete norepinephrine and make depression worse.

The main treatment for all of the neuroses is psychotherapy. A number of different techniques of psychotherapy are found to be effective. In most cases the treatment of choice is an expressive, investigative therapy based upon psychogenetic and dynamic concepts. Its purpose is to bring conflicts into conscious awareness so that they may be resolved. A trial of relatively brief therapy is usually indicated before intensive long-term therapies (e.g., psychoanalysis) are considered.

Behavior therapies, including systematic desensitization, are useful for certain phobic patients. Some object that these relieve the symptoms but do not resolve basic conflicts. Other investigators who have used these techniques believe that the role of conflict in the Phobic Disorders is overemphasized and that these symptoms are a result of learning or conditioning. However, even if they result from conflict, anything that relieves them is worth considering. If the underlying conflict remains, it is not necessarily disabling, nor is there necessarily a grave risk of recurrence or development of a more pathological set of defenses as a substitute. However, the patient's ego strength and risk, if any, of psychotic decompensation should be evaluated before such treatments are used and the overall mental health, not just the symptoms, must be evaluated at the end of treatment. The same considerations apply to the use of hypnosis and suggestion in the treatment of Conversion Disorders. Sometimes, when a hysterical symptom threatens life (e.g., hysterical vomiting) or prevents expressive therapy (e.g., aphonia, but not dysphonia; dissociative amnesia), symptomatic relief through hypnosis, or suggestion, sometimes with the use of amobarbital (Amytal) or thiopental (Pentothal) interviews, must precede other therapy.

Though long-term investigative psychotherapy is often the treatment of choice for patients with Obsessive Compulsive Disorder, behavioral therapies are also used. A number of medications, among them loxapine, clomipramine, tranylcypromine, and clonidine, have been reported as beneficial for this condition, but most of these reports are of small numbers of cases and lack adequate confirmation.

Hypochondriacs, because of preoccupation with symptoms, and in some cases a tendency to reject the possibility that psychotherapy can be helpful, often fail to respond to investigative and expressive psychotherapies, but they may be helped by nondirective counseling (cf. Chapter 19).

Most neurotic patients can be treated as outpatients. Only the most severely disabled require hospitalization. Some patients with dissociative symptoms require hospitalization for differential diagnosis. Severe obsessionals with impending psychotic breakdown are best treated as inpatients. Other neurotic patients may experience sufficient distress for hospitalization during the initial phases of treatment. Sometimes hospitalization is useful in removing the patient from contributing stress situations.

Neurotic patients who are depressed must be evaluated for suicide risk. The same considerations apply as in the study of suicide risk in other depressed people (cf. Chapter 10). One must not underestimate suicide risk because the patient occasionally appears cheerful. In acute cases the markedly suicidal patient must be hospitalized. In more chronic cases, when no special treatment can be offered in the hospital that cannot be given outside of it, a greater calculated risk in outpatient therapy is sometimes justified. If prognostic factors anticipate long-term therapy, and if the condition is not temporarily worse because of additional environmental stresses or internal crises, one would not expect the patient to improve or be less suicidal after brief hospitalization. The potential safety of long-term hospital care must be weighed against the effect on the self-esteem and social adjustment likely to result from removing the patient from occupational and family roles for a prolonged period. Neurotic patients are less likely to attempt suicide after a firm transference relationship with the therapist has been established.

REVIEW QUESTIONS

1. What is a neurosis? How does a neurosis differ from a psychosis? From a Personality Disorder?
2. What are the outward manifestations of anxiety? What system is responsible for them?
3. In what way and to what extent is anxiety useful?
4. What is meant by acting-out? Why is it called that?
5. Name some phobias. Can you think of any others that are not mentioned by name in this chapter?
6. Discuss differences and similarities in the psychogenesis and dynamics of Phobic and Obsessive Compulsive Disorders.
7. A woman of 30 comes as an outpatient with a moderately severe claustrophobia. Construct a hypothetical life history for this patient. How would you treat her? What other treatment might be considered?
8. What are the characteristics of a Factitious Disorder? How do Factitious Disorders differ from Somatoform Disorders? Malingering?
9. What is meant by an inhibiting obsession? Why is it called that? If the content of an inhibiting obsession relates to auto theft, how would this be different from a compulsion to steal cars?
10. How does insight help the patient with a neurosis?

SELECTED REFERENCES

1. Angyal, Andras: Evasions of growth. *Am J Psychiatry* 110:358–361, 1953.

2. Barsky, Arthur J., and Gerald L. Klerman: Overview: Hypochondriasis, bodily complaints, and somatic styles. *Am J Psychiatry* 140(3):273–283, 1983.

3. Eaton, Merrill T.: Psychoneurosis. In *Current Therapy.* Conn, Howard F. (Ed.). Philadelphia, Saunders, 1983, pp. 899–902.

4. Guze, Samuel B.: The validity and significance of the clinical diagnosis of hysteria (Briquet's syndrome). *Am J Psychiatry* 132(2):138–141, 1975.

5. Hoehn-Saric, Rudolf: Neurotransmitters in anxiety. *Arch Gen Psychiatry* 39(6):735–742, 1982.

6. Horowitz, Mardi J., Nancy Wilner, Nancy Kaltreider, and William Alvarez: Signs and symptoms of posttraumatic stress disorder. *Arch Gen Psychiatry* 37(1):85–92, 1980.

7. Insel, Thomas R., Dennis L. Murphy, Robert M. Cohen, Ina Alterman, Clinton Kilts, and Markku Linnoila: Obsessive-compulsive disorder. *Arch Gen Psychiatry* 40(6):605–612, 1983.

8. Jenike, Michael A.: Rapid response of severe obsessive-compulsive disorder to tranylcypromine. *Am J Psychiatry* 138(9):1249–1250, 1981.

9. Jobson, Kenneth, Markku Linnoila, John Gillam, and John L. Sullivan: Successful treatment of severe anxiety attacks with tricyclic antidepressants: A potential mechanism of action. *Am J Psychiatry* 135(7):863–864, 1978.

10. Kathol, Roger G., Russell Noyes, Donald J. Slymen, Raymond R. Crowe, John Clancy, and Richard E. Kerber: Propranolol in chronic anxiety disorders: A controlled study. *Arch Gen Psychiatry* 37(12):1361–1365, 1980.

11. Klein, Donald F., Charlotte Marker Zitrin, Margaret G. Woerner, and Donald C. Ross: Treatment of phobias. II. Behavior therapy and supportive psychotherapy: Are there any specific ingredients? *Arch Gen Psychiatry* 40(2):139–145, 1983.

12. Knesevich, John William: Successful treatment of obsessive-compulsive disorder with clonidine hydrochloride. *Am J Psychiatry* 139(3):364–365, 1982.

13. Mavissakalian, Matig, and Larry Michelson: Tricyclic antidepressants in obsessive-compulsive disorder: Antiobsessional or antidepressant agents? *J Nerv Ment Dis* 171(5):301–306, 1983.

14. Mavissakalian, Matig, Rosemarie Salerni, Mark E. Thompson, and Larry Michelson: Mitral valve prolapse and agoraphobia. *Am J Psychiatry* 140(12):1612–1614, 1983.

15. Merskey, Harold, and Michael Trimble: Personality, sexual adjustment, and brain lesions in patients with conversion symptoms. *Am J Psychiatry 136(2): 179-182, 1979.*

16. Morrison, James R.: Early birth order in Briquet's syndrome. *Am J Psychiatry* 140(12):1596-1597, 1983.

17. Morrison, James R.: Management of Briquet syndrome (hysteria). *West J Med* 128(6):482-487, 1978.

18. Raskin, Marjorie, Harmon V. S. Peeke, William Dickman, and Henry Pinsker: Panic and generalized anxiety disorders: Developmental antecedents and pre-cipitants. *Arch Gen Psychiatry* 39(6):687-689, 1982.

19. Rickels, Karl, W. George Case, Robert W. Downing, and Andrew Winokur: Long-term diazepam therapy and clinical outcome. *JAMA* 250(6):767-771, 1983.

20. Rivers-Bulkeley, Noel, and Marc H. Hollender: Successful treatment of obses-sive-compulsive disorder with loxapine. *Am J Psychiatry* 139(10):1345-1346, 1982.

21. Shader, Richard I., Melissa Goodman, and John Gever: Panic disorders: Cur-rent perspectives. *J Clin Psychopharmacol* 2(6):(Suppl.)2S-10S, 1982.

22. Sierles, Frederick S., JanJune Chen, Robert E. McFarland, and Michael Alan Taylor: Posttraumatic stress disorder and concurrent psychiatric illness: A preliminary report. *Am J Psychiatry* 140(9):1177-1179, 1983.

23. Sparr, Landy, and Loren D. Pankratz: Factitious posttraumatic stress disorder. *Am J Psychiatry* 140(8):1016-1019, 1983.

24. Steketee, Gail, Edna B. Foa, and Jonathan B. Grayson: Recent advances in the behavioral treatment of obsessive-compulsives. *Arch Gen Psychiatry* 39(12):1365-1371, 1982.

25. Zitrin, Charlotte Marker, Donald F. Klein, Margaret G. Woerner, and Donald C. Ross: Treatment of phobias: Comparison of imipramine hydrochloride and placebo. *Arch Gen Psychiatry* 40(2):125-138, 1983.

Chapter 9

PSYCHOLOGICAL FACTORS
AFFECTING PHYSICAL CONDITION

MIND AND BODY

In current nomenclature (see Chapter 4) the category (not a diagnosis itself) of Psychological Factors Affecting Physical Condition is applied to situations in which psychologically significant environmental stimuli, usually stresses, are temporally related to the onset or exacerbation of a nonpsychiatric disorder (an Axis III diagnosis). The category is used only when the nonpsychiatric condition is accompanied by pathological changes or has a known pathophysiological process. This is a rather narrow category that encompasses only a small part of the interrelationship between psychological factors, emotional and behavioral, and disease processes.

The older term, psychosomatic, still widely used, has broader application. Unfortunately, it implies a mind-body dualism which is incompatible with modern science. With a few notable exceptions (e.g., investigators in the field of parapsychology such as the late J. B. Rhine and his associates at Duke University) modern students of psychology and psychiatry find no evidence of a separate "mind" or of function independent of structure.

Neither the category of Psychological Factors Affecting Physical Condition nor the term psychosomatic is used for the Somatoform Disorders discussed in Chapter 8. Also note that physical symptoms and complaints may accompany many other psychiatric disorders, and if resulting directly from these disorders, do not require a separate diagnosis.

EMOTION, PHYSIOLOGY,
AND STRUCTURAL CHANGE

The experience of functional change in various organs and systems under the influence of emotion is so universal that the acceptance of the basic concept does not require experimental proof though experiments (e.g., observation of gastric mucosa in different emotional states) provide precise data. Anyone who has seen another person turn livid with rage, or whose heart has pounded with fear, or who has noted rapid respiration (among other things) while making love *knows* that emotions produce bodily changes. Perhaps one *might* feel that these changes represent normal physiology and are not necessarily related to disease. However, most people have experienced transitory psychophysiological disturbances of a more distinctly pathological nature (e.g., preexamination diarrhea).

The layman as well as the physician is aware of the effect of emotions on various systems. The person who describes something or someone as "getting under my skin," or observes that an experience "makes my blood boil," or that a situation "just makes me sick," or that when something happened, "I nearly defecated" is using a figure of speech, but it is a figure of speech related to consensually validated experiences.

If a transitory emotional change produces a temporary alteration in the function of an organ or system, then it appears logical that persistent or frequently recurring emotional states can produce chronic functional change. That this process can go on to structural change is only slightly less apparent. For example, one would expect an overworked heart to hypertrophy. One would expect recurring hyperacidity and hypermotility of the stomach and duodenum to interfere with healing of mucosal lesions.

These observations and deductions led investigators to search for emotional factors in many diseases. In certain diseases, clinical observations and psychological tests revealed a high incidence of emotional disturbance. Some emotional disturbance could be the result, not the cause of disease. However, histories often showed that emotional disturbance antedated systemic disease.

The exact relationship between emotional factors and some diseases has not been determined. In others, the relationship is relatively clear.

FACTORS IN THE ETIOLOGY
OF PSYCHOSOMATIC DISORDERS

There are many factors involved in the progress from emotional disturbance to systemic disease. These include the following.

Stress

The Post-traumatic Stress Disorders discussed in Chapter 8 result from grossly stressful circumstances such as civilian or military disasters or other calamities. However, milder stresses, things that create tension or tend to alter one's equilibrium, may have undesirable consequences. A stress is not necessarily perceived as unpleasant. Moving, taking a new job, getting married, or any major change in one's life situation, however desirable, creates some disequilibrium and tension. Stresses tend to have cumulative effects so that several mildly stressful events occurring at about the same time may have as much impact as a single major stress.

As has been noted, the category of Psychological Factors Affecting Physical Condition requires a temporal relationship with a psychologically significant environmental stimulus. The psychological significance of stress is variable, and since everyone encounters numerous stressful experiences in life, a history of stress occurring shortly before an illness can be merely coincidental. Still, stress has a higher correlation with psychosomatic illness than any other experiential or emotional factor. This still leaves an unanswered question of why a particular organ or system is affected rather than another. This may be related to the nature of the stress, a preexisting weakness or damage of an organ that makes it especially vulnerable, or interaction of the stress with other factors.

Somatization

With the ego defense mechanism of somatization, also commonly occurring in Somatoform Disorders, conflicts are represented by physical symptoms involving parts of the body innervated by the autonomic nervous system. Conversion involves parts of the body with sensory and/or motor innervation. However, there are other differences. Anxiety is not as well relieved by somatization as by conversion. Symbolism is often not as apparent in somatization. The milder manifestations of somatization (e.g., episodes of tachycardia) are distinguished from the physiological concomitants of free-floating anxiety in that only one organ or system is primarily involved. In more complex somatization reactions the symptom may relate to a conflicted emotional need (e.g., in some cases of arthritis there may be a connection with a hostile dependent interaction in which the symptom inhibits impulses to dissolve the relationship. "I can't get out of *this* joint, my *joints* won't let me; and besides, I need him to take care of me.")

Organ Language

Communication by way of symptoms is referred to as organ language. This is closely related to the symbolic element in some cases of somatization. Many illnesses communicate something to the effect of "take care of me" or "don't leave me" (this may represent primary rather than secondary gain). However, some communications are more specific. It was noted earlier that one may describe something as a nauseating experience; however, one can communicate this by actually being nauseated. Anyone who has had much experience at psychotherapy has encountered patients who express their disgust or anger by flatulence.

It is sometimes said, quite incorrectly, that one does not die of a broken heart. One can, not only by suicide, loss of concern for safety, or with the aid of strong drink, but also as a result of psychosomatic illness. One can communicate one's heartbreak by getting sick.

Emotional Specificity

The physiological concomitants of different emotions (e.g., fear, anger, grief, etc.) are not identical. One persistent recurring noxious emotional state might be expected to have a different result from another.

Undischarged Emotion

An emotional state represents a readiness for action, or at least for expression of feeling. Once the feeling is expressed (e.g., weeping) or actions are taken (e.g., fight or flight) a tension state associated with the preparation for action is eliminated or reduced. If there is no expression or action, the tension state remains and may affect the function of some system.

Some readers of popular psychology have misinterpreted a recognition of the consequences of undischarged emotions to be a prescription for "letting it all hang out" or "blowing one's stack" over trivia. Mounting, unexpressed anger, for example, can be harmful, but repeated episodes of anger are also harmful. One must do something about one's feelings before they reach a detrimental level. Even if crying does rid one of some excess neurotransmitters, as has been suggested, it may be preferable not to have generated the excess.

Personality Type

In one stage of research into psychosomatic disease, some investigators hoped that a personality type could be identified for each major disorder. This could be of use in predicting susceptibility, in diagnosis, and in treatment planning. Though personality profiles are described for many diseases, they are by no means consistent and many cases do not show the "typical" personality. However, character structures can certainly contribute to disease. For example, one often finds diseases of the upper gastrointestinal tract and some other diseases related to oral activities (e.g., obesity, diabetes) in persons whose major characteristics are derived from the oral stage of psychosexual development. Diseases of the lower gastrointestinal tract are often associated with anal character structure.

Alexithymia, a personality constellation including constriction of emotional life, difficulty in fantasizing, and trouble in finding appropriate words to describe emotions has been reported as sometimes occurring in patients with psychosomatic disease.

Life styles and personal habits, often influenced by character structure and sometimes by neurotic defenses, may contribute indirectly to a variety of illnesses.

The factors discussed above as being involved in the etiology of Psychosomatic Disorders are not mutually exclusive and are often interrelated. In a given case, one or several may be involved.

Mention that a certain factor is often associated with a particular syndrome does not imply that it is the only causative factor, or even the only emotional factor. Psychosomatic syndromes, like other manifestations of human behavior, are overdetermined; they have multiple causes. Likewise, it does not mean that the factor occurs in every case. Patients can have identical symptoms for unidentical reasons. For example, nonspecific diarrheas can be associated with fear, anger, unusually generous impulses (whether carried into action or at the level of fantasy) in some people with compulsive personalities, or any of a dozen or so other factors including a change in diet.

Some factors to consider in certain physical disorders, if there is reason to believe that emotional disturbances play an important role, are discussed below.

1. In the case of pruritus there is often a source of annoyance (or irritation?). Superficially the cause of annoyance may seem petty, but it is something that "gets under the patient's skin." The patient may be more or less conscious of the annoyance.

    In some other skin disorders, one looks for diffuse anxiety with excessive sweating (hyperhidrosis) as a contributing factor.
2. Some cases of asthma are related to fears of abandonment. Often there has been an experience of abandonment in childhood. The asthmatic wheeze has been likened to the cry of the abandoned child. In other cases, one may find suppressed or repressed grief; the asthmatic attacks often stop if the patient actually sheds tears. It has been reported that the need for steroids in the treatment of adult bronchial asthma is more directly associated with stressful life events than with the underlying pulmonary pathology.
3. Hypertension is sometimes related to suppressed or repressed rage. In cases of coronary heart disease a frequent finding is frustrated ambition or feelings of failure or impending failure in competitive situations (often encountered in the Type A personality described by Friedman and Rosenman).
4. Many patients with migraine place an unusual emphasis on intellectual achievement; their headaches may relate to guilt and to self-punishment "like beating one's head against a wall." The headache often follows periods of hard work or stress.

5.   Diseases of the upper gastrointestinal tract are usually associated with an oral character structure and are closely related to dependent needs. In peptic ulcer, one often finds a reaction formation against dependent needs. In the armed services it was noted that ulcer symptoms were less frequent in men in combat than in rest camps, though in combat there was great stress and often poor diet. However, in combat, men were with their units and met dependent needs in the relationship with their officers and fellow soldiers.

Obesity may also relate to dependent needs. Sometimes food is taken as a substitute for or symbol of affection; in such cases obesity results from a feeling of being unloved. In other cases obesity may represent a wish to be unattractive; this is usually related to a fear of sexual impulses. Depression is thought to be a frequent factor in morbid obesity, though some studies have failed to confirm this.

6.   Diabetics frequently have problems stemming from the oral stage of development. They too tend to feel unloved and unlovable. They find few pleasures and satisfactions in living other than in eating, and regard life as a dull grind.

7.   Diseases of the lower gastrointestinal tract are often related to problems arising in the anal stage of development. Patients subject to constipation, diarrhea, and colitis often have marked compulsive tendencies. Men who have ulcerative colitis sometimes are schizoid and occasionally periods of colitis alternate with psychotic episodes. Women with ulcerative colitis more often have an hysterical character structure; sometimes they have had conflicts over rectal masturbation.

8.   Some cases of rheumatoid arthritis are associated with hostile-dependent relationships.

9.   As might be expected, sexual conflicts are sometimes found in patients with genitourinary disorders. These are sometimes related to fears or guilt feelings concerning sexuality. In women, fears of pregnancy or fears of being inadequate to be a mother may be present. Disorders that interfere with satisfactory intercourse may be related to hostility toward the sexual partner (or to all members of the opposite sex).

10. There is often a major precipitating stress in cases of hyperthyroidism. Sometimes this is a loss. Often it is something about which the patient feels guilt or shame. Sometimes prior to onset the patient has had a frustrating overly dependent relationship with another person that has culminated in a breakup of the relationship accompanied by disturbing hostile feelings.

11. Emotional factors in convulsive disorder may relate to recurring stresses. Anger is sometimes involved. In some cases the convulsion follows a period of mounting tension. A convulsion may symbolize orgasm.

DIAGNOSING PSYCHOSOMATIC DISORDERS

Most psychophysiological disorders are diagnosed on the basis of the signs and symptoms of the particular syndrome. The psychiatric problem in diagnosis is that of evaluating the importance, if any, of emotional factors. Naturally, one suspects emotional factors in functional disorders without structural change; one also suspects their presence in certain syndromes in which they are frequently encountered. However, the emotional state of any patient, whatever the disease, should be evaluated. Emotional factors can contribute to almost any illness. On the other hand, few if any of the syndromes with structural change are exclusively psychosomatic. For example, there are emotional factors in many cases of peptic ulcer, but in a specific case these factors may be of little or no consequence, while in another they may represent the major etiological factor. In some cases of peptic ulcer, emotional factors play no part at all; peptic ulcer of the newborn is usually associated with congenital anomalies of the upper gastrointestinal tract. Asthma, along with other allergies, is usually thought of as having psychosomatic components, but in veterinary practice the variation in prevalence of asthma in different breeds of dogs suggests an important constitutional factor. (This does not exclude the emotional factors. The asthmatic Pekingese may be the neurotic pet of a neurotic master or mistress, but if the dog had had the good fortune to have been a Scotch Terrier, it might be less likely to wheeze.)

Remember that the presenting complaint of some patients with other psychiatric disorders (e.g., Generalized Anxiety Disorder, any type of depression, Passive-Aggressive Personality) may be one of physiological disturbance. This may be because it is the most disturbing symptom (e.g., the patient with a Generalized Anxiety Disorder may complain of palpitation), or it may be to some extent a rationalization, a socially acceptable reason for going to the doctor when one knows one is not feeling well but does not quite know how to describe the discomfort.

It is advisable to evaluate the possibility that psychological factors play a part in any disease in which the patient's failure to follow medical advice interferes seriously with treatment. There are of course many other possible reasons for noncompliance, ranging from failure of the physician to communicate adequately with the patient to the cost of medication.

PREVENTION OF PSYCHOSOMATIC DISORDERS

Though there are other psychological factors that affect physical conditions, stress is the one most amenable to preventive measures. Special attention may be given to this in industry. The individual may also be helped to minimize his or her exposure to stress, or at least to time such exposures so as to lessen the possibility of cumulative effects.

Persons apparently at risk for psychosomatic disturbance because of character structure, life style, a tendency to use somatization as a mechanism, a tendency to experience frequent noxious emotional states, or a difficulty in expressing and dealing with emotion may be candidates for a psychotherapeutic intervention.

COURSE AND TREATMENT

Most psychosomatic disorders can and should be treated by the generalist or internist. There are specific treatments for some syndromes. Many others respond to symptomatic medication.

If stress is an important etiological factor, recovery often rapidly follows the cessation of the stress or removal from an ongoing stress situation.

Failure to respond to usual treatments or apparent difficulty in cooperating with the physician may be an indication for greater emphasis on a psychotherapeutic approach. Examples: (1) A patient develops a peptic ulcer. He is given diet and medication and a short vacation is recommended. His symptoms subside quickly and the ulcer heals. He continues his diet more or less faithfully, but on his return to work his ulcer recurs. This pattern is repeated several times. Psychotherapy should be instituted before surgery becomes necessary. (2) An obese patient seeks treatment. She is given a diet and for a few weeks loses weight steadily. Then she begins to gain again. She finds it impossible to adhere to her diet.

Medication to reduce her appetite helps for a while, but again she finds excuses to make exceptions to her diet. Without psychotherapy she will stay fat.

For psychosomatic disorders an investigative or expressive therapy is usually used, but in selected cases other therapies, including behavior therapy, may be chosen. Biofeedback techniques are effective for some psychosomatic disorders.

In psychotherapy, one identifies emotional needs and helps the patient modify them or find less self-destructive ways of meeting them. However, in physical disorders, treatment may include meeting the emotional needs as they exist. Examples: (1) An ulcer patient shows a denial of oral dependent needs. When he is well he likes to be quite independent. He does not turn to his employer or his wife for help. He does not even enjoy eating. When he is busy he skips lunch or bolts it hastily. Medication and a simple diet fail to produce lasting results, but an elaborate diet which requires frequent eating and a number of prescribed activities which create dependence on his physician and on his wife meets the emotional need and allows the treatment to work. The patient may wonder what some instructions, such as having a nightly back rub given by his wife, have to do with relief of a pain in the epigastrium, but some unconscious awareness will probably keep him from asking embarrassing questions. (2) A mildly hypertensive minister suppresses a good bit of anger at members of his congregation. Antihypertensive drugs and diuretics fail to help adequately. His interest in sports is explored and it is found that he likes golf but rarely plays because he is too busy. He is instructed to play at least three times weekly. He assumes that this is for healthful exercise. His physician hopes the patient will express some aggression hitting the golf ball, and, hopefully, outplay a deacon or two who do not get as much practice.

A recognition of emotional needs may lead to modification of general medical management. For example, if weight reduction is considered for a mildly hypertensive patient, before prescribing a diet it is well to assess oral dependent needs.

The decision to include formal psychotherapy in the treatment program is not to be undertaken lightly. It is time consuming and difficult. In purely functional cases one evaluates:

1. The other manifestations of maladaption which might on their own merits require psychotherapy
2. The response to symptomatic medication

Tension headaches that respond to aspirin should be treated with aspirin, not analysis, unless the headaches are just one of several manifestations of disturbed living. Aspirin is cheaper and easier to take. However, some patients with psychosomatic disorders without structural change require psychotherapy by either the generalist or a psychiatrist. In cases with structural changes the addition of psychotherapy to the treatment program should not, initially at least, substitute for general medical management. Since combined treatment is needed, it is often better that the psychotherapy be done by the internist or generalist, but joint management is sometimes appropriate. The psychiatrist provides the psychotherapy; general medical management by the referring physician is continued.

In the presence of structural changes, failure to respond to general medical management is, as has been mentioned, an important consideration in evaluating the need for formal psychotherapy. If psychotherapy is to be part of the treatment program it must be started before changes become irreversible. If psychotherapy is to help a hypertensive, it should begin before the patient develops an Organic Mental Disorder.

Psychological factors affect physical illness, but physical illness is in itself stressful and affects the emotional and mental functioning of the patient. One must recognize and deal with the anxieties and fears, realistic or otherwise, of the sick. The effects of chronic illness, disability, or surgical procedures on the self-image are factors which must be taken into account. Signs of depression should not be overlooked.

Considering possible psychological factors in any illness, and furnishing appropriate treatment if they are present, is basic in a holistic or problem-oriented method of patient care. It is a part of treating patients, not just diseases.

REVIEW QUESTIONS

1. What is the difference between conversion and somatization?
2. Give an example of a cardiac disease without structural change in which psychological factors are contributory or causative. One with structural change.
3. Discuss emotional factors which might contribute to the etiology of pruritus ani. What would you look for first?
4. What is a common emotional factor in asthma? Rheumatoid arthritis?
5. Discuss the treatment of physical conditions with psychological factors.
6. Under what circumstances should a patient with a physical condition in which psychological factors play a part be treated by a psychiatrist? By a generalist or internist? By both?
7. The term anniversary reaction is sometimes used to describe an acute physical illness (e.g., coronary occlusion) which occurs on the anniversary of an important event in the patient's life. How would you explain such an occurrence? Why and how would you look for this possibility in taking a history? Would you expect the patient to be conscious of the fact that the illness occurs on an anniversary?
8. A patient with fracture has a history of being accident prone. How could character structure be a factor in this? What other psychological factors might be involved?

SELECTED REFERENCES

1. Alexander, Franz: *Psychosomatic Medicine, Its Principles and Applications.* New York, Norton, 1950.

2. Applebaum, Paul S., and Loren H. Roth: Patients who refuse treatment in medical hospitals. *JAMA* 250(10):1296-1301, 1983.

3. Blanchard, Edward B., and Larry D. Young: Clinical Applications of Biofeedback Training. *Arch Gen Psychiatry* 30(5):573-589, 1974.

4. Caplan, Gerald: Mastery of stress: Psychosocial aspects. *Am J Psychiatry* 138(4):413-420, 1981.

5. Chandrasena, Ranjith: Hypnosis in the treatment of viral warts. *Psychiatr J Univ Ottawa* 7(2):135-137, 1982.

6. Cousins, Norman: Denial: Are sharper definitions needed? *JAMA* 248(2):210-212 (Commentary), 1982.

7.   Derogatis, Leonard R., Gary R. Morrow, John Fetting, Doris Penman, Sheryl Piasetsky, Arthur M. Schmale, Michael Henrichs, and Charles L. M. Carnicke, Jr.: The prevalence of psychiatric disorders among cancer patients. *JAMA* 249(6):751-757, 1983.

8.   Dirks, Jerald F., Robert A. Kinsman, Herman Staudenmayer, and James H. Kleiger: Panic-fear in asthma: Symptomatology as an index of signal anxiety and personality as an index of ego resources. *J Nerv Men Dis* 167(10):615-619, 1979.

9.   Eaton, Merrill T., Jr.: Executive stresses do exist — But they can be controlled. *Personnel* 40(2):8-18, 1963.

10. Friedman, Meyer, and R.H. Rosenman: *Type A Behavior and Your Heart.* New York, Knopf, 1974.

11. Goldberg, Richard J.: Management of depression in the patient with advanced cancer. *JAMA* 246(4):373-376, 1981.

12. Jensen, Peter S.: Risk, protective factors, and supportive interventions in chronic airway obstruction. *Arch Gen Psychiatry* 40(11):1203-1207, 1983.

13. Kirkpatrick, Richard A.: Witchcraft and lupus erythematosus. *JAMA* 245(19):1937, 1981.

14. Kolb, Lawrence C., and H. Keith H. Brodie: *Modern Clinical Psychiatry.* 10th ed. Philadelphia, Saunders, 1982, pp. 535-592.

15. Lepore, Michael J.: The importance of emotional disturbances in chronic ulcerative colitis. *JAMA* 191(10):819-824, 1965.

16. Lowry, Michael R.: Frequency of depressive disorder in patients entering home hemodialysis. *J Nerv Men Dis* 167(4):199-204, 1979.

17. Miksanek, Tony: Dosteovsky's THE IDIOT and psychic disorders in epilepsy. *Perspect Biol Med* 25(2):231-237, 1982.

18. Rand, Colleen S. W., and Albert J. Stunkard: Obesity and psychoanalysis: Treatment and four-year follow-up. *Am J Psychiatry* 140(9):1140-1144, 1983.

19. Raskind, Murray, Richard Veith, Robert Barnes, and Gail Gumbrecht: Cardiovascular and antidepressant effects of imipramine in the treatment of secondary depression in patients with ischemic heart disease. *Am J Psychiatry* 139(9):1114-1117, 1982.

20. Schwab, John J., and Neal D. Traven: Factors related to the incidence of psychosomatic illness. *Psychosomatics* 20(5):307-315, 1979.

21. Slavin, Lesley A., John E. O'Malley, Gerald P. Koocher, and Diane J. Foster: Communication of the cancer diagnosis to pediatric patients: Impact on long-term adjustment. *Am J Psychiatry* 139(2):179-183, 1982.

22. Slawson, Paul F., William R. Flynn, and Edward J. Kollar: Psychological factors associated with the onset of diabetes mellitus. *JAMA* 185(3):166-170, 1965.

23. Smith, G. Richard, Jr.: Alexithymia in medical patients referred to a consultation liaison service. *Am J Psychiatry* 140(1):99-101, 1983.

24. Stanton, Babette, David Jenkins, Philip Denlinger, Judith Savageau, Ronald Weintraub, and Richard Goldstein: Predictors of employment status after cardiac surgery. *JAMA* 249(7):907-911, 1983.

25. Stunkard, Albert J.: The current status of treatment for obesity in adults. *Psychiatr Ann* 13(11):862-867, 1983.

Chapter 10

AFFECTIVE DISORDERS

MOOD DISORDERS

The Affective Disorders are those in which a prevailing disorder of mood, usually elation or depression, is the main symptom. The terms mood, affect, and emotion are often used interchangeably. If a distinction between mood and affect is made, mood applies to a more prolonged and basic state of feeling that influences all personality functions. *Mood* on a given day may be cheerful, but an untoward event may produce anger, grief, or some other unpleasant *affect*. In an Affective Disorder an abnormal mood may persist for days, weeks, or months. Many emotions, or affects, can be described (e.g., joy, sorrow, hate, fear, love) but in the context of a discussion of Affective Disorders, reference is primarily to that portion of the emotional state which can be represented somewhere on a continuum between depression and elation.

Affective Disorders are currently classified as follows:

1. Bipolar Disorder
    a. Mixed
    b. Manic
    c. Depressed
2. Major Depression
    a. Single Episode
    b. Recurrent
3. Other Specific Affective Disorders
    a. Cyclothymic Disorder
    b. Dysthymic Disorder (Depressive Neurosis)
4. Atypical Affective Disorders
    a. Atypical Bipolar Disorder
    b. Atypical Depression

In recording a diagnosis of a manic episode, qualifying terms that should be used, when appropriate, include: in remission, with mood-congruent psychotic features, with mood-incongruent psychotic features, without psychotic features. Qualifying terms used with diagnoses of major depressive episodes include: in remission, with mood-congruent psychotic features, with mood-incongruent psychotic features, with melancholia, without melancholia. Melancholia, in this context, refers to the presence of a severe depression believed to be endogenous rather than reactive. In melancholia there is usually early morning awakening and depression is worse in the morning; agitation or psychomotor retardation is likely to be present; and there may be significant weight loss with or without anorexia.

BIPOLAR DISORDER

This condition, formerly called manic-depressive illness, is manifested primarily by a period, or more often by recurring periods of marked depression or elation. Patients having manic-depressive illness may be subject only to periods of depression or elation or, during the course of illness may have both, but the diagnosis of Bipolar Disorder is used only for patients who have had at least one manic (elated) episode.

Cause

Among the causative factors, heredity is thought to be more important than it is in most other psychiatric disorders. Though other factors may be necessary for the disease to be manifest, the increased incidence of affective disorders among the relatives of patients with Bipolar Disorder (together with an increased incidence of persons having Alcoholism, Antisocial Personality, and possible color blindness and Xg^a blood type) leads to some speculation that Bipolar Disorder can be transmitted genetically. Types of transmission suggested for bipolar illness include single gene autosomal, X-linked, and polygenic inheritance. The depressed phase of Bipolar Disorder is sometimes spoken of as an endogenous depression in contradistinction to some other depressions which are regarded as exogenous, reactive, or psychogenic.

The disorder occurs most frequently in persons who have a cyclothymic personality. In this context, the term does not necessarily indicate a diagnosable Personality Disorder, but rather a tendency, often quite within normal limits, to experience greater than average mood swings. Such a person will have periods, usually of weeks or months, in which he or she is in exceptionally good spirits and is highly energetic and productive, and will have other periods of mild depression accompanied by reduced energy and productivity.

Generally speaking, people who have Bipolar Disorders are extroverts. They are outgoing, sociable people who are little given to introspection. People with this temperament are good salespersons. In some cases the description of the patient as an extrovert is accurate only to the degree that this is the way one is seen by casual acquaintances, and may appear on a brief interview. A closer study of the personality may show that the apparent extroversion conceals shyness and feelings of inadequacy; often the sociability is more compulsive than spontaneous. The *joie de vivre* is an act, a mask, a persona.

Many patients have pyknic body habitus. These are people with large body cavities and lots of fat. There is a tendency to baldness in men. The head is broad, the neck is short, and the trunk is barrel-like. The term pyknic was introduced by Kretschmer; it is roughly comparable to the habitus apoplecticus described by Hippocrates.

Bipolar Disorders are equally common in men and women. These disorders are more frequent in the upper socioeconomic classes (in contrast to Schizophrenia, which is more common among the poor).

Though hereditary and constitutional factors are important in the etiology of this disorder, experiential factors are thought to play a part in the development of many cases.

The loss of a significant person during childhood (e.g., the death of a parent), especially when there has been marked ambivalence to the lost person, is believed to play a part in the psychopathology of some patients with Bipolar Disorder, just as it does in the etiology of other depressions.

Most theories concerning the psychopathology of Bipolar Disorders give primary emphasis to the factors producing depression, and view the manic phases as a way of coping with depression, a reaction formation against depressed feelings, or a flight into activity.

Some of these patients come from families in which there is considerable disparity between the social standing, background, or education of the two parents. Often the parent who has the greater status in and out of the family is the less likeable, and a situation exists in which there are divided loyalties. This leads to marked ambivalence about both parents.

Families of patients with Bipolar Disorders have more than the usual concern about social approval. Often their status in the community is an uncomfortable one, and the child is expected, overtly or covertly, to change this through achievements. The patient who is to develop this illness often occupies a special place among the children and attempts to live up to the family's expectations despite feeling inadequate to do so. He or she is likely to feel different, alone, sensitive, and vulnerable.

The final common biochemical pathway for the production of Affective Disorders undoubtedly involves the neurotransmitters in the brain. Some research emphasizes the importance of the catecholamines (epinephrine, norepinephrine, and dopamine), and other studies emphasize the indoleamines (serotonin and histamine). The major hypotheses stated simply (perhaps oversimplified) are:

1. Catecholamine hypothesis: Catecholamines, especially norepinephrine, are decreased in depression and increased in mania.
2. Indoleamine hypothesis: Indoleamines, especially serotonin, are decreased in depression.
3. Combined hypothesis (biogenic amine permissive hypothesis): There is an indoleaminergic deficiency in both depression and mania with a decrease in catecholamines in depression and an increase in mania.
4. Depression heterogeneity hypothesis: There are two kinds of depression; in one kind there is a catecholamine (norepinephrine) decrease, and in the other an indoleamine (serotonin) decrease.

Symptoms and Course

The first attack of Bipolar Disorder usually occurs before the age of 30. In at least half of the cases there is an identifiable precipitating stress. The presence of a precipitating stress is generally a favorable prognostic sign. The first attack may be either a depression or a manic episode. Untreated, an attack will last from a few weeks up to a year (the condition rarely becomes chronic).

Though the disorder is described as having cyclic recurrences, an appreciable number of cases, perhaps as many as 20% have only one attack. However, patients who have a second attack will usually continue to have recurrences throughout life.

Recurrences are separated by periods ranging from a few months to several years. As patients grow older, the duration and the frequency of attacks tend to increase. However, those patients who have relatively short attacks and long periods of health between them can live quite normal lives, interrupted only by occasional periods of brief hospitalization.

Attacks of either form are characterized by a sudden onset. There is rarely more than a week between the onset of the first symptoms and the full development of the attack.

The mildest form of the depressed phase is referred to as simple retardation; the most severe as depressive stupor. The depressed phase of Bipolar Disorder usually differs from other depressions in that it is accompanied by psychomotor retardation. On mental examination, the patient's facial expression appears sad. Movements are slow. Speech shows underproductivity and slow reaction time. Feelings of depression, guilt, worthlessness, and hopelessness are expressed. The content of delusions and hallucinations, present in about half of the cases, is usually mood congruent (in keeping with the feeling tone of depression).

Sensorium is clear though it may be difficult to evaluate, since mental processes are slowed and the patient appears to lack the energy to answer questions calling for any effort or concentration. The patient usually has insight to the extent that she or he is aware of being ill.

Suicidal thoughts are frequent and suicide attempts are sometimes made. Often the suicide risk is greatest at the onset and during the period of recovery when psychomotor retardation is less severe.

Mild forms of the manic phase are called hypomanic; the most severe form is delirious mania (formerly called Bell's mania). The typical manic looks and acts cheerful. He or she is restless and overactive. Speech is overproductive and seems rapid. The patient moves quickly from one idea to another and often, in speaking, leaves out intermediate ideas. This flight of ideas differs from the looseness of associations of Schizophrenia in that:

1. The flight of ideas seems rapid and as if the speaker were experiencing a pressure of thoughts.
2. One can usually supply the connecting links and follow the chain of associations.

Actual measurements of manic speech suggest that the impression of rapid speech is based more on the patient's manner than on the number of words spoken.

Patients often joke and tease. Rhyming, punning, and clang associations are frequent.

The mood ranges from a sustained euphoria, cheerfulness, and optimism to elation or exaltation. Now and then there may be a transitory breakthrough of depressed feeling which quickly vanishes.

The patient's affect may also shift from elation to anger or rage; this is especially likely to happen if efforts are made to interfere with or control behavior. In some patients irritability rather than elation is the most prominent finding.

Except in hypomanic cases, delusions and hallucinations are usually present. The content of these is nearly always mood congruent and is usually grandiose. There is usually some apparent impairment of sensorium. The patient's attention span is short. If the patient cooperates at all with tests of retention and recall, or counting and calculation, they are done poorly, since the patient loses track of what he or she is doing and thoughts shift quickly to other things. In the same way, patients lose track of time and place, forget the names of recent acquaintances (or perhaps do not pay enough attention to them in the first place), and in general appear disoriented. The patient usually does not realize that he or she is ill.

Judgment is impaired by overoptimism, overconfidence, and inflated self-esteem. This is of greatest clinical significance in mild hypomanic cases in which excessive spending, poor business decisions, and socially unacceptable conduct may be the outstanding symptoms.

In very severe attacks, delirious mania, the patient neglects food and sleep and, as exhaustion develops, may become delirious or stuporous. Death from exhaustion may occur.

One may encounter patients with a mixture of manic and depressive symptoms (Bipolar Disorder, Mixed Type) or other variants of the illness (Atypical Bipolar Disorders). Among the variants of Bipolar Disorder are cases in which there is a continual alteration between the two phases, patients with underproductive mania (manic attacks with elation and hyperactivity without verbal overproductivity), those with akinetic mania (elation and flights of ideas without increased, or even with decreased activity), and various other mixtures of symptoms. These variants are rare, and, unless the patient has had a previous history of more typical manic-depressive attacks, cause considerable difficulty in differential diagnosis.

Diagnosis

Bipolar Affective Disorder must be differentiated from Schizophrenic Disorder (cf. Chapter 11). Though some authorities believe that one should not diagnose Bipolar Disorder if certain symptoms of Schizophrenia or Schizoaffective Disorder are present, one cannot always accept these arbitrary criteria as a guide for treatment planning. Actually, almost any symptom of Schizophrenia occurs in an appreciable number of patients with Bipolar Disorder. Diagnosis must be based on the total evaluation, not just on a few symptoms believed to be pathognomonic.

One might occasionally have difficulty in distinguishing depressive stupor from other forms of stupor or coma, and delirious mania from toxic deliria. Usually, one sees the patient before the attack reaches a level of severity sufficient to create these problems in diagnosis.

Mild cases present the greatest problems in differential diagnosis. While the distinction between a mild hypomanic attack and a period of mood elevation associated with a Cyclothymic Disorder is often a distinction without a difference, the differentiation between certain essentially *normal* character structures manifested by hyperactivity and high spirits, and a hypomanic attack, can be quite significant and is not always easy. Since the patient may not be aware of changes in behavior, an outside history may be necessary. Examples: (1) A college girl is referred by the Dean of Women. The immediate problem involves an episode of doing a strip tease at a campus party. On examination the girl is active, vivacious, and despite being in some difficulty with the Dean, cheerful. Her reports of her social life suggest that she may be a little wild. The examiner must decide whether the girl is normally this way and is making a satisfactory adjustment or whether she is hypomanic. If history shows that her intense involvement in social and extracurricular activities is recent, and that prior to this her general behavior had been more reserved, the probability that she is hypomanic should receive more serious consideration than if there had been no personality change. (2) An employer refers a junior executive. The patient has been quite successful in the firm, but there is concern because he is urging expansion and financial commitments that older colleagues feel are unwise. He appears in high spirits, radiates optimism and self-confidence, and describes doing a great deal of overtime work and formulating a variety of new plans. The clinician's problem is similar to that in the first example.

Failure to diagnose the hypomanic attack can have serious consequences. The hypomanic may run up debts that cause personal and family hardship. A hypomanic student may jeopardize an academic record not only by boisterous behavior but also by inattention to studies. The behavior may involve some risk of accidents. Alcohol consumption may increase. The hypomanic may have increased sexual activity, and the optimism and disregard of consequences that go along with high spirits can lead to impulsive marriages, undesirable affairs, and unplanned pregnancies. Moreover, after an attack is over the patient may feel guilt or shame about the activities while sick; even relatively innocuous pranks may be embarrassing as they are recalled, and a depression may be precipitated.

Mild depressions are often overlooked clinically, but they can account for academic and vocational failures. Though the term simple retardation can be applied, there is really no term for a bipolar depression of comparable severity (or mildness?) to the hypomanic state. Some cases are confused with Depressive Neuroses. Differences include:

1.   The cyclothymic premorbid personality of the patient with the depressed type of Bipolar Disorder
2.   The psychomotor retardation which is usually present to some extent in even mild cases of bipolar depression
3.   The absence of the mercurial, fluctuating character of the Depressive Neurosis

Situational euphoria, and perhaps more often grief, may pose a problem in differential diagnosis if the patient for some reason conceals the cause of the altered mood.

Occasionally, diseases of other systems require differentiation. Hypothyroidism, malignant diseases of the gastrointestinal tract, and sometimes other debilitating diseases may simulate mild endogenous depression. Hyperthyroidism, the euphoria which sometimes accompanies multiple sclerosis, and occasionally the effect of medications (e.g., steroids, stimulants) may simulate the hypomanic state.

In the future, measurements of catecholamine or indoleamine metabolites in spinal fluid, blood, or urine may contribute to the differential diagnosis of Affective Disorders. At present, such tests have limited usefulness.

Attempts have also been made to utilize the fact that severe depression is accompanied by excessive cortisol secretion in developing a diagnostic test for depression. In the dexamethasone suppression test, 1 mg of dexamethasone is given orally at 11 PM and serum cortisol levels are determined at various times the following day. Depending on the laboratory procedures used, a serum cortisol level of greater than 4.5 to 5.0 µg/dL at any time the day after the dexamethasone is administered is viewed as a positive test. The test identifies a subgroup of depressed patients that does not suppress cortisol. Unfortunately, there are many sources of false positive and false negative results. The test is not recommended for routine screening of depressed patients, and its usefulness is as yet unproven.

Prevention

At present there is little that can be done to prevent Bipolar Disorder. Perhaps as community psychiatry develops it will be possible to identify children and adolescents who may be susceptible (e.g., those who have family histories showing several cases of the disorder; ones who show marked cyclothymic tendencies; those whose family situation is the type that can contribute to the illness). It may be that counseling or treatment of such youngsters could reduce the incidence of the disease. As hereditary factors are better understood, genetic counseling may play some role in prevention. Prevention of recurrences will be considered in the discussion of treatment.

Evaluating Suicide Risk

In the management of bipolar depression, as in any other depressive illness, however mild, one must evaluate the risk of suicide. In the United States suicide ranks ninth among causes of death in the population as a whole; one of every 100 persons dies from suicide. Suicide rates are probably underestimated, since there is no way of knowing how many apparently accidental deaths are concealed suicides, and some suicides are not reported as such because families and friends choose to conceal the cause of death.

Factors to consider in the evaluation of suicide risk include the following.

1. Degree of depression. Generally speaking, the greater the depression, the greater the suicide risk.
2. Feelings of hopelessness. The extent to which such feelings are present may be an even more important measure of suicide risk than the degree of depression itself.
3. Amount of agitation. Though most patients with Bipolar depression show decreased activity (psychomotor retardation) rather than agitation, some are agitated, and agitation is common in other forms of depression. The more agitated and restless the patient is, the more likely the suicide attempt. Agitation would add to one's concern over possible suicide in even a mildly depressed patient.
4. Attitudes toward suicide. Direct questioning about the extent to which the patient is troubled by thoughts of suicide is indicated. Some clinicians are reluctant to ask the questions lest it suggest suicide as a way for the patient to end the discomfort, or add to fears by implying that the doctor considers the illness severe enough for this to be a major risk. Wording the question so that it refers to troubling thoughts and also asks for an estimate of degree overcomes some of the objection. Almost everyone has thoughts of suicide on occasion, and certainly one expects a depressed person to have at least an occasional thought of suicide. If the patient acknowledges such thoughts but indicates an ability to dismiss them, and to control suicidal impulses, one is more optimistic than if the patient claims to have never even thought of doing such a thing. On the other hand, the patient who is greatly troubled by suicidal ideas should be regarded as a potential suicidal risk. Previous threats of suicide, or attempts, even if these are regarded more as suicide gestures than genuine self-destructive efforts, add to the risk. The idea that a previous failure indicates that the patient consciously or unconsciously does not really want to commit suicide is often erroneous. A better interpretation is that the patient is considering suicide but is ambivalent about it, and a shift in degree of depression or in external circumstances may provoke a more serious and possibly successful attempt. The successful suicide rate is 100 times greater among persons who have attempted suicide than in the general population.
5. Impulsivity. Impulsive people are more likely to commit suicide. The person who stops to think it over will often decide against a suicide attempt. Impulsivity can be determined from interview behavior and from history. Short courtships, sudden decisions to drop out of school, to change jobs, or move suggest that the patient is impulsive. The fact that a patient appears to be compulsive and ruminates for a long time before making decisions does not always mean that these decisions are deliberate and well considered. Some compulsives will ruminate for months over a decision and actually make the decision at the spur of the moment.

6. Use of alcohol or sedatives. Any use of alcohol beyond one or two drinks with meals, at bedtime, or in social situations adds to suicide risk. Intoxication, even mild intoxication, lessens cortical control and adds to the chance of impulsive behavior. The same applies to the effects of sedatives.

7. Family history of suicide. Any family history of suicide or suicide attempts adds to risk. If the suicide occurred in the patient's household during his or her formative years, the risk is even greater. It seems to set a pattern, or suggests a way of coping with troubles. To a lesser extent, any death in the patient's immediate environment during the formative years may be a risk factor.

8. Recent stresses (especially losses). A recent divorce, separation, loss of job, or other major stress adds to the suicide risk.

9. General health. Poor general health, chronic illness, or handicap may add to suicide risk.

10. Attitude toward responsibilities. The patient who feels needed by a family and takes this obligation seriously is less a suicide risk than the person who is not as concerned about playing a role in maintaining the welfare of others. However, suicide risk is greatly increased if the patient begins to feel that she or he is doing more harm than good to loved ones.

11. Religion. Some religious beliefs are a deterrent to suicide. Religion carries with it an element of hope even in a hopeless situation, and many religions teach that there is a virtue in tolerating discomfort. Also, certain religions regard suicide as sinful. However, membership without strong convictions in a particular denomination offers no protection.

12. Reality situation. If the patient can expect upon recovery to have a reasonably comfortable and satisfactory life situation, one is less likely to commit suicide than if one will return to a situation involving numerous stresses and discomforts. Also, the interest, support, and concern of family members may help reduce risk of suicide, both because of the psychological effect on the patient and also because such people can better be relied upon to notify the physician of changes in the patient's condition, and to minimize the opportunities for suicide.

13. Future plans. Questioning the patient about his or her plans for the future may sometimes be helpful in evaluating the likelihood of a suicide attempt. A patient who has some specific plans for the future is less likely to commit suicide than a person with none.

14. Constricted thinking. A depressed person may attribute his or her depression to a problem. While the healthy person can usually see several options for dealing with a problem, the thinking of a depressed person sometimes becomes constricted, so that suicide is seen as the only way out. Another manifestation of constricted thinking is to see suicide as the alternative in an either-or situation (e.g., "Either I pass the examination, or I must kill myself;" "If I don't get an abortion, I will have to die"). One should look for this sort of thinking, as when present it adds materially to suicide risk.

Treatment

The form and severity of the attack governs the mode of treatment:

1. Severe depressive attacks require hospitalization. Electric shock therapy is usually effective in producing a remission and is the treatment of choice if the patient is highly suicidal. Otherwise, antidepressant drugs may be used initially. If a severely depressed patient is not eating well, one must keep in mind the possibility of nutritional deficiencies and take steps to correct them

if necessary. Suicidal tendencies often persist after some of the other signs of depression become less marked. Premature discontinuation of treatment or relaxation of precautions against suicide is to be avoided.

2.   Mild depressive attacks, especially those at a level of severity comparable to the hypomanic, can often be treated on an outpatient basis. However, if there is an appreciable suicide risk, the patient should be hospitalized and treated as one would treat a severe depressive. Mild depressives with minimal suicide risk can be treated as outpatients with the use of antidepressant drugs. Lithium carbonate, usually used in the treatment of manic attacks, may be used in depressions that do not respond adequately to other antidepressants. Sleep deprivation and/or efforts to change sleep patterns have been used experimentally in the treatment of depression, and one should be alert to new developments in the literature on this subject.

Differentiating these cases from Depressive Neuroses is especially important, since the endogenous depressions respond well to medication and slowly, if at all, to psychotherapy, while the Depressive Neuroses respond minimally to medication and often benefit greatly from investigative psychotherapy or cognitive therapy.

If tricyclic antidepressants are to be used for either severe or mild depressive episodes and one can obtain amine metabolite levels (not yet practical in most settings), the depression heterogeneity hypothesis may help one select medication as patients with low 3-methoxy-4-hydroxyphenolglycol (MHPG), a norepinephrine metabolite, in a 24-hour urine specimen may be imipramine or desipramine responders, while those with high pretreatment MHPG are more likely to be amitriptyline responders. There is also some evidence that patients who experience mood elevation when given methylphenidate tend to respond to imipramine or desipramine but not to amitriptyline or nortriptyline, and patients who do not have improved mood after taking methylphenidate are more likely to respond to amitriptyline or nortriptyline than to desipramine or imipramine. One may at least bear in mind that some tricyclics (e.g., amitriptyline) are most effective in blocking serotonin reuptake at the synapses and others (e.g., desipramine) are most effective in blocking norepinephrine. If one type of tricyclic does not help the patient, the other might.

3.   Severe manic attacks require hospitalization. Lithium carbonate is the drug of choice. Since there is a period of 10 days to 2 weeks or more between the start of lithium treatment and significant reduction of agitation, tranquilizing medication or sedation is needed early in treatment. A few cases of serious reaction to the combination of lithium and haloperidol have been reported. Though it is unlikely that these drugs are actually incompatible, it may be preferable to use another major tranquilizer. The therapeutic level for lithium is so near the toxic that close observation, together with obtaining frequent determinations of plasma lithium level or tests of saliva if these prove reliable, is necessary. For patients who do not respond to lithium, or for whom it is contraindicated, a phenothiazine or haloperidol may be used, though it is generally believed that these serve only to control certain of the symptoms and do not have the overall effect on the illness that lithium has. In rare cases, electric shock therapy may be considered; it is not as effective in the treatment of manic attacks as it is for depression.

4.   Hypomanic attacks must be evaluated carefully. Sometimes hospitalization of a relatively mild case is necessary to protect the patient from the consequences of activities resulting from overoptimism and overconfidence. Lithium or tranquilizers can be used in both inpatient and outpatient treatment.

5. Follow-up therapy, usually short-term, is desirable for patients who have recovered from episodes of Bipolar Disorder. Psychotherapy helps the patient understand and accept the illness, deal with the readjustments that must be made in returning to normal activities, and cope with any feelings of embarrassment that behavior during illness has caused. This follow-up period is also helpful in permitting early recognition of relapse. If a relapse is recognized promptly it can often be treated on an outpatient basis and rehospitalization can be avoided. The patient who has a good relationship with the therapist will, if there is a recurrence at a later date, seek help promptly and will require less treatment. Subsequent hospitalization may be avoided or at least reduced in frequency and duration.

6. Interval treatment may be used to prevent recurrences. Since prolonged administration of the medications used carries with it the risk of undesirable side effects, the decision to keep a patient on medication at a maintenance level following an attack is weighed carefully, taking into account the severity and frequency of attacks. Lithium carbonate has proven effective in reducing the incidence of recurrence of Bipolar Disorders. Alternatively, if the patient is subject only to attacks of depression, antidepressants may be used prophylactically, or if only manic attacks occur, tranquilizers may be used. Patients on prophylactic medication must be seen frequently because of the risks of side effects and complications and in order to support their continued use of medications that they may feel they no longer need.

Long-term intensive psychotherapy is sometimes recommended. If emotional factors appear to play an important role in causing or precipitating attacks, this can be recommended without hesitation.

MAJOR DEPRESSION

Severe depressions, other than those which occur in Bipolar Disorders, are classified as:

1. Major Depression, Single Episode
2. Major Depression, Recurrent

Since the diagnosis of Bipolar Disorder is not made unless, or until, the patient has had a manic episode, some patients that fall into this classification actually have manic-depressive illness and can be reclassified after a manic episode occurs. Other patients may never have a manic episode; there are various types of these unipolar depressions. Some of these are apparently endogenous, and are indistinguishable clinically from depressed episodes of Bipolar Disorder, though there may be subgroups characterized by differences in norepinephrine metabolism.

Other unipolar depressions appear to have more psychogenic elements in their etiology. The psychopathology in these cases is often closely related to emotional turmoil surrounding a precipitating event, usually a loss. Guilt feelings, also present in 20 percent or more of other major depressions, are a prominent finding in most cases. The level of depression tends to fluctuate. These patients do not respond as well to antidepressant medication and electroconvulsive therapy as do other patients with Major Depressions. They usually require psychotherapy along with other treatments.

Depression at the Change of Life

Involutional melancholia is a Major Depression usually having its onset in women between the ages of 45 and 55 and in men between 50 and 65. Its main symptom is agitated depression. Otherwise similar cases in which the chief manifestation is paranoid thinking are classified among the Paranoid Disorders.

Cause

The cause is unknown and, as is the case with most psychiatric disorders, it is believed that multiple factors are involved. The disorder was first recognized in women (three times more women are affected than men), and since it occurs at about the time of the menopause (clinical cases may begin before the cessation of menstruation or considerably after it) it was first attributed to endocrine changes. Though a male climacteric has been described, it is doubtful that men go through a sequence of physiological changes actually comparable to the menopause. If endocrine changes play a part in some or all cases, the specific deficiency or pathological metabolite has yet to be identified.

Emotional factors which influence a person's reaction to the involutional period include:

1. Attitude toward the climacteric itself
2. Attitudes toward middle age
3. Losses occurring during this period of life
4. Factors related to the premorbid personality and its defenses

To a woman, the menopause means the cessation of childbearing ability. This can be a source of disappointment and distress if, consciously or unconsciously, she wants to have children and does not have them, or wants more children than she has. However, the ability to bear children may be psychologically important even if one does not want to have them. The ability is part of being a woman; without it some women feel incomplete.

Misinformation concerning the menopause leads some women to fear it. Some erroneously believe they will lose their own desire for or pleasure in sexual activity at that time; others, equally incorrectly, feel that the endocrine changes in themselves lessen sexual attractiveness.

A fear of loss of sexual capacity may be augmented by failures in extramarital relationships. When these are undertaken to prove one's continued attractiveness and "ability," they are likely to be unsatisfactory. The level of sexual desire, the feelings concerning the partner, and concern over complications that could arise from the relationship contribute to this. It is a bit like testing a declining capacity for food by trying to eat something one does not especially like, at a time when one is not particularly hungry, under circumstances that would get one into trouble if one were discovered eating.

The attitude toward middle age is as important in the problems of men and women at this time of life as are the sexual changes themselves. Advertisements feature beautiful young women and handsome, athletic young men. Employers discriminate against the middle aged. The individual's ability to accept middle age, despite cultural attitudes toward it, depends to a large extent on sources of self-esteem. Examples: (1) A woman who feels that she is attractive to others, in social situations as well as sexually, and is admired largely because of her appearance and figure, is going to be more upset by middle-age spread, wrinkles, and graying hair than is the woman who sees herself admired because she is friendly, sincere, a good conversationalist, witty, intelligent, successful in a career, a good house-keeper, or some combination of factors which may improve rather than fade with the passing years. (2) A man whose ideas of being a real man are based on physical strength and skill in sports will lose more of the support to his self-esteem as he grows older than will a man who places more emphasis on the value of experience, maturity, and judgment.

Loss plays an important role in the dynamics of all types of depressive illness. A number of losses may occur at about the time of the climacteric. The death of a parent, or both parents, often occurs when one is in this age range. Children grow up and leave home.

The usual premorbid personality of those who develop involutional melancholia is compulsive, often sufficiently so to have justified the diagnosis of Compulsive Personality, though the diagnosis may never have been made. The Compulsive Personality is conforming, hard-working, and tends to defer pleasure, and at the time of involution is subject to feelings that hard work and good behavior have gone unrewarded, and that it is too late for deferred pleasures. There is a breakdown of fantasy as a defense mechanism. A person who tolerates (rather than corrects) an unhappy life situation with the aid of fantasies of future wealth, a new career, or a better marriage is likely to become aware at middle age that the dreams simply are not going to come true.

The various emotional factors combine to make the involutional period an especially stressful time. When the stresses lead to a breakdown of ego defenses, it is not surprising that reactions to losses, actual and symbolic, cause the illness to take the form of a depression, or that an effort to blame others, to overutilize projection as a defense, leads to paranoid manifestations.

No matter how various primary factors combine to produce involutional melancholia, there is no doubt a final common biochemical pathway. As in other depressions, this probably involves a depletion of the biogenic amines which serve as neurotransmitters in the brain.

Symptoms and Course

Involutional melancholia has a gradual onset. During the first few weeks, symptoms are usually limited to insomnia, irritability, and worry. The last is often an exaggerated concern over a real problem that has been accepted with equanimity in the past. There are frequently vague somatic complaints.

Depression is at first mild and gradually becomes more severe. The patient expresses feelings of sadness, hopelessness, and guilt. Guilt feelings are sometimes reality based (concern over things of relative consequence that one has done or failed to do) but may be over trivial matters.

Delusions, if present, are mood congruent. They may be of guilt (e.g., "I am going to be sent to the penitentiary for life because I once failed to include some poker winnings in my income tax report"); poverty (e.g., a patient with sufficient income from property and investments to ensure a comfortable living for his family may say that he is penniless and that he and his family are going to starve); disease (e.g., "my internal organs are rotting away"; "My brain is full of maggots"); or something else of an equally unpleasant nature. Nihilistic delusions, ideas of nonexistence, are common.

Patients are overactive, agitated, often pace the floor, wring their hands, or weep. They usually seek help from others in a way that can be described as "clinging" or "sticky."

Suicidal thoughts are frequent. Prior to the introduction of electroconvulsive therapy up to 25 percent of patients with involutional melancholia committed suicide, often despite intensive hospital precautions.

In involutional paranoid states, depressive symptoms, though usually present to some degree, are less prominent. Rather than turning hostility toward the self, it is turned outward toward others. Instead of worrying about losing sexual attractiveness and capacity, the patient accuses the spouse of infidelity. Instead of worrying about becoming poor, one suspects others of stealing. Instead of thinking of the body as being diseased, one has delusions of being poisoned.

In the absence of treatment, patients with involutional melancholia who have had a relatively healthy premorbid personality gradually reestablish ego defenses and some clinical improvement begins. Improvement is often noted in 6 to 9 months and recovery occurs in 1 to 2 years. Suicide risk continues for some time after clinical improvement is apparent. In the past, up to 20 percent of the cases became chronic and required hospitalization for the remainder of life.

Diagnosis

Depressive symptoms appearing for the first time in middle age should suggest the possibility of involutional melancholia. However, diagnosis should not be made on the basis of age alone. Early and/or mild cases must be distinguished from:

1.   Normal menopause
2.   Systemic diseases
3.   Adjustment Disorders
4.   Dysthymic Disorders
5.   Atypical Depressions that are primarily neurotic in character

Some subjective complaints of nervousness or irritability coupled with vasomotor symptoms, including hot flashes, sweating, headache, and vertigo, often accompany the normal menopause. At this time one might expect to find some more or less realistic concern about what can be done with the remainder of life and how anticipated problems are to be met; one would not be surprised to elicit some regret over acts and omissions from the first half century of living. All this must be differentiated from incipient involutional depression. The distinction is vital because of the suicidal propensity of the involutional. If the patient is obviously cheerful despite the symptoms observed, there is no diagnostic problem. However, an early involutional may not show gross signs of depression and a socially adept person who believes it bad manners to reveal unpleasant affective states may conceal mild depression effectively by responding appropriately to the amenities and smiling at the proper times. Direct questioning is indicated. In doubtful cases, questions concerning future plans (e.g., "What do you and your husband plan to do after he retires?"; "Where are you going for vacation next summer?") are often helpful. An active interest in planning for the future is rarely, if ever, encountered in the involutional depressive.

Periodic complete physical examination, desirable at any age, is especially indicated at this time of life. When the person of middle age complains of poor appetite, disturbed sleep, weight loss, fatigue, and poor spirits, one must rule out systemic disease, especially malignancies, including pancreatic carcinoma, as well as involutional melancholia.

Adjustment Disorders manifested by depression are distinguished on the basis of the presence of a stress sufficient to produce symptoms in a healthy person, and by the fact that perspective in reality testing is not lost. Differential diagnosis is not always possible and, if in doubt, the condition should be regarded as involutional.

The depression of involutional melancholia is relatively consistent, and it lacks the labile, mercurial character of many of the depressive neuroses. More severe and/or advanced cases are to be distinguished from:

1.   Depression Accompanying an Organic Mental Disorder
2.   Bipolar Disorder
3.   Schizoaffective Disorder

Recognition of the severe advanced case of involutional melancholia is relatively easy, but the differential diagnosis presents a few problems. Difficulty in evaluating possible sensorium impairment may make it hard to rule out an Organic Mental Disorder when the patient is unable or unwilling to cooperate in sensorium examination. Also, at the upper limit of the age range, especially in men, one may be misled by minimal sensorium changes associated with early senile brain disease or arteriosclerosis unrelated to the main psychiatric symptoms.

Though some authors regard involutional melancholia as a variant of manic depressive illness, there are some marked differences. Recurrences of bipolar depression do occur during the involutional period. In these cases there is a history of previous attacks. The premorbid personality of the involutional is usually compulsive and introverted; that of the person with Bipolar Disorder, cyclothymic and extroverted. The onset of involutional melancholia is gradual, with several weeks between the first symptoms and the fully developed illness; the comparable early stage of the Bipolar Disorder usually occupies less than a week. Bipolar depressions are accompanied usually by psychomotor retardation; patients are hypoactive, have slow movements, and slow reaction time. Involutionals are agitated, hyperactive, and move quickly.

Prevention

The physician can contribute to the prevention of involutional melancholia:

1.   In contacts with involutional patients.
2.   By participation in public education.

Goals include:

1.   Dispelling misinformation concerning menopause and climacteric.
2.   Encouraging a positive attitude toward middle age.
3.   Helping people accept, rather than defer, satisfactions in daily living.
4.   Modifying compulsive character structure.

Dissemination of accurate information concerning the menopause and sexual activity in middle and late life can be accomplished in part through community mental health programs. Also, in routine examinations of people approaching middle age, a history by systems should include sufficient discussion of sexual function to elicit misinformation, worries, and fears related to climacteric, and to enable the physician to offer appropriate help.

In some cases, discussion of sexual technique is indicated; more active participation in foreplay by the spouse may be helpful if either partner is concerned by reduced frequency of intercourse or by declining potency. In other cases, helping patients accept changed patterns of sexual activity as normal and not as a sign of impending total loss of sexual function is sufficient.

Attitudes toward middle age can also be influenced by public education. Efforts can be made to minimize discrimination against the middle-aged by employers and educational institutions. Youth has desirable attributes; so does maturity.

The family physician should be aware of the psychological makeup of his or her patient. When patients derive an inordinate proportion of self-esteem from evanescent qualities of youth they should be guided into finding new ways of self-appraisal and self-esteem.

Patients should be helped to anticipate and prepare for some of the usual stresses of middle life. For example, a mother who has devoted much of her energies and obtained most satisfaction through care of her children should be helped to find new outlets before her family grows up and leaves home.

A concern of public mental health activity is encouraging the development of recreational and social facilities which encourage the pursuit of satisfaction. Public education can help make the use of such facilities ego-syntonic. The physician, in dealing with an individual patient, can emphasize the desirability of devoting some energy to seeking satisfaction.

Because the Compulsive Personality is the usual premorbid personality for involutional melancholia, it should be modified. This may require formal psychotherapy; however, in some cases the physician can influence patients' attitudes and activities by comments and suggestions made while managing other medical problems.

Treatment

Most patients with involutional melancholia require hospitalization. However, in some early or mild cases outpatient treatment may be feasible. Because of the high incidence of suicide in this disorder, a careful evaluation of suicide risk is necessary before the election of outpatient treatment (or treatment on a general medical ward).

Many involutional patients express a reluctance to accept a recommendation for hospitalization. They give a variety of reasons and rationalizations, including concern over the cost of hospital care. With the involutional patient it is important to remember that this concern may be symptomatic rather than reality based.

Despite expressed reluctance to accept hospitalization, most patients who come voluntarily and alone to seek consultation will be amenable to persuasion to enter a hospital. Those who are brought by relatives are less likely to accept the recommendation. In this case, the recommendation for hospitalization should be given to the accompanying relatives. This is best done in the patient's presence, since handling it otherwise may impair the future doctor-patient relationship. If a patient who presents a real suicide risk cannot be persuaded to accept hospitalization voluntarily, and if the relatives decline to arrange commitment, it is imperative that the patient and family be advised to seek additional consultation with other physicians. This should usually be followed by a registered letter to the patient stating the recommendation for hospitalization in definite terms.

If the suicide risk is not too great, an attempt may sometimes be made to treat the early case on an outpatient basis. Since the disorder progresses for several weeks before reaching the maximum severity, it is important that the early outpatient case be seen at frequent intervals, usually no less than three times weekly. Patient and relatives should be instructed to contact the physician at once should the patient's condition change for the worse. Psychotherapy dealing with some of the emotional problems of this age range may be useful in the early stages of the involutional illness, and medication can also be used to help prevent the development of more severe symptoms. Tricyclic antidepressants (especially amitriptyline) are frequently effective.

Outpatient treatment may also be considered for patients with relatively mild involutional illnesses that have gone on for several months (long enough for maximum severity to have developed) before the patient starts treatment. In history-taking, one must be alert to the possibility of retrospective falsification on an unconscious basis. A patient who has actually been ill only a few weeks may sometimes claim to have felt the same way for several years. If one is in doubt, it may be necessary to obtain information from the family.

The relatively mild case (without great suicide risk) who has been ill for several months can be treated expectantly, since spontaneous improvement and recovery may be anticipated in a fair percentage of cases. Psychotherapy and antidepressant drugs are used. Sometimes tranquilizing or sedative medications may be considered for insomnia, restlessness, or mild agitation. These are used with caution, since they may increase depression or interfere with the effect of antidepressants. Rauwolfia derivatives are contraindicated. The possibility that sedative medication might be used in a suicide attempt should also be kept in mind. These patients do not need to be seen as often as the early cases; weekly interviews often suffice.

A patient well enough to be treated on an outpatient basis should continue to work (the housewife should maintain responsibility for her home). Work helps the patient keep in contact with reality and reduces preoccupation with symptoms and worries. Vacations, leaves of absence, and travel should not be prescribed as they are likely to make symptoms worse and may take the patient away from needed medical help. The involutional who is too sick to work probably belongs in the hospital.

The severely ill patient or the patient with a major suicide risk must be hospitalized. In the hospital, the best treatment is electroconvulsive therapy. A favorable response is usually noted after four treatments, and a total of six to 12 treatments often is sufficient. Up to 90 percent of patients with involutional melancholia will recover with electric shock treatment (results are not quite as good in patients with involutional paranoid states). When there is a relative contraindication to electric shock therapy, or when the suicide risk is not too great, antidepressant drugs may be tried prior to starting shock treatment.

Treatment must be instituted promptly after admission, since any prolonged period of observation carries an increased suicide risk even in the hospital.

Before the advent of modern treatment, elaborate suicidal precautions were taken in hospitals. Patients were placed on locked wards and all belongings that could be used in a suicide attempt were taken away from them, including belts and shoe laces. Often, such patients found a way to end their lives despite these precautions. Now, with the prompt administration of modern treatment, elaborate precautions are no longer needed. Patients may be cared for on an open ward; however, close nursing observation is essential. It is desirable that the patient be on the ground floor, or on a ward with detention screens. The patient should not leave the hospital unaccompanied until the suicide risk is diminished.

The suicide risk does not abate during treatment as rapidly as do some of the most obvious symptoms. Therefore, precautions should not be relaxed during the early stages of clinical improvement. If a patient reaches a decision to commit suicide, the symptoms often abate, and the apparent dramatic improvement must not mislead the clinician and cause her or him to allow a premature visit home or discharge.

Outpatient visits should be arranged following hospitalization so that if there is a relapse shortly after treatment it will be recognized promptly. Needs for follow-up psychotherapy can also be evaluated.

OTHER SPECIFIC AFFECTIVE DISORDERS

Official nomenclature (DSM-III) classifies two conditions under the heading of Other Specific Affective Disorder:

1.   Dysthymic Disorder (Depressive Neurosis)
2.   Cyclothymic Disorder

Dysthymic Disorder (Depressive Neurosis)

The diagnosis of Dysthymic Disorder is used for chronic depressions that are not severe enough to meet the criteria for a Major Depressive Episode. The diagnosis is applied only when the depressed mood has been present all or most of the time for at least 2 years (1 year in children or adolescents). The depression may be interrupted, at times, by periods of a few days or weeks during which the mood is normal (but not elevated as in the Cyclothymic Disorders).

Though Dysthymic Disorder is often regarded as synonymous with depressive neurosis, there are two distinct groups of patients who meet the criteria for this diagnosis. One group consists of patients whose symptoms are, though milder, very much like those of the Depressed Episodes of Bipolar Disorder and most other Major Depressions. The condition may be endogenous and history may fail to show neuropathic traits in childhood or signs of intrapsychic conflict, though a Personality Disorder may have been present prior to the illness. The level of depression is relatively consistent. Along with feelings of depression, these patients lose interest in the usual activities, complain of fatigue or lack of energy, and are self-critical. There may be complaints of sleep disturbance, loss of appetite or overeating, and/or sexual dysfunction. Other findings may include mild psychomotor retardation or restlessness, social withdrawal, crying spells, and suicidal preoccupation. There are no delusions nor hallucinations.

The onset of this type of Dysthymic Disorder is often in adolescence or early adult life. Other cases, often with a later onset, may follow a Major Depression and represent partial remission or residual symptoms of that condition. A person with a chronic Dysthymic Disorder may have superimposed episodes of Major Depression, a situation sometimes spoken of as double depression.

More typically neurotic depressions usually occur in persons who have shown neuropathic traits in childhood, and have been troubled with anxiety at various times during life, though often not sufficiently to require medical attention. During interview, and in psychological testing, they show evidence of having significant intrapsychic conflicts.

These depressive neuroses follow a precipitating stress which is almost always a loss of some sort. The loss may be:

1.   The loss of a significant person from the patient's life. Examples: (1) the death of a family member or friend, (2) a close friend moving away, or (3) the breaking-up of a relationship as the result of a quarrel.
2.   Loss of money or material possessions. Examples: (1) loss of personal belongings in a fire, or (2) a bank failure.
3.   Loss of status. Examples: (1) being fired from a job even though an equally good position is found promptly, or (2) being involved in a scandal which affects social standing.

Rarely, the loss is not elicited during history taking. Sometimes, it is something the patient is reluctant to discuss (e.g., gambling losses which the patient has concealed from the family; the break-up of an extramarital affair).

The patient feels sad, "blue," unhappy. Guilt feelings, feelings of inadequacy and unworthiness, and feelings of hopelessness are usual.

The depression is not accompanied by psychomotor retardation, nor is it usually accompanied by agitation. There are no delusions. One of the main observed differences between these depressive neuroses and other depressions is the tendency of the neurotic depression to fluctuate markedly in intensity. Depressive neuroses are often described as mercurial. The patient may appear in the depths of depression, weeping, and totally pessimistic; a few hours later that patient may be engaged in social activity, animated, laughing, and acting as if there were not a care in the world.

This can be seen in the clinical interview. The patient may express sorrow and guilt with appropriate facial expression and tone of voice. Later in the interview, when led to discuss a topic that is pleasant, the patient can brighten up and for the moment seem to forget all troubles, and then suddenly he or she thinks of them again and is plunged into grief. The changes are not inexplicable, as may be the case in emotional lability associated with brain disease, but are clearly related to activities and manifest thought content.

The sudden shifts of mood may be misinterpreted. The degree of illness may be underestimated. There is a risk of suicide in these depressive neuroses and this must be evaluated carefully, even though much of the time the patient appears cheerful and continues to function well at work and in social activities.

Often, the history of the patient with a depressive neurosis reveals a significant loss in childhood (e.g., the death of a parent or sibling). It is felt that in many cases the person lost is one about whom the patient had ambivalent feelings. The hostile element in the feeling about the lost person gives rise to guilt. This may be compounded by the magical thinking of the child who sometimes believes that the death wishes caused the loss. These feelings are effectively repressed, but they remain as a source of intrapsychic conflict and are reactivated by another loss in adult life.

The Dysthymic Disorders that are similar to Major Depressions often respond to antidepressant medication. If the patient also has a personality disorder, the treatment plan must take this into account. The neurotic depressions which appear to be primarily psychogenic are less likely to respond to antidepressant medication, but a clinical trial may be warranted. Investigative psychotherapy or cognitive therapy, with or without concurrent medication, is nearly always indicated for both types of Dysthymic Disorder.

One sees many mild depressions of less than 2 years duration. When these follow a loss, or other precipitating stress, the role of the precipitating stress and the extent of underlying neurotic conflict must be evaluated to determine whether they are best classified as Adjustment Disorders with Depressed Mood or as Atypical Depressions.

Cyclothymic Disorder

This condition, formerly classified with the Personality Disorders, differs from Bipolar Disorder only in degree. The diagnosis requires a duration of at least 2 years during which the patient has recurring periods of depression and hypomania not severe enough to meet the criteria for Major Depression and Manic Episode. Many cases have a lifelong pattern of abnormal mood swings.

During mild hypomanic periods a person may not be greatly disabled. The optimism and impulsivity that go with elation impair judgment and this interferes to some extent with vocational and domestic adjustment. Patients tend to get into stress situations by making commitments they cannot fulfill and starting things they cannot finish. The good spirits and effervescence of such people may be trying to friends and family, especially in the early morning hours. In more markedly hypomanic episodes, frivolous spending, increased sexual drive, and risk-taking behavior may lead to significant problems. Of course, in markedly hypomanic episodes, the patient may meet the criteria for the diagnosis of a Manic Episode.

The depressed periods are accompanied by definite disability and discomfort. Some motor retardation often accompanies this depression. The patient's work rate is slowed. He or she lacks energy and enthusiasm. Motivation for accomplishment is lost; nothing seems worth the effort. Social activities and recreation are not enjoyed. The patient has feelings of guilt, inferiority, unworthiness, and hopelessness.

Differential Diagnosis

The diagnosis should not be made in cases in which mood swings remain within normal limits and have no maladaptive effects. One can have prolonged periods of cheerfulness, even in modern society, without being sick! On the other hand, not all pessimists are psychiatric invalids.

The characteristic cyclic changes in affective states may be overlooked if some deviant behavior accompanies either the "up" or the "down" phase. The person who drinks when depressed may be viewed as just an alcoholic; the person who shows mildly antisocial behavior when "high" may be thought of as neurotic with acting-out tendencies, a Histrionic Personality, or even an Antisocial Personality.

Metabolic disorders, including thyroid disease, sometimes produce symptoms suggestive of one of the phases of the Cyclothymic Disorder.

Treatment

If symptoms are severe enough to warrant its use, lithium may be the treatment of choice for Cyclothymic Disorders. Otherwise, when necessary, major tranquilizers can be used during hypomanic periods and antidepressants during the depressed phases. Milder cases may not require medication and may be taught to live with the disorder. With help, some patients can recognize the maladaptive behavior accompanying altered mood states and modify it. Being mildly hypomanic is rather pleasant if one can keep out of trouble, and being mildly depressed is tolerable if one recognizes that the episode will pass and can make oneself continue functioning appropriately during it.

ATYPICAL AFFECTIVE DISORDERS

Categories of Atypical Bipolar Disorder and Atypical Depression provide flexibility. Some cases are really not very atypical. The symptoms and findings are present and one anticipates the correct diagnosis, but cannot use it because the patient has not been sick long enough! There are other cases in which specific diagnosis would be made save that the patient does not meet quite all of the criteria.

There are patients that really do not quite fit any of the standard classifications. For example, there is the disorder sometimes called bipolar-II. It consists of having Major Depressive Episodes along with hypomanic episodes that are too mild or do not last long enough to be Manic Episodes. It is classified as an Atypical Bipolar Disorder. Likewise, the patient who would be diagnosed as having Cyclothymic Disorder, but who has only hypomanic episodes or is chronically hypomanic but has never had a period of depression falls into this classification.

REVIEW QUESTIONS

1. Discuss the possible role of catecholamines in the production of depression and elation.
2. How does the onset of an episode of Bipolar Disorder differ from the onset of Schizophrenia?
3. Discuss the role of experiential factors in the etiology of Bipolar Disorder.
4. Under what circumstances would you hospitalize a hypomanic patient?
5. How does a Dysthymic Disorder differ from a Major Depressive Episode? From an Adjustment Disorder with Depressed Mood?
6. Is Bipolar Disorder more common among the lower or higher socioeconomic classes? To what extent is this different from other psychiatric conditions?
7. Describe the usual premorbid personality of patients with involutional melancholia. From what stage of psychosexual development are the most prominent traits derived? How is involutional melancholia classified in current nomenclature?
8. What factors influence a person's attitude toward the climacteric?
9. Suggest ways in which the physician's contribution to public education and community mental health activities can reduce the incidence of involutional disorders.
10. Discuss the treatment of Bipolar Disorder.
11. A patient is hospitalized with severe involutional melancholia. After four electric shock treatments, he is no longer agitated, smiles appropriately at times, and is free of delusional content. Careful questioning elicits some depressive ideation. He wants to be discharged from the hospital and continue treatments as an outpatient. What will you probably recommend? Why? What factors will influence your recommendation?
12. A young adult patient has been mildly depressed except for brief intervals ever since graduating from college, getting married and going to work. How would you decide whether this patient has a Dysthymic Disorder, Cyclothymic Disorder, or Adjustment Disorder with Depressed Mood? How would the treatment for these three conditions differ?

SELECTED REFERENCES

1. Akiskal, Hagop S., (Guest Ed.): Recent advances in the diagnosis and treatment of affective disorders. *Psychiatr Clin North Am* 6:1, 1983.

2. Baldessarini, Ross J.: *Biomedical Aspects of Depression and Its Treatment.* Washington, D.C., American Psychiatric Press, 1983.

3. Bank, Robert L., and R. Harlan Bridenbaugh: Clinical reliability of tricyclic antidepressant levels. *Psychiatr For* 11(1):30-31, Summer-Fall, 1982.

4. Brown, J. Trig, and Alan Stoudemire: Normal and pathological grief. *JAMA* 250(3):378-382, 1983.

5. Brown, Richard P., John Sweeney, Erica Loutsch, James Kocsis, and Allen Frances: Involutional melancholia revisited. *Am J Psychiatry* 141(1):24-28, 1984.

6. Calobrisi, Arcangelo: The case for involutional melancholia. *Psychiatr For* 8(1):34-38, Winter, 1978-1979.

7. Cavenar, Jesse O., James L. Nash, and Allan A. Maltbie: Anniversary reactions masquerading as manic-depressive illness. *Am J Psychiatry* 134(11): 1273-1276, 1977.

8. Charney, Dennis S., and J. Craig Nelson: Delusional and nondelusional unipolar depression: Further evidence for distinct subtypes. *Am J Psychiatry* 138(3):328-333, 1981.

9. Davis, John M., and James W. Maas (Eds.): *The Affective Disorders.* Washington, D.C., American Psychiatric Press, 1983.

10. Dunner, David L., Vijayalakshmy Patrick, and Ronald R. Fieve: Life events at the onset of bipolar affective illness. *Am J Psychiatry* 136(4B):508-511, 1979.

11. Gibson, R. W.: *Psychotherapy of Manic-Depressive States.* Psychiatric Research Report 17, American Psychiatric Association, 1963, pp. 91-102.

12. Hirschfeld, Robert M. A., Stephen H. Koslow, and David J. Kupfer: The clinical utility of the dexamethasone suppression test in psychiatry: Summary of a National Institute of Mental Health Workshop. *JAMA* 250(16):2172-2174, 1983.

13. Keller, Martin B., Philip W. Lavori, Collins E. Lewis, and Gerald L. Klerman: Predictors of relapse in major depressive disorder. *JAMA* 250(24):3299-3304, 1983.

14. Kovacs, Maria, and Aaron T. Beck: Maladaptive cognitive structures in depression. *Am J Psychiatry* 135(5):525-533, 1978.

15. Lieberman, Paul B., and John S. Strauss: The recurrence of mania: Environmental factors and medical treatment. *Am J Psychiatry* 141(1):77-80, 1984.

16. Murphy, George E., Anne D. Simons, Richard D. Wetzel, and Patrick J. Lustman: Cognitive therapy and pharmacotherapy. *Arch Gen Psychiatry* 41(1):33-41, 1984.

17. Rasmussen, Kathlyn L. R., and Martin Reite: Loss-induced depression in an adult macaque monkey. *Am J Psychiatry* 139(5):679-681, 1982.

18. Rosenthal, Norman E., David A. Sack, J. Christian Gillin, Alfred J. Lewy, Frederick K. Goodwin, Yolande Davenport, Peter S. Mueller, David A. Newsome, and Thomas A. Wehr: Seasonal affective disorder: A description of the syndrome and preliminary findings with light therapy. *Arch Gen Psychiatry* 41(1):72-80, 1984.

19. Roy, Alec: Family history of suicide. *Arch Gen Psychiatry* 40(9):971-974, 1983.

20. Roy, Alec: Role of past loss in depression. *Arch Gen Psychiatry* 38(3):301-302, 1981.

21. Rush, A. John, and Donna E. Giles: Cognitive therapy: Theory and research. In *Short-Term Psychotherapies for Depression.* A. John Rush (Ed.). New York, Guilford Press, 1982.

22. Sabelli, Hector C., Jan Fawcett, Javaid I. Javaid, and Sushil Bagri: The methylphenidate test for differentiating desipramine-responsive from nortriptyline-responsive depression. *Am J Psychiatry* 140(2):212-214, 1983.

23. Schatzberg, Alan F., Paul J. Orsulak, Alan H. Rosenbaum, Toshihiko Maruta, Ellen R. Kruger, Jonathan O. Cole, and Joseph J. Schildkraut: Toward a biochemical classification of depressive disorders. V: Heterogeneity of unipolar depressions. *Am J Psychiatry* 139(4):471-475, 1982.

24. Schildkraut, Joseph J., Saul M. Schanberg, George R. Breese, and Irwin J. Kopin: Norepinephrine metabolism and drugs used in the affective disorders: A possible mechanism of action. *Am J Psychiatry* 124(5):600-607, 1967.

25. Silverman, Joseph Shepsel, Julia Ann Silverman, and David A. Eardley: Do maladaptive attitudes cause depression? *Arch Gen Psychiatry* 41(1):28-30, 1984.

26. Weissman, Myrna M., Brigitte A. Prusoff, Alberto DiMascio, Carlos Neu, Mahesh Goklaney, and Gerald L. Klerman: The efficacy of drugs and psychotherapy in the treatment of acute depressive episodes. *Am J Psychiatry* 136(4B):555-558, 1979.

Chapter 11

SCHIZOPHRENIA: SCHIZOPHRENIC, SCHIZOPHRENIFORM, AND SCHIZOAFFECTIVE DISORDERS

DISORDERED THOUGHT PROCESSES

Schizophrenia represents a major mental illness, or possibly a group of illnesses, manifested chiefly by disordered thought processes. The thinking disturbance leads to difficulties in communication, in interpersonal relationships, and in reality testing.

Patients with Schizophrenia make up about 36 percent of admissions to state and county mental hospitals, and because of the chronicity of many cases, 50 percent of the patients in such institutions. As a cause of human suffering, or lost productivity, and of public expense for health care, Schizophrenia is a major public health problem in modern society.

CLASSIFICATION OF SCHIZOPHRENIA

Persons suffering from the symptoms of Schizophrenia are classified according to the current system (see Chapter 4) under five major headings:

1. Brief Reactive Psychosis
2. Atypical Psychosis
3. Schizophreniform Disorder
4. Schizophrenic Disorders
5. Schizoaffective Disorder

Classifying a patient's condition in one of the first four of these categories is based on criteria primarily relating to duration of illness. If the patient has been sick for less than 2 weeks, and the illness follows an experience which would be regarded as highly stressful by the average person, the category of Brief Reactive Psychosis is used. If the illness has lasted less than 2 weeks, and does not follow a major stress, the diagnosis is Atypical Psychosis. If it has lasted longer than 2 weeks but less than 6 months, the term Schizophreniform Disorder is used. Only disorders that persist 6 months or longer are now called Schizophrenic Disorders.

The Schizophrenic Disorders are subclassified on the basis of the most prominent symptoms. Most patients show a mixture of symptoms. The subclassification of Schizophrenic Disorders includes:

1. Disorganized
2. Catatonic
3. Paranoid
4. Undifferentiated
5. Residual

Schizoaffective Disorder was formerly regarded as a subtype of Schizophrenia, and though it is now separately classified, for convenience it will be described along with the Schizophrenic Disorders listed above.

WHAT IS/ARE SCHIZOPHRENIA(S)?

Scientific investigation of Schizophrenia, and likewise any meaningful discussion of causes, symptoms and course, or treatments, is hampered by the unanswered question: How many schizophrenias are there?

Prior to 1896 a number of syndromes now classified as schizophrenic had been described. In 1896 Kraepelin grouped these together under the name dementia praecox, a term first introduced by Morel in 1860. Etymologically, dementia praecox implies an onset early in life and a loss of intellectual capacities. The term schizophrenia, meaning a splitting of the mind, was introduced by Bleuler in 1911 and has largely supplanted dementia praecox in contemporary psychiatric usage.

Conflicting findings in studies of different groups of schizophrenic patients have led some investigators to feel that Schizophrenia represents several basically different disorders having certain primary symptoms in common.

Others believe that there are two major disorders: process and nonprocess (remitting, reactive, schizophreniform) Schizophrenia; the former probably biologically caused and unlikely to respond to presently available treatments, and the latter experiential and offering a more favorable prognosis. An objection to this concept is that it may be based on an artificial weighing of prognostic factors not directly related to the disease(s).

Another factor which complicated research on Schizophrenia is that many of the patients most readily available for intensive study have experienced long-term hospitalization which in itself may alter findings.

THE CAUSES OF SCHIZOPHRENIA

The etiology of Schizophrenia includes:

1. Biological factors
2. Social factors
3. Experiential factors

There is little doubt that biological factors play an important role in the etiology of Schizophrenia. How important the role is, and what factors are most significant, is controversial.

Studies of the incidence of Schizophrenia among the biological relatives of index cases, together with data from twin studies, provides strong evidence that genetic factors operate significantly in the transmission of Schizophrenia; these data do not prove Schizophrenia to be a unitary disorder and are compatible with a concept of multiple etiologies and different modes of genetic transmission. One cannot, on the basis of presently available information, call Schizophrenia a hereditary disease, but one can say that a hereditary predisposition is present in many, if not all, cases.

Biochemical abnormalities, resulting from hereditary factors or caused in some other way, are likewise present in many, if not all, cases. Numerous studies report abnormal substances, including various metabolites, in the cerebrospinal fluid, blood, and urine of Schizophrenics, and these findings taken along with the effect of neuroleptics on schizophrenic symptoms, leave little doubt that there is something downright unhealthy going on in the brain chemistry of the Schizophrenic. Whatever it is, probably it is part of the cause of Schizophrenia, though it may be simply the mechanism by which symptoms are produced (a final common biochemical pathway), or even a result of having Schizophrenia (i.e., just as abnormal metabolites found in patients with a febrile illness may be the result of the illness and not part of its etiology).

There are two main groups of theories about what the basic abnormal chemical process is in Schizophrenia. These are:

1. Hypotheses relating to abnormal methylation
2. Hypotheses relating to excessive dopamine activity

The two groups of hypotheses are not mutually incompatible. Abnormal methylation hypotheses suggest that the brain of the Schizophrenic contains an endogenous hallucinogen, possibly produced by enzymes causing an abnormal transmethylation of an endogenous amine (tryptophan? norepinephrine? dopamine?).

Dopamine hypotheses, supported by the fact that neuroleptics which control the symptoms of Schizophrenia, though they do not cure it, are dopamine blockers, suggest that there is:

1. An excess of dopamine in some parts of the brain and/or
2. Hypersensitivity of postsynaptic dopamine receptors, and/or
3. A deficiency in other neurotransmitters (e.g., gamma-aminobutyric acid — GABA) which normally inhibit the effects of dopamine, and/or
4. Abnormal functioning of the enzyme dopamine-beta-hydroxylase (DBH) that converts dopamine to norepinephrine, resulting in an imbalance of transmitters

Some newer chemical hypotheses, for which there is as yet less evidence, are based on the existence of opiate receptors and endorphins (endogenous peptides) that bind them. Whether an abnormal morphinelike peptide has anything to do with causing Schizophrenia, and whether this substance is involved with dopamine systems remains to be seen.

While most psychiatrists are convinced that hereditary predisposition and chemical imbalance are involved in the production of Schizophrenia, a number of other possible biological causative factors have been suggested by the findings of various researchers, but none of these has confirmed significance. They include: vitamin deficiencies, intolerance for cereals (gluten) in the diet similar to that found in celiac disease, an association with the presence of human histocompatibility antigens (HLA), various allergies, endocrine disturbances, and infections.

Recent studies report that structural abnormalities in the cerebral cortex of chronic schizophrenic patients have been identified by computerized tomography in up to two-thirds of cases and lateralized neuropsychological dysfunctions (dominant hemisphere) may be detected in an appreciable number of Schizophrenics. Findings suggest that there is a subgroup of chronic Schizophrenics in which ventricular enlargement associated with cerebral atrophy produces cognitive impairment.

Social and cultural factors may play a role in the cause of Schizophrenia. It would be an oversimplification to say that poverty causes Schizophrenia, but the fact is that Schizophrenic Disorders, like most diseases, are several times more common in the lower socioeconomic groups than in the upper.

Studies showing that the distribution of socioeconomic class among the parents of Schizophrenics is about the same as in the population as a whole suggest that the greater prevalence of Schizophrenia among the poor may result from a downward drift prior to or after the onset of the disease. However, some psychiatrists still believe that poverty together with other social and cultural factors contributes to the etiology of some cases of Schizophrenia.

There are several possible ways in which poverty might contribute to the etiology of Schizophrenia. Crowding may be a factor. A human being's need for space may be likened to territoriality of the other species. Poverty may affect the ability of mothers to give adequate care to children. It may be that poorer schools and limited recreational facilities in slum areas are contributing factors. One likely factor is related to the stress experienced during adolescence and early adult life when one realizes that social and economic factors are a bar to achieving fundamental gratifications. Ambition is lost and the regressive process of Schizophrenia begins.

The higher incidence of broken homes in the lower socioeconomic groups is probably not in itself a factor in the etiology of Schizophrenia.

The relatively stable prevalence of Schizophrenia over time and in various cultures makes it unlikely that the pressure of modern life (if, indeed, life today in an industrial society is really more stressful than life in a more "primitive" society) is an important factor in the majority of cases, though it may be in individual ones.

Experiential factors in the etiology of Schizophrenia include a number of circumstances that may occur during psychosocial development. Hypotheses concerning psychological factors have been formed on the basis of data obtained from patients' life histories, from the study of families of schizophrenic patients, and to a limited extent from animal experimentation. In regard to the last, isolation and maternal deprivation during infancy have produced in experimental animals not only some of the behavioral symptoms suggestive of Schizophrenia but also some of the metabolic abnormalities.

Possible etiological significance has been attached to:

1. Maternal deprivation, or inadequate mothering, during the oral stage of development
2. Disturbed family relationships
3. Repeated exposure to double bind situations
4. Stresses during the phallic stage of development with reactivation of sexual fears at the time of adolescence

The ability to test reality and to think logically is acquired. Expectations concerning the effect of one's behavior in an interpersonal situation, the beginning of an ability to communicate and to interpret the communications of others (verbal and otherwise), and a general idea of cause and effect which is essential to logical thinking have their inception quite early in life. If a mother or mother surrogate is highly inconsistent in her attitudes toward the child and responses to the child's behavior, a serious gap in personality development may occur.

Though the behavior of the mother is thought to be important in the development of the preschizophrenic personality, the personality of the father is also consequential. If one grows up in a household where either parent has a psychosis, a serious alcohol problem, or a major personality disturbance, one's risk of becoming Schizophrenic may be increased. If the parents quarrel constantly and the family situation is chaotic the risk is further increased. Some schizophrenic patients have a history of having one parent who is unusually domineering and aggressive and another who is passive and withdrawn. In such a situation a child has difficulty in identifying with either parent and developing a sound self-concept.

Basic needs are met through interaction with others; successful dealing with others requires an ability to communicate. Much of the Schizophrenic's disorder involves the inability to communicate meaningfully. Repeated "double bind" experiences interfere with learning effective communication and at the same time create frustration and anxiety.

The double bind, as described by Bateson and his associates, involves a recurring situation in communication in which there is a primary negative injunction and a secondary injunction in conflict with it. The basic idea of two opposite communications may be illustrated by motioning someone to come toward you and saying "go away"; by placing ash trays by the chairs in a room with a "no smoking" sign; or by a girl puckering her lips, snuggling close, and saying "don't kiss me." In addition to these simple situations are more complex and subtle ones in which a person is told or asked to do two conflicting things. Examples: (1) A professor urges her students to ask questions, but if questions are asked she appears annoyed, brushes the questions off, or criticizes the student for not already knowing the answers. (2) An employer urges his staff to use initiative and make decisions for themselves, but he favors and promotes those employees who adhere rigidly to standard procedures and consult him about all situations not covered by these procedures. (3) A person urges a friend to "drop in any time" and complains that "you never come to see me," but if the friend does visit, seems surprised and acts as if the visit were inconvenient.

The dilemma produced by such ambiguous situations may be resolved by:

1. Seeking to ascertain which communication is actually meant
2. Electing to respond to one communication and ignore the other
3. Combining the apparently conflicting communications so that they make sense (e.g., interpreting "do it" plus "do not do it" as "do it, but not just now," or even "coax me")
4. Extricating oneself from the ambiguous situation

The double bind hypothesis, however, involves more than conflicting communication. It implies that either response will meet with rejection, disapproval, punishment, or some threat to well-being (i.e., the injunctions have a negative quality — you are damned if you do and damned if you don't). It also implies that the double bind occurs repetitively in a situation in which escape is impossible. An infant, a small child, or even Lolita has nowhere else to go.

It is suggested that after enough double bind experiences, the total environment begins to be perceived in double bind patterns, and that one learns to react to any part of what seems to be a double bind sequence with panic, rage, or apathy.

Peculiarities in sexual behavior and attitudes in schizophrenic patients suggest that sexual conflict may play some part in the production of the disorder. That the sexual difficulty is not merely a symptom of the disease is suggested by histories of sexual maladjustment prior to illness. Fears of sexuality probably arise in the phallic stage of development and are reactivated during adolescence. Homosexual panic, based on an actual situation or an imagined one which evokes fears of becoming involved in homosexual behavior, is a precipitating event in some cases of Schizophrenia.

Reference has previously been made to the possible role of stresses resulting from poverty and those associated with growing up and assuming adult responsibilities. The role of specific individually experienced stresses is even less clear. Animal experiments suggest that some stresses can produce a condition resembling Catatonic Schizophrenia. For humans, acute stress can produce Schizophrenia-like symptoms, but these are usually transitory. Some but by no means a majority of schizophrenic patients have been exposed to ongoing stress in the period immediately prior to the onset of illness. Whether stress is an etiological factor, a precipitating factor, a coincidence, or even a consequence of behavior during the prodromal phases of illness must be evaluated on a case by case basis.

MULTIPLE CAUSATIVE FACTORS

Combining the causative factors for which evidence exists, and assuming Schizophrenia to be one disease, a typical case formulation can be offered.

The patient was born with a constitutional predisposition to Schizophrenia. He had an inconsistent, frustrating mother and had difficulties in the oral stage of development. Inconsistency led to some difficulty in learning the meaning of usual human communication and grasping cause and effect relationships. As he grew older, his mother was aggressive and dominating and his father extremely passive. He was unable to identify with his father and had difficulty in assuming a masculine role. He found women frightening. Efforts to obtain closeness and tenderness from his parents were rebuffed, so that needs for affection began to be experienced as threatening rebuff, as anxiety-provoking.

Communication problems were worsened by repeated double bind experiences; these experiences also caused any ambiguous situation to become threatening.

Sexual conflicts and fears, some stemming from the Oedipus situation and some based upon ongoing exposure to his mother's inconsistency and hostility, increased when he reached adolescence. His awareness of sexual drive was stressful to him. He wanted to have dates but was shy and uneasy around girls.

Poverty, which may have contributed to a lack of adequate mothering in childhood, limited opportunities for socialization, advanced education, and a rewarding career.

Faced with the stresses of late adolescence and early adult life, with relationships threatening, communication difficult, and opportunities limited, the patient gave up. He stopped trying to cope with his environment. He substituted fantasy for reality. He withdrew. He regressed.

It should be emphasized that in an actual case, some, perhaps all, of the factors listed in this formulation may be absent (e.g., the patient may come from a wealthy family). Factors not included in this formulation may be important in some cases. The only safe generalization is that few, if any, Schizophrenics are people who have enjoyed childhood and adolescence.

Symptoms and Course

The onset of Schizophrenia is usually in late adolescence or early adult life. Among the current criteria for the diagnosis of Schizophrenia is an onset of prodromal or active symptoms before the age of 45. Seventy-five percent of first admissions of Schizophrenics to mental hospitals are patients between 15 and 44 (median age: 33). Because of the gradual onset of the illness, and in addition because some first admissions are patients who have been chronically ill prior to hospitalization, the median age of onset is somewhat lower.

The disease usually begins gradually and prodromal symptoms are present for weeks or months before all of the major symptoms are apparent.

During the early stages the patient feels anxious, worried, and unhappy. He or she often hesitates to seek professional help because of shyness and distrust of others; if help is sought, the complaints are likely to be vague and discussion of them is guarded. The patient may complain of nervousness but usually does not show the physiological concomitants of anxiety.

He or she gradually withdraws from social activities and contacts with others. Performance on the job or school work becomes inefficient; ambition is lost. There may be fantasies of, or even aspirations for, socioeconomic betterment (often wealth, power, or notable achievement), but the patient does not take active steps toward attaining these goals. She or he sits at the bottom of the ladder, dreams of being at the top, but does not actually attempt the first step up.

Often the patient becomes careless of personal appearance. He or she ruminates about various problems, including sex (most often fears of homosexuality) and religion.

By this time the family, those friends he or she has not alienated, and the employers or teachers know that the patient is ill. The patient feels desperately unhappy but sometimes does not admit being sick.

The primary symptoms described by Bleuler (the four As) are apparent. These are:

1.   Affective disturbance
2.   Associative disturbance
3.   Autism
4.   Ambivalence

The affective disturbance usually takes the form of a flatness of affect, a lack of outward display of emotion. Inappropriate affect, or an apparent dissociation between affect and thought content (e.g., laughing when describing a tragedy in one's life or that of a member of one's family) may be present. The inappropriateness of affect is often more apparent than real, more a matter of outward display than actual feeling. The patient feels that people in the environment, including the physician, are hostile and threatening. The patient's words and manner are used to conceal than to reveal feeling.

Looseness of associations (derailment) is one of the manifestations of the disorder in thinking and communicative ability of the Schizophrenic. The healthy person, when talking, maintains a fair continuity of ideas and a relatively orderly movement from one group of thoughts to another. There is a pause before a change of subject, and if the new topic is entirely unrelated, an introductory phrase of some sort usually calls attention to the impending change. In the Schizophrenic's speech, successive ideas appear to be unrelated or only slightly related to each other. The Schizophrenic does not indicate the intention to change the subject nor does he or she explain the transition.

The associative disturbance is easily recognized when it is severe. The patient may give totally irrelevant answers to questions. Example: Q. How old are you? A. First Baptist Church. Thoughts can be so disconnected as to be obviously incoherent. Example: "I want to talk to you about my wife — have you ever seen the

circus — blue is my favorite color — how's your liver today?" However, the looseness may be much less obvious and can be missed in interview. It is necessary to
ask some questions that allow for fairly long answers and to listen to them closely.
Encountering minimal looseness, the examiner has a natural tendency to assume
that she or he missed something that was said which would relate the subjects to
each other or account for the transitions; also, one supplies connecting links mentally, so that the patient's communications seem to make sense. Normally, one
writes more coherently than one speaks; however, the clinician is sometimes surprised in seeing a letter a patient has written in which a looseness of associations,
missed during interview, is clearly apparent.

Autism refers to a subjective, self-centered, unrealistic type of thinking. It is
manifested by a preponderance of fantasy, daydreaming, which substitutes for reality in wish fulfillment. It is also manifested by a tendency to apply personal and
private meanings to situations and to words rather than consensually validated ones.
An example of autistic language in the healthy person is the use of a private nick-
name or pet name for a person. This name, however, is used in speaking to the person, usually, and has some meaning or special reference that is shared. Schizophrenic humor is often autistic; no one gets the joke besides the patient. In ordinary humor irony involves a situation in which the speaker says something that may be
taken at face value by one (or more) listener but has a second, humorous meaning
to at least one other listener. Schizophrenic humor is irony without the other
listener.

Ambivalence refers to having two opposite feelings or emotions toward the
same person, thing, situation, or goal (e.g., wanting and not wanting; love and hate).
Everyone has a number of ambivalent feelings. However, the Schizophrenic is ambivalent toward almost everything; the ambivalent feelings tend to be almost
equal, not 90 percent in favor of something and 10 against as is more usual in the
ambivalence of the healthy person.

The primary symptoms are the ones that permit one to recognize Schizophrenia
in its early phases, and are the ones that are most helpful in differential diagnosis.
However, the actual diagnoses of Schizophreniform Disorder, used for patients who
have been sick longer than 2 weeks but less than 6 months, and Schizophrenic Disorder, used for patients who have been sick longer than 6 months, usually requires
the presence of secondary or accessory symptoms, though the diagnosis can be made
in their absence if there is a marked looseness of associations accompanied by flat
or inappropriate affect and/or grossly disorganized behavior.

The main accessory symptoms are:

1.   Delusions
2.   Hallucinations
3.   Ideas of reference

If the Schizophrenic is delusional, the false beliefs are numerous and are not
systematically organized. They are usually quite out of keeping with reality. Often
the content is dissociated from the affect accompanying it. One would expect the
lack of systematization because of the prevailing looseness of associations. The
content of delusions is understandable in two ways:

1.   The delusion often amounts to a daydream that is treated as if it were real.
2.   Some delusions are in fact communications in the form of metaphor or analogy
     (the metaphor is not easily grasped because of its autistic qualities and the ac-
     companying associative disturbance).

Though a delusion is by definition a false belief that is not amenable to logical persuasion (and not a part of the patient's cultural beliefs), most Schizophrenics have at least a partial insight into the unreality of their delusions. While it is useless to argue with a patient about delusions or to try to convince him or her that they are not true, it is detrimental to the formation of a working relationship with the patient to act as if one assumes the patient believes the delusions implicitly.

Hallucinations occur in about two-thirds of schizophrenic patients. They are most often auditory, but they may involve any of the other senses. (In contrast, hallucinations in Organic Mental Disorders are most often visual.)

Ideas of reference are an advanced manifestation of autistic thinking. The patient is likely to take almost anything that is said as referring to him or her personally. On seeing people in conversation, the patient thinks that they are talking about him or her. The patient may feel that items in the newspaper or on television refer to him or her personally.

In advanced Schizophrenia there is increasing difficulty in communication. The patient may create new words, neologisms, frequently by fusing two words, somewhat like the "portmanteau words" from Lewis Carroll's *Alice in Wonderland*. The fantasies and delusions tend to become increasingly bizarre. The thinking becomes perceptual and concrete rather than conceptual and abstract. Though the patient may speak in metaphors, he or she interprets another person's metaphors quite literally. There are psychological tests which will show this concreteness in thinking, but since this is a relatively late manifestation of schizophrenia, they are seldom needed diagnostically. In the clinical setting, the patient's interpretation of several proverbs will usually demonstrate it (e.g., Q. What does the proverb People who live in glass houses shouldn't throw stones mean? A. Glass breaks). Caution: If this technique is used diagnostically, remember to give several proverbs; a healthy person may give one or two concrete answers (or even an autistic one), and a Schizophrenic may give some conventional interpretations from memory. Sometimes it helps to use some foreign proverbs that will not be familiar to the patient.

Descriptions of schizophrenic language and communication sometimes refer to formal thought disorder. This refers to abnormalities in the form, as distinguished from the content, of thought.

In cataloging the symptoms of Schizophrenia, Kurt Schneider felt that a group of first rank symptoms were most important in the diagnosis of the Disorder. These symptoms are: (1) audible thoughts (hallucinations in which one hears one's thoughts spoken aloud); (2) hallucinations of voices arguing; (3) hallucinations of voices commenting on one's actions; (4) feelings of external influences playing upon the body (attributing sensations to radio waves, hypnosis, etc.); (5) thought withdrawal (the idea that one's thoughts are being extracted from one's mind); (6) thought insertion (thoughts ascribed to others); (7) illusions that one's thoughts are being broadcast; (8) made feelings (feelings attributed to an external source); (9) made impulses; (10) made volitional acts; (11) delusional perception (delusions based on a perception which seems entirely normal to the patient). While Schneider's first rank symptoms are no more helpful in the diagnosis of Schizophrenia than are other criteria and do not have established diagnostic specificity, they may identify a subgroup of Schizophrenics.

Other authors emphasize a distinction between the significance of positive symptoms (e.g., delusions, hallucinations, bizarre behavior) and negative symptoms (e.g., flatness of affect, withdrawal), and describes three types of Schizophrenia: positive, negative, and mixed.

Intellectual functions are apparently preserved in early Schizophrenia. The original concept of deterioration implying dementia, or a loss of mental function comparable to that in extensive brain disease, has not been widely accepted in recent years. Abnormal findings on intellectual testing of chronic Schizophrenics have been attributed in part to lack of cooperation, anxiety, loose associations, and autistic meanings attached to words in test situations, and partly, especially in hospitalized Schizophrenics, to the effect of long periods of social isolation, withdrawl, and lack of use of intellectual capacities. However, recent studies do suggest that some cognitive impairment may be found in a majority of chronic Schizophrenias.

While there are a few spontaneous remissions, untreated Schizophrenia usually becomes chronic and gradually becomes worse during middle life. Variations in the symptoms and course occur in the subtypes.

Literature concerning the outcome of treated Schizophrenia is difficult to evaluate because of differences in patient populations and in treatments used. Some studies do not distinguish between Schizophreniform Disorders and Schizophrenic Disorders. Probably 20 to 30 percent of patients recover fully and permanently. Fifty percent or more improve significantly or have a course marked by remissions and relapses. Only 20 or 30 percent remain severely symptomatic. Even among these, recovery can occur late in life. Despite earlier reports of Schizophrenic deterioration, and recent evidence of brain damage in many Schizophrenics, some symptoms, especially positive symptoms, tend to disappear in late life.

SYMPTOMS OF THE SUBTYPES OF SCHIZOPHRENIA

Schizophrenic Disorder, Disorganized Type, formerly called the hebephrenic type, is usually a variant that appears in relatively chronic cases. That is, a patient does not begin as a hebephrenic, but he or she shows the symptoms of some other type of Schizophrenia first and then develops this form. Affect is superficial. The patient displays a great deal of schizophrenic humor, frequently laughs inappropriately, and behaves in a way that would generally be described as silly. He or she shows numerous peculiar mannerisms. Delusions and hallucinations, if present, are often grotesque or bizarre, and are fragmentary rather than systematized.

Schizophrenic Disorder, Catatonic Type, differs in onset from other types of Schizophrenia in that an abrupt onset without prodromal symptoms may occur. An abnormality of motor behavior is the finding which distinguishes this from the other types. This may take one of two forms (a patient may display either or both of these in the course of the illness):

1. Catatonic Type, withdrawn (catatonic stupor)
2. Catatonic Type, excited

The patient in catatonic stupor is mute. He or she is likely to stay in one place, and if permitted to do so will probably remain in bed. On getting up (or being required to get up) the patient will usually stand or sit in one position and may remain immobile long enough to develop hypostatic edema. The patient is negativistic and passively uncooperative. One form of passive uncooperativeness sometimes present is automatic obedience (there is a passive-aggressive quality in doing exactly what one is told and *only* that). Echolalia (repeating the examiner's words) and echopraxia (repeating the examiner's actions) are closely related to automatic obedience. Sometimes for purposes of differential diagnosis in the apparently mute patient it is helpful to elicit these findings. If one looks at the patient closely and repeats in a clear voice a series of nonsense syllables several times, the patient is likely to repeat them and then will repeat any other words or phrases the examiner uses. If the examiner then goes through some motions and postures, the patient will copy them.

The patient's body and extremities may show a patchy cyanosis. Moving the patient's arms or legs reveals a waxy flexibility. If the patient is placed in a particular posture, even an uncomfortable one, she or he is likely to retain it for a long period of time. The patient may refuse to eat.

Catatonic excitement is characterized by hyperactivity. The patient often gives the impression of being enraged and may be destructive.

Schizophrenic Disorder, Paranoid Type usually has an onset later in life than other types of Schizophrenia. The loss of attention to personal appearance seen in most types of Schizophrenia rarely is present in the paranoid type. Hostility, suspicion, and distrust of others are even more marked in this type than in the other forms of Schizophrenia. Ideas of reference are nearly always present. Patients have delusions of persecution, delusions of grandeur (the idea of being a very important person, a king, a millionaire, a messiah, or a significant political leader is utilized to explain the ideas of persecution), or delusional jealousy.

Schizophrenic Disorder, Undifferentiated Type is the diagnosis used for patients with mixed schizophrenic symptoms, none of which are predominant enough to justify inclusion in any of the foregoing categories. Patients who would formerly have been diagnosed as having simple schizophrenia or latent schizophrenia are classified with the Undifferentiated Type if they meet the criteria for Schizophrenic Disorder. Otherwise, the diagnosis of Schizotypal Personality may be appropriate (cf. Chapter 7).

The Classification of Schizophrenic Disorder, Residual Type is used for patients who have had acute Schizophrenia and who, either as a result of treatment or spontaneous remission, show material improvement, have no prominent psychotic symptoms, and usually are able to make a satisfactory adjustment in the community, but still display some of the primary symptoms of Schizophrenia.

Schizoaffective Disorder is currently classified separately from the Schizophrenic Disorders. In the past there has been some disagreement about whether patients showing both schizophrenic symptoms and clear-cut signs of depression, or less frequently, elation, are suffering from a variant of Schizophrenia, a variant of manic-depressive illness, or a separate disease. The preponderance of evidence suggests that two populations are involved:

1. Schizophreniform and Schizophrenic Disorder with atypical affective symptoms (the usual affective disturbance in schizophrenia being flat or inappropriate affect)
2. Manic-depressive illnesses with concurrent schizophrenic symptoms

Classifying all such patients as Schizoaffective contributes to an orderly system of nosology, but is not much help in determining prognosis and planning treatment. The clinician's problem is to determine which syndrome is predominant and treat the patient accordingly. If the patient fails to improve, or gets worse, the choice must be reinspected.

DIAGNOSIS

Advanced cases of Schizophrenia are usually easy to diagnose, but some difficulty may be encountered in diagnosing the milder cases. Diagnosis is aided by the identification of the primary symptoms.

Near the time of onset Schizophreniform Disorders can be mistaken for Adjustment Disorders. With the onset in adolescence, or in early adult life, a number of stresses are identified; when an adolescent or young adult shows a gradual decrease in efficiency or in school performance, and a tendency to withdraw from social contacts, the possibility of Schizophrenia should be considered. This is an important differential diagnosis. An Adjustment Disorder resulting from an apparently self-limited stress may be treated symptomatically and expectantly, but incipient Schizophrenia requires a more definitive treatment program.

Catatonic stupor must be differentiated from a number of nonpsychiatric conditions manifested by stupor or coma. The waxy flexibility is helpful as a diagnostic sign. Echolalia and echopraxia, if elicited, and automatic obedience may be helpful in differential diagnosis. When conditions that would contraindicate its use have been ruled out, an amobarbital (Amytal) or thiopental (Pentothal) interview may be helpful. Catatonic patients will usually communicate under the influence of intravenous barbiturates and the procedure may be helpful in eliciting a significant history and symptoms. Benzodiazepines may also temporarily relieve catatonic symptoms.

Catatonic excitement must be differentiated from the Manic phase of the Bipolar Disorder. The presence of bizarre mental content and exitement without an apparent elevation of mood are suggestive of a Schizophrenic rather than a Manic Episode.

Schizoaffective Disorders which are primarily schizophrenic in character are to be differentiated from those which are variants of manic-depressive illness. The premorbid personality of the Schizophrenic is more likely to be introverted, and that of the manic-depressive extroverted. The onset of Schizophrenia is usually much more gradual than that of manic-depressive illness. Schizoaffective depressions do not show the psychomotor retardation characteristic of manic-depressive depressions. However, the presence or absence of the *primary* symptoms of Schizophrenia is the most important point in the differential diagnosis.

Schizophrenic Disorder, Paranoid Type is to be distinguished from other disorders in which delusions of persecution occur. In addition to the presence of the primary symptoms of Schizophrenia, one finds a poorly organized and poorly systematized quality to Paranoid Schizophrenic delusions, and this is helpful in establishing and confirming the diagnosis.

Occasionally there is a problem in differentiating Schizophrenia from Organic Mental Disorder. Since intellectual functioning, memory, and the fund of general information are preserved in early Schizophrenia, this should not be a difficult differential. Actually, problems in obtaining an adequate sensorium examination in the Schizophrenic can make it troublesome. In doubtful cases, psychological testing may be helpful. In addition, a careful search can be made for evidences of the causes of Organic Mental Disorders. Also, it should be borne in mind that Schizophrenic Disorders and Organic Mental Disorders can coexist. In chronic Schizophrenia, if one finds signs of sensorium impairment, one has to decide whether these are a feature of the schizophrenic process or are signs of another, superimposed illness.

Drug intoxication (hallucinogens; amphetamine) sometimes results in schizophrenic symptoms. Differential diagnosis may be difficult until an adequate history is available and one has had an opportunity to observe the patient over a period of time.

PREVENTION

The physician should recognize emotional disturbances in mothers that interfere with their rendering adequate maternal care to small infants and should refer these mothers for treatment. He or she can also recognize pathological interactions in families that tend to create recurrent double bind situations for children, and recommend corrective interventions. Children and adolescents with family histories of Schizophrenia require ongoing observation.

When one encounters an older child or adolescent who is introverted, shy, withdrawn, and unhappy, one can see that treatment is instituted before Schizophrenia begins. It should be borne in mind, of course, that introversion in itself is not pathological. It is the unhappy introvert who is at risk.

Participation in community mental health programs aimed at correcting social and environmental conditions which may contribute to the etiology of Schizophrenia is also important.

PROGNOSIS

There are several factors which influence the prognosis of Schizophrenia. These include:

1. *Onset:* The more rapidly Schizophrenia develops, the better the prognosis. An insidious onset covering a period of longer than 6 months is a poor prognostic sign.
2. *Duration:* The earlier in the illness any form of treatment is started, the better the prognosis. Best results are obtained when treatment is started within the first 6 months. After 2 years of illness, prognosis is generally poor, though recovery can occur even after many years of illness.
3. *Precipitating stress:* Prognosis in Schizophrenia is better when the onset follows an external precipitating stress situation. The greater the stress, the better the prognosis.
4. *Premorbid personality and level of attainment:* The more schizoid the premorbid personality, the worse the prognosis. The more successful the patient has been in school, at work, and in personal and social life, the better the prognosis.
5. *Subjective discomfort:* The presence of, or perhaps the willingness to admit to, subjective discomfort is a favorable prognostic sign in Schizophrenia. As a prognostic factor this is closely related but not identical to motivation. The patient who seeks treatment on a voluntary basis has a better prospect than the patient who is brought to treatment.
6. *Types of symptoms:* Overt manifestations of anxiety are usually favorable prognostic signs. The presence of depressive elements in the illness is favorable. Schizoaffective Disorders and Schizophrenic Disorders of the Catatonic and acute Paranoid Type offer the best prognosis, and Schizophrenic Disorders of the Disorganized and Undifferentiated Type the worst.
7. *Home environment:* The less stressful and unpleasant a home environment, the better the chance for recovery. The home environment also influences the risk of relapse. A home in which the patient does not experience hostility, frustration, and recurring double bind situations is necessary for recovery to be maintained. Understanding and acceptance of the patient are important. However, the patient retains improvement better when not overprotected, and those patients who are expected to resume their usual activities, duties, and obligations do better than those who are treated as invalids.

TREATMENT

In the last few years there has been a strong emphasis on drug treatment for Schizophrenia. While medications have been helpful to many patients, medication alone has apparently not significantly affected the long-term social adaptation of schizophrenic patients. It is generally more effective in relieving positive symptoms than negative ones. There is no basis for advocating the use of medication to the exclusion of psychotherapy, or the use of psychotherapy to the exclusion of medication.

Treatment of early Schizophrenia is imperative. Most early cases showing only prodromal and/or primary symptoms can be treated as outpatients. Hospitalization may be necessary if there is a need for differential diagnosis or if the patient's behavior represents a danger to general well-being. Examples: (1) Preoccupation with fantasies while driving or engaging in other activities in which this creates an accident risk; (2) Peculiar dietary habits leading to possible deficiency disease. If secondary accessory symptoms are already present, the possibility of actions based on delusional material must be evaluated, since these might make the patient dangerous to self or others. The fact that a patient believes that people are persecuting him or her does not make the patient dangerous to them, but if the patient is aggressive and/or is expressing aggressive ideation about them, the possibility becomes more serious. The patient who is securing weapons for self-defense against presumed persecutors can be a danger to a trespasser, or even to a door-to-door salesman. The vast majority of Schizophrenics are of course in no way dangerous to others.

In early cases hospitalization may be elected to remove the patient from a pathological home situation or to permit special treatment.

When practical, if a patient is able to continue to work, go to school, or keep up housekeeping activities, an attempt at outpatient treatment is generally preferable to hospitalization. The usual activities limit withdrawal and fantasy and help to keep the patient in contact with reality. If the patient is not working, hospitalization, or partial hospitalization, often offers a better environment for treatment. The activity programs of the hospital take the place of work in directing the patient's attention outward.

Psychotherapy is often effective in the early stages of Schizophrenia even if some of the secondary symptoms are present. A number of techniques of dynamically oriented, investigative, and/or expressive therapy can be adapted for work with the Schizophrenic. In the older literature, certain conclusions that Schizophrenic Disorders are not treatable by psychotherapy are based on:

1. The tendency to regard the patients who recover as not having been Schizophrenic in the first place.
2. Freud and other early investigators in the field of psychoanalysis believed, on a reasonable theoretical basis, that Schizophrenia could not be treated by psychoanalysis or analytically oriented techniques. Since the interpretation of transference is an essential feature of the psychoanalytic method, and since schizophrenic patients do not form the usual types of transference relationships with therapists, this appeared logical. Sullivan recognized that ignoring the therapist, or not relating to the therapist, could also be seen as a transference manifestation and this has opened the way to the application of analytically oriented techniques in the treatment of Schizophrenia.
3. Academic rather than practical questions as to whether the successful psychotherapy of the schizophrenic patient leads to a true remission or to an ability to live with the disease.

In any technique of therapy chosen for work with the Schizophrenic, a recognition of the patient's distrust of others and difficulty in tolerating closeness in relationships must be kept in mind. Also, in an expressive therapy, it is important that the patient not spend the time "practicing" some of the symptoms of the disorder in communication. Long periods of expressing loose and highly symbolic associations without questions that help clarify the communication may be undesirable. Usually more is accomplished by focusing on the patient's real problems in day-to-day living, in interpersonal realtionships, and in planning for the future than in attempting to explore some of the more bizarre ideation.

Medication is often used in outpatient treatment as an adjunct to psychotherapy. Some clinicians use antipsychotics (major tranquilizers; neuroleptics; dopamine blocking agents) routinely; they believe these relieve inner turmoil even if outward signs are absent. Others use medication only when there are positive symptoms and believe that even though statistical studies show antipsychotics to be helpful to some withdrawn apathetic patients as well as to agitated ones, psychotherapy may be more effective if medication can be avoided, or at least used conservatively. Also, side effects associated with the long-term use of antipsychotics, including tardive dyskinesia, cause some clinicians to prefer to avoid using these drugs when possible.

Treatment of the hospitalized schizophrenic also includes psychotherapy. Good results have been obtained even with brief psychotherapy in a sufficient number of cases to justify its use. In addition to adaptations of techniques of psychotherapy in general use, some specialized methods have been developed. High percentages of remission have been reported with some of these techniques, but most of them require special training and have not yet been widely enough used for full confirmation of the results reported from them.

Medications are more likely to be used in the treatment of the hospitalized schizophrenic than the outpatient. Medications and other somatic therapies are discussed in Chapter 20.

As important as the specific therapies is the overall program of the hospital, including the milieu, the attitudes toward patients, the activity programs, group experiences (including but not limited to group therapies), and remotivation programs. These serve to draw the patient away from fantasies and autistic thinking, help him or her learn to communicate effectively with people, and develop greater self-confidence in the ability to cope with interpersonal situations.

As has been noted, the more chronic the condition, the poorer the prognosis. However, a fair number of chronic patients can be rehabilitated sufficiently to function adequately in the community. Many of these need follow-up care and some require continued medication.

As an alternative to prolonged hospitalization or to frequent readmissions (the revolving door syndrome), day hospital programs and sheltered living arrangements can add materially to the number of chronic patients who can make it in the community. Such facilities not only contribute to patient well being, but reduce costs as well.

The chronic ambulatory Schizophrenic often does not need intensive treatment. In fact, investigative therapy is contraindicated in some cases. The prognosis is at best poor, and efforts to explore conflictual material may stir up anxiety which the patient is unable to handle without the development of more severe psychotic defenses. Unduly vigorous efforts to get the patient to participate in new activities can also be detrimental. Often, such patients can be offered little more than symptomatic medication and an occasional (perhaps monthly) brief visit with someone with whom they can discuss problems and who shows some interest in their well-being. This sort of service, though limited, often makes the difference between a satisfactory outpatient adjustment and a relapse.

Some Schizophrenics require long-term maintenance on antipsychotic drugs. From time to time one encounters patients who respond well to medication while hospitalized, but who have frequent relapses. Often the relapses result from patients' stopping taking medication or beginning to take it irregularly. If one can form a good therapeutic alliance with the patient, this is unlikely to happen. One wants the patient to understand the need for continuing medication and at the same time to understand that the physician does not want to prolong the use of medication unless it is necessary. Patient and physician can determine jointly when to test the patient's ability to function without medication and plan for close observation while medication is being withdrawn so as to detect signs of relapse early. Medication should be withdrawn gradually to avoid withdrawal, or rebound, exacerbation of psychotic symptoms.

Patients who have been kept in follow-up therapy and other chronic ambulatory Schizophrenics who are not in treatment often need help at times of situational crisis. It is important to recognize that the patient's need for help is with the immediate situational problems and not with the chronic underlying illness. A common mistake in such situations is to increase medication and then not to decrease it when the crisis is over.

A few chronic ambulatory Schizophrenics do need intensive psychotherapy and in these cases the calculated risks associated with doing it must be taken. In deciding to undertake intensive psychotherapy in the chronic outpatient Schizophrenic, one takes into consideration the patient's motivation for change, the degree of discomfort being experienced, and the extent to which the condition is progressive.

REVIEW QUESTIONS

1. What are the primary symptoms of Schizophrenia?
2. Describe the onset of a typical case of Schizophrenia.
3. What is meant by a double bind? Give two or more original examples.
4. Discuss the relationship between Schizophrenia and socioeconomic status.
5. How does a patient's expression of delusional content serve as a communication or attempt at communication?
6. What factors are taken into consideration in deciding whether to hospitalize a schizophrenic patient?
7. List and describe the subtypes of Schizophrenic Disorder.
8. A 50-year-old woman is clearly schizophrenic. History suggests that she has had this disorder for 25 years. She has never been hospitalized. She has earned her living doing part-time domestic work. Recently, she lost a job and since then she has had an increase in intensity of delusions and hallucinations (she says that "sex devils come to my room every night and talk about me"). What else do you need to know about the case to plan treatment? Are you likely to hospitalize her? Why or why not? If not, how will you treat her?
9. How does a Schizophreniform Disorder differ from a Schizophrenic Disorder?
10. Why do some patients with Schizoaffective Disorder respond to medications generally used for Major Affective Disorders, whereas others get worse when given such drugs?

SELECTED REFERENCES

1. Andreasen, Nancy C., and Scott Olsen: Negative v positive schizophrenia. *Arch Gen Psychiatry* 39(7):789-794, 1982.

2. Andreasen, Nancy C., Michael R. Smith, Charles G. Jacoby, James W. Dennert, and Scott A. Olsen: Ventricular enlargement in schizophrenia: Definition and prevalence. *Am J Psychiatry* 139(3):292-296, 1982.

3. Andreasen, Nancy C., Scott A. Olsen, James W. Dennert, and Michael R. Smith: Ventricular enlargement in schizophrenia: Relationship to positive and negative symptoms. *Am J Psychiatry* 139(3):297-302, 1982.

4. Arieti, Silvano: An overview of schizophrenia from a predominantly psychological approach. *Am J Psychiatry* 131(3):241-249, 1974.

5. Bateson, Gregory: Minimal requirements for a theory of schizophrenia. *Arch Gen Psychiatry* 2(5):477-491, 1960.

6. Bleuler, Eugen: *Dementia Praecox; or, The Group of Schizophrenias.* New York, International Universities Press, 1950.

7. Chandrasena, R.: Schneider's first rank symptoms: A review. *Psychiatr J Univ Ottawa* 8(2):86-95, 1983.

8. Dunham, H. Warren: Society, culture, and mental disorder. *Arch Gen Psychiatry* 33(2):147-156, 1976.

9. Goodman, Ann B., Carole Siegel, Thomas J. Craig, and Shang P. Lin: The relationship between socioeconomic class and prevalence of schizophrenia, alcoholism, and affective disorders treated by inpatient care in a suburban area. *Am J Psychiatry* 140(2):166-170, 1983.

10. Group for the Advancement of Psychiatry: *Research and the Complex Causality of the Schizophrenias.* Report No. 116. New York, Brunner/Mazel, 1984.

11. Hollingshead, August, and Frederick C. Redlich: *Social Class and Mental Illness.* New York, Wiley, 1958.

12. Kendler, Kenneth S., Alan M. Gruenberg, and Ming T. Tsuang: Outcome of schizophrenic subtypes defined by four diagnostic systems. *Arch Gen Psychiatry* 41(2):149-154, 1984.

13. Kendler, Kenneth S., and C. Dennis Robinette: Schizophrenia in the National Academy of Sciences – National Research Council Twin Registry: A 16-year-update. *Am J Psychiatry* 140(12):1551-1563, 1983.

14. Lowing, Patricia A., Allan F. Mirsky, and Robert Pereira: The inheritance of schizophrenia spectrum disorders: A reanalysis of the Danish adoptee study data. *Am J Psychiatry* 140(9):1167-1171, 1983.

15. Mackay, Angus V. P., Leslie L. Iversen, Martin Rossor, Ernest Spokes, Edward Bird, Alberto Arregui, Ian Creese, and Solomon H. Snyder: Increased brain dopamine and dopamine receptors in schizophrenia. *Arch Gen Psychiatry* 39(9):991-997, 1982.

16. McEvoy, Joseph P., and James B. Lohr: Diazepam for catatonia. *Am J Psychiatry* 141(2):284-285, 1984.

17. Pope, Harrison G., Jeffrey M. Jonas, Bruce M. Cohen, and Joseph F. Lipinski: Failure to find evidence of schizophrenia in first-degree relatives of schizophrenic probands. *Am J Psychiatry* 139(6):826-828, 1982.

18. Rieder, Ronald O., Lee S. Mann, Daniel R. Weinberger, Daniel P. van Kammen, and Robert M. Post: Computed tomographic scans in patients with schizophrenia, schizoaffective, and bipolar affective disorder. *Arch Gen Psychiatry* 40(7):735-739, 1983.

19. Salzman, Carl: The use of ECT in the treatment of schizophrenia. *Am J Psychiatry* 137(9):1032-1041, 1980.

20. Schulz, S. Charles, Miriam M. Koller, Pulla R. Kishore, Robert M. Hamer, Jerome J. Gehl, and Robert O. Friedel: Ventricular enlargement in teenage patients with schizophrenia spectrum disorder. *Am J Psychiatry* 140(12): 1592-1595, 1983.

21. Silverstein, Marshall L., and Martin Harrow: Schneiderian first-rank symptoms in schizophrenia. *Arch Gen Psychiatry* 38(3):288-293, 1981.

22. Taylor, Michael Alan, and Richard Abrams: Cognitive impairment in schizophrenia. *Am J Psychiatry* 141(2):196-201, 1984.

Chapter 12

PARANOID DISORDERS

A KIND OF MADNESS

By derivation, the noun paranoia and the adjective paranoid refer simply to mental derangement. In modern usage, referring to a person's behavior or attitude as paranoid implies suspiciousness, wariness, sensitivity, jealousy, hostility, and a tendency to accuse or blame others.

Though paranoid symptoms occur in many psychiatric disorders, the classification of Paranoid Disorders is reserved for those patients with major mental illness, psychosis, manifested primarily by delusions of persecution or delusional jealousy. Four types of Paranoid Disorders are recognized:

1.   Paranoia
2.   Shared Paranoid Disorder (folie à deux)
3.   Acute Paranoid Disorder
4.   Atypical Paranoid Disorder (a residual category for Paranoid Disorders not otherwise classifiable)

A paranoid psychosis which has been present for more than a week but less than 6 months is called *Acute Paranoid Disorder.* After 6 months the diagnosis becomes *Paranoia.*

PARANOIA

Though any patient with Paranoid Disorder who has had a chronic stable persecutory delusional system lasting at least 6 months can be diagnosed as having Paranoia, a number of patients in this group are ones whose illness had had an insidious onset and is manifested by a single delusional system that is internally consistent and logical. The delusional system is compartmentalized and dissociated from the remainder of conscious activity. The condition is usually described as being extremely rare. This is undoubtedly true if the diagnosis is restricted to those patients with elaborate and complex delusional systems. However, many persons harbor feelings of jealousy of or enmity toward individuals or groups accompanied by thoughts about them which reach the delusional level (persistent false beliefs, not amenable to logical persuasion, and not a part of the culture). Few such persons regard themselves as sick or seek professional help. Paranoia is rarely fully developed before the age of 30.

SHARED PARANOID DISORDER

The diagnosis of Shared Paranoid Disorder (folie à deux) is used when two persons (or, rarely, more than two persons) have a delusional system in common. These persons may be a husband and a wife, two other persons who are related and live together (e.g., a pair of spinster sisters), or may less frequently be formed of two people who are not related and do not live together. One is usually obviously paranoid and delusional. The other is a suggestible person, often with a Histrionic or Dependent Personality Disorder, who gradually comes to believe the delusions and treat them as real.

ACUTE PARANOID DISORDER

Acute Paranoid Disorder is a descriptive classification that may be used for any patient who has persistent delusions of persecution or delusional jealousy with behavior and emotional reactions compatible with the delusional content. The diagnosis is used for patients who have had these symptoms for more than 1 week and less than 6 months. Of course, it is not used for patients whose paranoid delusions result from other mental illnesses (e.g., Organic Mental Disorders; Schizophrenia; Major Affective Disorders).

Some patients in this category are in the early stages of true Paranoia. They show an insidious onset, well-systematized delusions, and preservation of the remainder of the personality. Also in this category are patients with involutional paranoia of under 6 months duration. These cases represent a variant of involutional melancholia, occur in the same age range, and have a similar premorbid personality and psychopathology. Depressive symptoms, if present, are not prominent. Some agitation may be present.

Another group of Acute Paranoid Disorders includes patients who have experienced major stresses often involving cultural shock or some stress associated with environmental change. These have an abrupt onset and rarely become chronic. Finally, there are paranoid states that are sometimes described as intermediate between Paranoia and Paranoid Schizophrenia. These patients, rather than having one systematized group of delusions have several loosely connected or unconnected delusions. There is often an acute onset and a relatively short duration.

CAUSE OF PARANOID DISORDERS

The main causative factors for the Paranoid Disorders are believed to be experiential. The conditions most often arise in persons who have had a Paranoid Personality at the clinical, or at least at a borderline, level.

Nearly always the patient has some basis for suspiciousness and sensitivity in early life experiences. There were reasons for feeling insecure and viewing the environment as hostile and threatening. Often there was mistreatment by a critical parent. A capacity for trust and confidence in others, sometimes called basic trust, normally begins to be acquired early in infancy (in the oral stage of psychosexual development), but if the task of establishing this basic trust is continuously frustrated, a state of chronic mistrust becomes a part of the developing personality.

Sullivan described a malevolent transformation in the personality that occurs when needs for tenderness encounter repeated rebuffs and become associated with felt anxiety. Patients who have experienced this malevolent transformation feel threatened and angry whenever they experience a need for affection.

There is usually a precipitating stress. In true Paranoia the patient misinterprets or overreacts to an actual occurrence. In some Acute Paranoid Disorders the precipitating situation is an environmental change, or a threat to sexual identity or role.

The main ego-defense mechanism involved in Paranoid Disorders is projection.

Freud, beginning with his report on the Schreber case in 1911, elaborated a theory that Paranoid symptoms result from a projection of repressed homosexuality. This represents a way of dealing with the unacceptable thought that I, a man, love him, another man.

From this formulation the delusion that one is being persecuted by a man (or a group led by a man) would be explained as follows:

1.   The patient is sexually attracted to the man (I love him).
2.   The feeling is unacceptable and a reaction formation takes place (I do not love him, I hate him).
3.   This feeling is also unacceptable in part for lack of logical basis and is projected (I don't hate him, he hates me).

Delusions of grandeur, which also sometimes occur in Paranoid Disorders, require a fourth step, rationalization (He hates me because I am someone very important). An alternate formulation for delusions of grandeur begins with the second step which becomes I do not love him or anyone else, I love only myself, and is then justified by rationalization.

Another type of paranoid delusion, the idea that a person of the opposite sex is in love with the patient, or is attempting seduction, can be explained as a simple projection (i.e., I, a married woman, am not attracted to another man, he is attempting to seduce me). However, the formulation based upon repressed homosexuality would be as follows:

1.   The person is sexually attracted to a person of the same sex (I, a woman, love her, another woman).
2.   This feeling is unacceptable and is displaced (I do not love her, I love him).
3.   This feeling, though less unacceptable, still produces discomfort and is projected (I do not love him, he is trying to seduce me).

A delusion that the spouse is promiscuous can also be explained on the basis of repressed homosexuality. The mechanism is projection (I am not attracted to other men, she is).

Many clinicians agree that repressed homosexual feelings are responsible for some Paranoid Disorders, but they are not present in all cases and many other factors can be involved. Sometimes the projected material is based upon feelings of sexual inadequacy; in other cases unacceptable impulses of a nonsexual nature are projected.

Symptoms and Course of Paranoia

In the early stages of Paranoia, after a precipitating event which often involves some feeling of failure or loss of self-esteem (e.g., failure to obtain an expected promotion; loss of a girlfriend to a rival; discovery that a supposed friend has been disloyal) there is frequently an initial period of depression, of blaming oneself for the situation, before projective mechanisms appear. At this time there may be some hypochondriacal symptoms.

The tendency to blame others does not at first reach a delusional level. For example, the person who fails to receive a promotion may feel that an employer has discriminated against him or her or that a rival has been unscrupulous; but while one may exaggerate and overemphasize certain incidents, there are no fixed beliefs that are clearly contrary to fact. One may suspect that a rival has told lies, altered documents, or bribed the boss's secretary without being convinced that such things have really happened.

Gradually the patient does become convinced of things contrary to fact. The delusional system slowly becomes more intricate and complex. The delusions are not bizarre. Hallucinations do not occur. There may be ideas of reference.

The patient's delusional ideas may not be known to many acquaintances. The premorbid personality is usually reserved and sensitive; the patient is unlikely to discuss personal matters spontaneously and resents questioning. If, as the delusions develop, there has been displacement to something relatively impersonal (e.g., feelings about the menace of some political or religious group) that the patient will discuss willingly, the delusional character may not be recognized. In a social setting the hostility being expressed makes listeners uneasy; they tend to change the subject and avoid it in future contact with the patient. While the patient is recognized as prejudiced or bigoted, he or she does not usually get a chance to express the most "far out" ideas.

There are several types of delusions. The most usual are the delusions of persecution, which take the form of:

1. Belief that some particular person, nearly always someone of the same sex, is in some way trying to harm the patient. The "enemy" may be accused of spreading lies, of trying to prevent the patient from attaining success or recognition, of harassing the patient in various ways, or of actually attempting physical harm.
2. Belief that a group rather than a specific individual is responsible for persecuting the patient. This is sometimes simply an elaboration of the idea that an individual is the persecutor. Others are thought of as associated with that person; they are part of the gang. If the persecuting group is thought to be a political, religious, fraternal, or ethnic group, the principal persecutor is believed to be their leader. However, in some cases, there is no leader or specific individual persecutor in the patient's delusional scheme. This can represent displacement of feelings about an individual and in some cases careful history-taking will elicit delusions of persecution by a specific person which preceded the main delusional system.
3. Jealousy in which suspicion of the spouse or lover reaches a delusional level. The mate is believed to be in love with someone else, or to be promiscuous. Later, ideas develop that he or she is spying, or attempting to gain control of property, or trying to drive one into a psychosis, or even putting poison in the soup (a slow poison, of course; one cannot keep being logical and accuse a mate of many attempts with fast-acting poisons).

Grandiose delusions, when present, usually accompany or follow delusions of persecution. However, they are sometimes found in the absence of any history of persecutory ideas. They occur as:

1. Belief that one is wealthy, powerful, or important. Examples: (1) A patient believes he is heir to the Russian empire. He realizes that this empire is non-existent, but he feels that if it were not for his enemies, he would be recognized as a member of royalty, might claim money and property in various parts of the world, and could perhaps some day lead a counter revolution. (2) A woman believes that she is the next Messiah. She feels that she receives signs from God that direct her in the formation of a new religion. She believes that she has special powers such as being able to heal the sick — if they believe. (3) A man believes that he has a new economic theory that will, if only he could find a publisher who is not afraid of the wrath of the establishment, revolutionize the world. (4) A young woman claims to be working on an important invention. She feels that her task will soon be completed. She spends hours assembling various electrical circuits and bits of machinery — that do exactly nothing.
2. Belief that someone of the opposite sex is in love with or is attempting to seduce the patient. This is sometimes called erotomania. Usually the person involved in the delusion is prominent or is unusually attractive. The patient may not actually be acquainted with the person; or it may be someone with whom he or she has had a few dates. Sometimes the patient believes that many people, rather than just one, are overcome by his or her near fatal charms. The patient may believe that the various things that the supposed lover does and says are secret messages. If the patient writes to or telephones the person and is rebuffed, the rebuff is interpreted as testing or being discreet. The patient may prove annoying and occasionally frightening to the person who is the object of the delusion.

Paranoid patients are sometimes litigious. Also, when they feel persecuted by a religious or political group they are inclined to join groups and movements opposed to their supposed enemies. As happens with the Paranoid Personality, the patient with a Paranoid Disorder who joins a political or quasipolitical group usually does not get far. He or she cannot trust the other members and they react with a reciprocal distrust. If the group is composed largely of more or less sane citizens, though they may welcome the patient at first as an ally or fellow traveler, they soon become aware of the delusional ideas and find their new chum more a liability than an asset. Paranoid individuals are a shade more successful when they form a new religion, a political group, an organization to reform something or even a professional organization. It is *against* something. Its leader generally feels persecuted, demands absolute loyalty from followers, tolerates no deviation, and suspects subversion.

Sometimes it is suggested that various notable political leaders were paranoid (e.g., Hitler; Stalin). This is largely speculative. Sometimes the writing and actions of the individual provide inferential data; but adequate clinical evaluations simply are not available.

In addition to being attracted to more or less legitimate political groups that are against something, and to forming new political, religious, and reform movements, paranoids are often attracted to hate groups and eccentric organizations composed chiefly of emotionally disturbed people. The groups are small; they have a common enemy; they feel discriminated against or persecuted. They may have grandiose ideas of their importance, virtue, and mission.

If beliefs about a common enemy or persecutor reach the delusional level, the diagnosis of Shared Paranoid Disorder becomes appropriate.

It is usually said that in Paranoia, aside from the delusional system, the personality remains intact. This is not always entirely true. Many patients in addition to the delusional system retain, or develop, the characteristics of the Paranoid Personality. In addition to behavior in situations relevant to their delusions, they are often hostile and contentious. Even if this is not the case, the energy and attention given to the delusional material is taken away from other activities. One rarely sees a paranoid whose sense of humor is intact.

In true Paranoia, once paranoid delusions are fully developed, they remain relatively unchanged for the remainder of the patient's life. There is some fluctuation in intensity which depends in part upon the level of stress in the environment. Spontaneous remissions are rare. When Paranoia coexists with Alcoholism, a change in the alcohol problem may lead to changes in the Paranoia. If there is a remission of Alcoholism as a result of psychotherapy, participation in Alcoholics Anonymous, or independent efforts to quit drinking, the Paranoia usually improves. If drinking is made impossible by the use of disulfiram or by confinement, the Paranoia often becomes worse. The paranoid patient who stops drinking because of religious conversion may show an increase in paranoid symptoms and tend to incorporate the new beliefs into the delusional system.

Much that has been said about the symptoms and course of Paranoia is also applicable to the Acute Paranoid Disorders that have a remission in less than 6 months. The differences are as follows:

1. These patients are less likely to have had diagnosable Paranoid Personalities. Some degree of suspiciousness and sensitivity is usual prior to illness in both groups, but those who have an early remission are less likely to have had a Personality Disorder. They may have been more Schizoid or Passive-Aggressive than Paranoid. Often they have had feelings of sexual inadequacy or inferiority in the masculine or feminine roles.
2. The precipitating stress is usually a more serious and direct threat to well-being and self-esteem.
3. Onset is more abrupt.
4. They may not show one internally logical system of delusions, but they may have several delusions. Though hallucinations are not a prominent feature of any of the Paranoid Disorders, these patients occasionally have auditory hallucinations.
5. Spontaneous improvement or remission may occur following lessening of environmental stress.

Diagnosis

The diagnosis of Paranoia is nearly always difficult. In part, this results from the circumstances under which examination usually takes place. The paranoid rarely seeks treatment. If the patient is seen, it is because of referral from a court or an employer, or because of pressure from family members. He or she is suspicious and relatively unwilling to supply information. However, this cannot be used as a diagnostic clue; it may be appropriate to the situation as the patient sees it.

Since the chief, and perhaps only symptom, is the delusional system, it is necessary to establish that the patient's beliefs are false. This is a problem peculiar to the diagnosis of Paranoia; if one were making a diagnosis of Schizophrenia, paranoid type, for example, a diagnosis could be made on the basis of the presence of the primary symptoms of Schizophrenia, and the assumption that certain of the patient's ideas were delusional would not require validation. Since the paranoid's delusions are not bizarre or impossible, proof that they are false beliefs may be difficult. This is often compounded by the fact that they are based on some actual experiences. However, as the patient elaborates upon the delusional ideas, the diagnosis can usually be made on the basis of the number of improbabilities, the patient's failure to take appropriate steps to ameliorate interpersonal problems, and the minimal evidence on which some of the beliefs are based (e.g., a man believes that his wife is unfaithful; she denies it. The clinician cannot be sure that the patient is incorrect, but when the patient "knows" her lover visited her because he found a cigarette butt in the yard, one can be fairly sure that sick thinking is involved).

Still, one must remember that at times a person who reports harassment or persecution or even states that attempts are being made to kill him or her may be reporting facts and not delusions.

Evaluation of the patient whose possible delusions are related to religious or political beliefs is especially difficult. Suppose one is asked to evaluate a candidate for the legislature who insists that a governor, despite a conservative record, is a member of the Communist underground? Or suppose you are asked to examine the leader of the local antimental health group who believes that certain psychiatrists are part of a conspiracy to undermine public morality. In such cases the examiner may be satisfied that the patient's beliefs are incorrect, but it is hard to establish that they are delusions.

Differentiation from Paranoid Personality is largely a matter of degree and duration. The Paranoid Personality, by definition, is not accompanied by delusions, and Personality Disorders are generally lifelong.

Differentiation from paranoid Schizophrenia, more common than the Acute Paranoid Disorders, is based on identification of the primary symptoms of Schizophrenia. Presence of hallucinations suggests some illness other than the Paranoid Psychoses, though an occasional patient with an Acute Paranoid Disorder or an Atypical Paranoid Disorder believes that he or she hears the voice of God, receives messages by telepathy, or has some similar experience.

Paranoid symptoms also occur in amphetamine-induced psychoses, various other Organic Mental Disorders, and, though not at a delusional level, in some Adjustment Disorders. Grandiose delusions in Manic Episodes can usually be distinguished from those of Paranoia easily because of the elation and hyperactivity of the Manic.

WHEN IS THE PARANOID DANGEROUS TO OTHERS?

The mentally ill are sick people. They are people with personal problems who deserve sympathy, understanding, and treatment rather than confinement. Like other sick people, they usually have the right to refuse treatment. There are exceptions to these generalizations. Most, though not all, clinicians would deny the depressed patient's right to commit suicide. There is no question that the rights of some patients with Antisocial Personalities to interfere with the welfare of others must be abridged.

The paranoid's right to hate people he or she regards as persecutors is an even more difficult problem for clinical evaluation. Most paranoids are harmless to others. The average paranoid's idea that an individual or a group is persecuting him or her causes subjective discomfort; it may cause litigiousness or give rise to unfounded complaints to law enforcement agencies or employers, but it does not cause the patient to attack the "persecutors." However, some paranoids do attack.

They may kill or attempt to kill a supposed enemy; or they may do real harm by false accusations arising from projection. The clinician must try to find out what the patient intends to do about the supposed enemies. The risk is greatest when the paranoid has a delusion of being endangered in a way that an aggressive act would seem to be needed for self-defense. The patient's level of agitation and history of overt aggressive behavior is helpful in evaluation of risks.

If one's patient appears to be dangerous to another person, and refuses hospitalization, involuntary hospitalization must be considered, and one may need legal advice in resolving the dilemma over one's obligation to maintain confidentiality and one's duty to warn the intended victim.

Sometimes one is consulted by the object of the paranoid's delusions. Examples: (1) An employer receives letters from a former employee who accuses him of discharging the employee unfairly and of sending false reports to other employers. The letters are vaguely threatening. The employer barely remembers the case; his files show the employee was discharged for some appropriate cause and reveal no reports that should keep the individual from finding other work. (2) A wife consults her physician because of her husband's extreme jealousy. (3) A young woman reports that a man with whom she talked a few times at a bus stop is writing her love letters that sound as if she and he had been quite intimate and as if she reciprocated his feelings; she says she has given him no encouragement. He calls her and expresses jealousy of her male friends. She believes he sometimes follows her when she has dates.

These people need legal as well as medical advice. They may need special police protection. The possibly paranoid patient must be investigated and potential danger assessed (preferably by someone other than the person the "victim" has consulted). The victim should be advised to be courteous but distant in any contacts with the paranoid. There are several things which the victim may consider doing which are not advisable:

1. One may elect to ignore the situation. This is not safe if the accusations are persistent and if the accuser has not been adequately evaluated.
2. One may attempt to win over the paranoid by being kind. This is potentially dangerous. Often a transformation of unacceptable feelings underlies the paranoid delusional system. Friendly gestures may make the symptoms worse instead of better.
3. One may try to frighten the paranoid or at least reject him or her forcefully. This is also potentially dangerous.
4. Less frequently, one may be tempted to admit the things of which one is being accused. This does not work and may create complications. For example, a husband who writes his wife a letter (perhaps at her request) admitting a series of indiscretions that did not take place puts himself in an awkward situation if he decides later that she should be committed to a hospital, or if he seeks a divorce.

Prevention

There is little that can be done on the basis of present knowledge to reduce the incidence of Paranoid Disorder. Some advice to parents, teachers, and others concerning attitudes toward children may be helpful.

The degree to which children are suspicious, sensitive, and tend to blame others for their troubles should be observed, and if this is disproportionate or inappropriate, it should be modified by early treatment. Children do blame others. Example: A small child falls down. No one is near him. An adult rushes to help him to his feet. More often than not he cries and says, "You pushed me." However, if this sort of reaction is frequent, intense, and persistent in the school-age child, it is an indication for professional evaluation. Parents may foster a paranoid tendency by critical attitudes toward others. They may also foster it by a tacit or active approval of maladaptive projective mechanisms. The parent who blames the bad influence of other children when a youngster gets into trouble, or joins the child in criticizing a teacher as unfair, may be doing the child a disservice even if there is some basis for the viewpoint. The child should be helped to see his or her own role in interpersonal reactions and to deal with them constructively rather than by attaching blame to someone. If is usually better for a child to learn to cope with a difficult teacher than to get the teacher in trouble or get transferred to another class.

Like other attitudes, suspiciousness and wariness are acquired. One needs them, but only in proportion to the real dangers in the environment. Growing up to distrust everyone's motivation is indeed unfortunate. It is equally unfortunate to be too trusting. The woman who cannot trust any man is unlikely to have a happy marriage; however, the woman who believes everything any man tells her will spend most of her life pregnant, barefooted, and very likely single.

The industrial consultant may prevent some cases of Paranoid Disorder. An employee who is making a poor adjustment and who is being passed over for a promotion is likely to be under considerable stress. One may tend to blame either oneself or others. Failure of management to give the employee a candid work evaluation may contribute to this. Sometimes an administrator may feel that he or she is being considerate by not being frank in giving a work evaluation and by retaining an employee despite a poor adjustment. The reverse may be the case. An honest appraisal may be disturbing and may cause the employee to change jobs, but this is better for the employee and the organization than it would be to allow resentment and suspicion to grow.

Social action to eliminate prejudices and hate groups, together with the inculcation of social attitudes which make suspicion and enmity less ego-syntonic, can be helpful if constructive attitudes are substituted and if prejudices are not simply driven underground.

Treatment

Psychotherapy is the treatment of choice for the Paranoid Disorders. Outpatient treatment can be used if the patient is willing to accept it and if evaluation fails to indicate a danger to others.

The therapist must be able to tolerate the paranoid's suspiciousness, hostility, and tendencies to accuse and blame those who are trying to help. It must be remembered that the paranoid is a lonely, frightened, and unhappy person. One must not add to the discomfort. At the same time there are sound theoretical and clinical reasons for believing that the paranoid cannot tolerate a great deal of closeness or warmth in the treatment relationship. The therapist must, initially at least, maintain a somewhat more distant and reserved attitude than would be appropriate for most other patients.

The therapist must prove consistent, reliable, and trustworthy. However, to do this one must rely on actions over a period of time rather than words of reassurance which will not be believed. One does not need to go to great lengths to answer more or less delusional accusation; trying to prove that one is not in league with the patient's "enemies" is futile and indicates something approaching a folie a deux as does attempting to take sides with the patient against the world. Reality is emphasized gently and without argument.

One assumes that the patient harbors certain suspicions about the therapist whether these are expressed or not. Many paranoids believe that their appointments are being recorded. Sometimes they talk more freely if a tape recorder is actually in use. They are more comfortable knowing the recorder is there than suspecting a hidden one.

The unwilling patient in an inpatient setting may eventually enter into therapy if the physician is consistent in attempts to form a working relationship and becomes neither angry nor oversolicitous when rejected by the patient.

Since family crises play a role in the etiology of some Acute Paranoid Disorders, an interview with the spouse, usually by someone other than the therapist may be helpful in treatment planning, and in some instances family therapy or case work with the spouse may be an important part of the management of such cases. These Acute Paranoid Disorders have a much better prognosis than true Paranoia for which effective therapeutic intervention is always difficult and often impossible because of the patient's lack of basic trust.

REVIEW QUESTIONS

1. What is the principal ego-defense mechanism shown by patients with Paranoid Disorders? What other ego-defense mechanisms are frequently present?
2. Discuss the Schreber case. Did Freud actually examine Schreber?
3. What is the difference between Paranoia and Shared Paranoid Disorder? Acute Paranoid Disorder? Atypical Paranoid Disorder?
4. Paranoid symptoms sometimes arise in patients with alcohol problems (alcoholic paranoia). What common etiological factors are there that may contribute to both the alcohol problem and the paranoid ideation?
5. What is meant by the phrase well-systematized delusions?
6. What is the malevolent transformation? What is its role in the etiology of paranoid behavior?
7. Discuss the relationship between delusions of grandeur and delusions of persecution.
8. For a number of years a man showed no tendency toward suspiciousness of his wife. In fact, she feels that he tacitly and at times actively encouraged her interest in other men. Suddenly, he becomes extremely jealous and makes many accusations of infidelity, which his wife denies. What factors might account for the change in the patient's personality? Could this be Paranoia? What other diagnoses would you consider? In attempting to account for this patient's symptoms, how would it help you to know his age? Would you have to know for sure whether the wife had been having any extramarital affairs in order to make the diagnosis?
9. What is a folie à deux?
10. Discuss the prognosis in Acute Paranoid Disorders.

SELECTED REFERENCES

1. Blumenthal, Monica D.: Resentment and suspicion among American men. *Am J Psychiatry* 130(8):876-880, 1973.

2. Bruch, Hilde: Mass murder: The Wagner case. *Am J Psychiatry* 124(5):693-698, 1967.

3. DiBella, G. A. Williston: Educating staff to manage threatening paranoid patients. *Am J Psychiatry* 136(3):333–335, 1979.

4. Freedman, Robert, and Paul J. Schwab: Paranoid symptoms in patients on a general hospital psychiatric unit: Implications for diagnosis and treatment. *Arch Gen Psychiatry* 35(3):387–390, 1978.

5. Freud, Sigmund: The case of Schreber; papers on technique and other works. In: *The Standard Edition of the Complete Psychological Works of Sigmund Freud.* Vol. 12, 1911–1913. London, The Hogarth Press, 1958, 12–82.

6. Higdon, John F.: Paranoia: Power conflict or homosexual projection? *J Oper Psychiatry* 7:1, 1976.

7. Janosko, Rudolph E. M.: Therapy for paranoia. *Psychiatr Ann* 9(12):28–35, 1979.

8. Kendler, Kenneth S.: Demography of paranoid psychosis (delusional disorder): A review and comparison with schizophrenia and affective illness. *Arch Gen Psychiatry* 39(8):890–902, 1982.

9. Modlin, H. D.: Psychodynamics and management of paranoid states in women. *Arch Gen Psychiatry* 8(3):263–268, 1963.

10. Mullahy, Patrick: *Oedipus (Myth and Complex), a Review of Psychoanalytic Theory.* New York, Hermitage Press, 1948, 304.

11. Oxman, Thomas E., Stanley D. Rosenberg, and Gary J. Tucker: The language of paranoia. *Am J Psychiatry* 139(3):275–282, 1982.

12. Sacks, M.H., William T. Carpenter, Jr., and John S. Strauss: Recovery from Delusions. *Arch Gen Psychiatry* 30(1):117–121, 1974.

Chapter 13

PSYCHOSEXUAL DISORDERS

SEX IS NOT ALWAYS JOYFUL

On the basis of the Pleasure Principle, one might expect sexual activity, like the satisfaction of other instinctual (biological) drives, to be enjoyable as, indeed, it is *most* of the time for *most* healthy people. However, worries about sex, guilt feelings, frustrations, and sexual dysfunction are major causes of human discomfort. Help with these problems as with other sources of discomfort, is often sought from the family physician.

To deal effectively with human sexual problems, the physician must be thoroughly informed about sexual development and function, including the basic anatomical, physiological, and endocrine (and other biochemical) factors together with sociological and psychological factors which help shape attitudes and behaviors.

Until relatively recent times precise information about the frequency of occurrence of various types of sexual behavior and some of the physiological changes occurring during sexual activity was unavailable. Since the publication of studies by Kinsey and his associates, beginning in the late 1940s, and the work of Masters and Johnson, which began to be available in the 1960s, the physician has been able to deal with sexual problems more objectively, and most medical schools now offer courses in human sexuality.

TYPES OF SEXUAL PROBLEMS

The physician must utilize a knowledge of both human sexuality and of psychiatry in a variety of ways including:

1. Furnishing information in answer to specific questions or requests for instruction.

2.   Helping healthy persons who are worried about some aspect of sexual behavior.
3.   The diagnosis and treatment of Psychosexual Disorders.

In responding to requests for information or advice (e.g., at the time of a pre-marital examination), one needs to be alert to the possibility that the questions may relate to a source of concern that is not immediately obvious. When concern is voiced by the apparently healthy person who is worried about some sexual feeling or activity, it may represent a relatively minor problem that will be solved by furnishing information, simple advice, or reassurance, or it may be a clue to more serious psychopathology. Before assuming that one is dealing with a member of the "worried well" one must be sure that the sexual problem is not causing other symptoms that would merit a diagnosis of an Adjustment Disorder, and on the other hand, one must be sure that the sexual problem is not symptomatic of a Neurosis or other psychiatric disorder.

From the medical rather than the statistical or moral point of view sexual behavior is clinically significant when it is a source of concern, discomfort, or unpleasant consequences to the person indulging in it. One might add a reference to harm to society or to other individuals, but this is already implicit in the definition, since it is one of the things that leads to unpleasant consequences for the individual.

Psychosexual Disorders are divided into four categories: (1) Gender Identity Disorders, (2) Paraphilias, (3) Psychosexual Dysfunctions, and (4) Other Psychosexual Disorders. Sexual problems that are secondary to another disease, psychiatric or otherwise, are not diagnosed under these headings.

Gender Identity Disorders are conditions in which the individual rejects his or her biological (anatomical) sex and believes that he or she is really a member of the opposite sex.

The term Paraphilia is used to describe sexual behavior patterns that would have formerly been classified as forms of sexual deviation or as perversions. The paraphiliac obtains sexual gratification from acts not associated with normal coitus (or masturbation) or from coitus performed in bizarre ways. The paraphiliac may be able to obtain sexual gratification solely through deviant behavior or may engage in such behavior in addition to normal sexual activities. The terms normal and deviant as used in this chapter refer to the usual, or modal, patterns of sexual behavior within the culture and do not in themselves imply value judgments. Obviously, a person engaging in an unusual, even bizarre, sexual activity with another consenting adult is not for this reason alone to be regarded as sick. The diagnostic classification is relevant only to compulsive or impulsive behavior patterns that cannot be controlled and that cause discomfort (dysphoria) for the person, create consequential problems for the person through their effects upon relationships with significant others (including sexual partners), or lead to illegal acts (e.g., sexual activities involving children or nonconsenting adults).

The third group, Psychosexual Dysfunctions, are manifested by lack of sexual desire (when this is a source of concern to the patient) or impairment in some portion of the sexual response cycle (excitement, plateau, orgasm, resolution). Lastly, included under the category Other Psychosexual Disorders are Ego-Dystonic Homosexuality and Psychosexual Disorders Not Classified Elsewhere.

TYPES OF PSYCHOSEXUAL DISORDERS

People seek assistance for many varieties of sexual behavior. The conditions classified in the four major groups of Psychosexual Disorders are:

1.   Gender Identity Disorders
      a. Transsexualism
      b. Gender Identity Disorder of Childhood
      c. Atypical Gender Identity Disorder of Adolescence or Adult Life
2.   Paraphilias
      a. Fetishism
      b. Transvestism
      c. Zoophilia
      d. Pedophilia
      e. Exhibitionism
      f. Voyeurism
      g. Sexual Masochism
      h. Sexual Sadism
      i. Atypical Paraphilia
3.   Psychosexual Dysfunctions
      a. Inhibited Sexual Desire
      b. Inhibited Sexual Excitement
      c. Inhibited Female Orgasm
      d. Inhibited Male Orgasm
      e. Premature Ejaculation
      f. Functional Dyspareunia
      g. Functional Vaginismus
      h. Atypical Psychosexual Dysfunction
4.   Other Psychosexual Disorders
      a. Ego-Dystonic Homosexuality
      b. Psychosexual Disorder Not Elsewhere Classified

GENDER IDENTITY DISORDERS

Transsexualism

A transsexual is a person who feels he or she was born the wrong sex. During the development of gender identity between 18 months and 3 years of age the child accepts the identity of the sex opposite to its biology. Although there is an occasional person with Schizophrenia, as a general rule these patients are relatively healthy except for their dissatisfaction with their sexual identities. Sex change operations, done in stages and preceded by hormone therapy, have yielded satisfactory results in some cases and have been disappointing in others. Surgeons at one major medical center where pioneering work in this treatment was done have discontinued using it. However, it is still being done in several other facilities, and a physician approached by a transsexual patient desiring a sex change operation should not dismiss the possibility without having consultation from someone experienced in evaluating patients with this disorder. Individuals seeking the sex change operation have been preponderantly male.

Gender Identity Disorder of Childhood

The category of Gender Identity Disorder of Childhood is used for cases of Transsexualism diagnosed before puberty. The diagnosis should not be used for behavior which mimics the opposite sex, but for those children who, despite the evidence of their genitalia, believe themselves to be of the opposite sex.

PARAPHILIAS

Fetishism

Some people are sexually stimulated by parts of the body not generally experienced as erotogenic (e.g., the feet), or by articles of clothing or other objects. Fetishism varies in degree and clinical significance. For a man who has a generally satisfactory heterosexual adjustment to have an erection at the sight of black lace panties, on or off, or for a woman to be aroused in foreplay only after she has kissed her lover's feet, is in a limited sense deviant; but it is less pathological than obtaining sexual gratification only when using the fetish in masturbatory activity (e.g., having an orgasm while handling feet, with or without additional manual stimulation of the sex organs; a man masturbating while handling women's underwear). Often, when the fetish is an article of clothing, the patient has certain additional requirements concerning it (e.g., it must have been used; it must be stolen).

Symbolization, complex formation, and perhaps conditioning play a part in the development of the fetish.

Whether the fetish is a part of the body or an inanimate object (in official nomenclature [see Chapter 4] the diagnosis is limited to the use of inanimate objects), and the fetish is used in sexual activity with another person, fetishism is unlikely to be distressing to the patient or to produce secondary symptoms (e.g., feelings of frustration; anxiety; depression) so long as there is a willing and available partner.

Transvestism

The transvestite's sexual gratification is associated with wearing clothing of members of the opposite sex. Transvestite behavior varies in nature and degree. It is sometimes associated with other Paraphilias. Most transvestites are heterosexual rather than homosexual.

During childhood and preadolescence most youngsters dress up a few times in the clothing of the opposite sex, either in parent's or sibling's clothing at play, at costume parties, or to act a role in a play. Unusual or extreme expressions of parental approval or disapproval at such times, or other concomitant events, may possibly contribute to complex formation. Parental preference, expressed or implied, for having a child of the opposite sex may play some part in certain cases, as may envy of the other gender's social role.

Transvestism is to be distinguished from Transsexualism. The transvestite is sexually excited by cross dressing; the transsexual is not. The transvestite accepts his or her biological gender; the transsexual does not.

Zoophilia (Sexual Activity with Animals)

Occasional sexual activity with animals (bestiality) by adolescent boys in rural communities is probably not clinically significant beyond the degree to which it may give rise to guilt feelings or fears. This activity in adult life is relatively unusual. It is sometimes done by patients with Antisocial Personalities and, rarely, by Schizophrenics; and these conditions should be considered in differential diagnosis.

Pedophilia

Sexual behavior with children of the same or opposite sex, whether limited to "indecent liberties" or including definite sexual practices, is of more serious social consequence than most other Paraphilias because of its possible adverse effects on the emotional development of the children involved. Though sexual experiences during or before adolescence with underdeveloped partners, as described in the novel *Lolita,* may play a part in the development of Pedophilia, the majority of patients showing this symptom are people with gross feelings of sexual and general inadequacy. They are afraid of attempting sexual activity with adults. This type of behavior usually begins early in life, but one occasionally sees an onset in elderly patients. Diminished sexual capacity coupled with brain damage and weakening of cortical controls is responsible for this.

Sometimes pedophilic behavior is limited to incest. When this occurs it is usually but one feature of a disturbed family situation. Often the uninvolved marriage partner seems consciously or unconsciously to be encouraging it, or at least doing things that make it possible (e.g., initiating sleeping arrangements that facilitate it). The most commonly reported incestual situation is father–daughter. Incest between siblings is usually not pedophilic in origin.

Not all sexual behavior with persons below the age of consent is pedophilic. For an adult to become involved with "jail bait" is illegal and reflects poor judgment. It is not Pedophilia if an adolescent who has fully developed secondary sex characteristics is involved.

The diagnosis of Pedophilia is used for activities with prepubertal children. The diagnosis is not used unless the adult is at least 10 years older than the child. This difference in age is not necessarily applicable to adolescent patients; one considers the sexual maturity of the child, and the adolescent, as well as the ages of each. Pedophilia may be either heterosexual or homosexual. An isolated episode of sexual behavior with a child would not be diagnosed as Pedophilia, but if the patient is in trouble over such an incident and denies previous involvement or fantasies about children, one must keep in mind the possibility that the patient is not furnishing an accurate history.

Exhibitionism

The exhibitionist, the person who displays his sexual organs to strangers of the opposite sex, is usually an inadequate, insecure individual who has failed to attain an adult heterosexual adjustment. He is more likely to be a nuisance to society than a menace. It is rare for the exhibitionist, even if encouraged, to make physical contact with his "victims." Closely related to the exhibitionist is the individual who makes obscene phone calls to strangers or sends them obscene letters or pictures. Often the exhibitionist seems to want only to shock or frighten the observer. It may be a way of showing hostility toward the opposite sex.

Exhibitionistic tendencies are closely related to scopophilia (Freud viewed these two things as a paired instinctual phenomenon). Some exhibitionistic impulses generally arising in little boys during the phallic stage of development are subsequently repressed. Sublimations in later life include various ways of showing off or gaining attention (e.g., driving a red sports car; lecturing).

It is sometimes said that there are no women exhibitionists. This is not altogether true, though women are rarely arrested for exhibitionistic behavior. There are women who, consciously or unconsciously, make a habit of disrobing near windows through which they can be readily observed. Sometimes this is not so much exhibitionism as indifference to the possibility of being seen (if they don't want to look, let them pull their own shades), but in other cases, exhibition is intended, and is a source of sexual excitement. Differential diagnosis includes mental retardation, Schizophrenia, and Antisocial or Histrionic Personalities.

Some believe that the relative infrequency of exhibitionism in women is related to feelings about not having a penis (castration complex). However, an alternate hypothesis is that our society offers more opportunity for aim-inhibited exhibitionistic behavior (e.g., wearing revealing garments) for women. The tendency does not have to be as rigidly repressed and, hence, is not as likely to occur in the form of clear-cut acting-out.

Voyeurism

The peeping Tom represents a type of Psychosexual Disorder by any definition. Some scopophilic impulses are usual in men, while according to some authorities, visual stimulation is less likely to arouse women sexually. For the healthy man, voyeuristic impulses are usually sublimated (e.g., enjoyment of art, bird watching, scientific curiosity) or aim inhibited (e.g., enjoyment of shows featuring scantily clad chorus girls, watching women in bathing suits on the beach, or looking at pictures of nude or seminude models in magazines). Scopophilic impulses are also gratified by seeing the marital partner in the nude (unless her inhibitions, conflicts, or hostilities lead her to dress and undress in the closet). There is probably something of a continuum between this normal masculine scopophilia and the voyeur who habitually attempts to peer into the bedroom windows of strangers. Occasionally, an adolescent, or less frequently an adult is arrested for peeping when there is reason to suspect as much provocation on the part of the "victim" as pathology on the part of the peeper. The woman who undresses without pulling her shades should not be too surprised if someone stops to look. However, if she is frightened, she may call the police. Clinical evaluation of such cases is often difficult, since an habitual voyeur who has not accumulated a police record is likely to lie when asked about a history of previous episodes.

Recurring voyeuristic practices are usually associated with a lack of satisfactory adult heterosexual adjustment and with overall feelings of inadequacy. Curiosity about parental sexual activity arising in the phallic stage of development is sometimes implicated in the etiology of voyeurism. The voyeur is usually a timid, inadequate individual who is very unlikely to "graduate" to more serious forms of sexual deviation.

Sexual Masochism

Sexual Masochism is the need to have the partner inflict pain in order to perform sexually and to obtain gratification. One finds mild cases which have borderline or no clinical significance. Examples: (1) A woman enjoys sexual relations with her husband most of the time, but she finds that intercourse is most pleasant when her husband's behavior is rough rather than tender or affectionate. (2) A man prefers that his wife dig her fingernails into his back and bite his shoulder hard enough to make a mark during foreplay. (3) A woman achieves orgasm only occasionally in her marriage, but she usually attains it in extramarital affairs, often with men whom she picks up in taverns. She says, "I like it when they treat me like a prostitute. You know, talk rough to me and use four-letter words."

Other masochistic persons obtain satisfaction through wearing uncomfortable garments (e.g., painfully tight girdles or belts; tight shoes with spiked heels) while engaging in or fantasying sexual activity. Others like to be whipped or beaten. Self-mutilation sometimes occurs. Complex formation associating pain with sexual gratification may be a factor in the etiology of this form of Paraphilia. A view of the primal scene as a violent attack may also be a contributing factor.

Rape victims are rarely masochistic. A person who is raped may experience an Adjustment Disorder and may require psychiatric attention as a part of medical care (which also includes treatment of injuries, venereal disease prophylaxis, and possible steps to prevent an unwanted pregnancy). In evaluating the emotional problems of the rape victim, tact must be used (e.g., direct questions about the patient's own possible role in precipitating the occurrence are to be avoided until the patient introduces the topic). In some communities there are social agencies specifically established to counsel rape victims.

Occasionally one encounters a woman who has repeated experiences of being raped. Sometimes she seems to invite this by provocative or at least careless behavior. In some instances this may be masochistic. It may be different only in degree from the woman who virtually insists that her husband use force. As well as being masochistic, it has the element of engaging in sexual activity without being or feeling responsible for it, so that any belief that sexuality is wrong may be rationalized with the thought that she is being forced to participate against her will.

Sexual Sadism

Sadism is the need to inflict pain in order to achieve sexual gratification, just as masochism is the need to have the partner inflict pain. Sadism and masochism were viewed by Freud as paired instinctual components. Sometimes sadists and masochists form groups in which members refer to one another as dominants or submissives and practice bondage. These practices, involving consenting adults, and usually not leading to serious injuries, are relatively benign. However, there are groups in which the activities are sufficiently dangerous that the possibility of serious injuries or even death must be considered.

Though most sadists are relatively harmless to others, there are some who inflict suffering on nonconsenting partners, and some who assault, rape, mutilate, or even murder to obtain sexual gratification.

Just as most rape victims are not masochistic, most rapists are not sadists. However, in evaluating a rapist, the possibility that sexual gratification is obtained only through the violent assault or humiliation of another person must be considered.

Atypical Paraphilias

There are a number of other Paraphilias, most of them relatively rare, for which the diagnostic category of Atypical Paraphilias can be used. These include Frotteurism (sexual arousal from rubbing one's body against another clothed person), and Necrophilia (sexual activity with a corpse).

In addition to the recognized Paraphilias one may be consulted about other sexual behaviors that are of concern to patients or their sexual partners. For example, fellatio (sexual stimulation of the penis with the mouth), cunnilingus (sexual stimulation of the clitoris and labia with the tongue), and anal stimulation as a part of foreplay or as an occasional substitute for coitus by heterosexual partners are all relatively common practices. When they are a source of worry or guilt feelings, or when one partner desires them and the other rejects them, they may become clinically significant, but they are not diagnosed as Paraphilias. However, such variant behavior may be the only way in which a person can be sexually aroused or gratified. It may be habitually substituted for coitus. It may be compulsive or may result from impulses that cannot be controlled. In such cases, classification with the Paraphilias may be warranted. Whether diagnosable as Paraphilias or not, the evaluation, and if necessary the treatment, of these conditions is the same as for the other Paraphilias.

In the description of each of the common types of Paraphilias, a few notes have been made about common etiological factors. However, most cases are highly complex, and stem from multiple causes. A discussion of the etiology of a Paraphilia, to be complete, would cover almost all aspects of psychopathology. In studying the causes of a Paraphilia in a given patient, one may look for some of the following:

1. Reasons why the patient fails to achieve a pattern of healthy adult sexual behavior or fails to find this sufficiently gratifying.
    a. Biological deficiencies. These may include an inadequate development of the sex organs, endocrine abnormalities, and/or failure to develop secondary sex characteristics. Other constitutional factors which tend to make the person unattractive to members of the opposite sex or make one unable to assume the social role appropriate to the anatomical sex may also contribute.
    b. Feelings of sexual inadequacy in the socially appropriate role, based upon experiential factors but fundamentally unrealistic.
    c. Fear of sex. This includes strong feelings that normal sexual activity is wrong and/or guilt feelings over normal sexual impulses.
    d. Fear of the opposite sex.
    e. Fixation, regression, complex formation or conflict involving sexual impulses arising at any stage of psychosexual development.
2. Factors influencing the type of disordered sexual behavior.
    a. Symbolization and complex formation.
    b. Acting-out of neurotic conflict.
    c. Development of behavior patterns in a manner similar to the development of the Personality Disorders.
    d. Conditioning, or at least learning, through gratifying or rewarding experiences.

Symptoms and Course

Sexually disordered behavior is generally a lifelong process having its onset in adolescence or very early in adult life. Patients showing minor disorders rarely become worse or "graduate" to more severe sexually disordered behavior. However, before offering a prognosis on this basis that the voyeur, for example, is more likely to be a nuisance than a menace to society, one would want to feel reasonably sure that the patient has not concealed the history of another type of disordered behavior and that he does not have an Antisocial Personality.

Since aberrant sexual behavior is usually a lifelong process, its apparent development in middle or late life requires careful study. Sometimes this reflects only an inadequate history. If the onset is indeed acute, one might suspect the behavior of being symptomatic of another psychiatric illness. Patients may act out otherwise controlled impulses in stress situations at the time of intrapsychic crisis or in connection with any of a number of psychiatric disorders. Also, an apparently isolated episode of aberrant behavior may be accounted for in part by provocative activity on the part of the "victim." Most persons have a number of fairly well-repressed impulses and some of these may come into the open when such things as opportunity and alcohol mix. Most Paraphilias do not lessen in late life, but if there are aggressive components these may be less marked following involution.

Diagnosis

Paraphilia is a descriptive diagnosis. Some patients so diagnosed show a preponderance of neurotic conflict and might equally appropriately be regarded as Neurotic. Some authors use the term paraphilic neurosis to describe such patients. In other patients, the clinical picture and history are similar to one of the Personality Disorders. When appropriate, one may make another diagnosis in addition to that of a Paraphilia. One does not, however, diagnose a Paraphilia when deviant sexual behavior is the direct result of another psychiatric condition.

Diagnosis is rarely difficult when the patient comes voluntarily for help with a symptom. Usually, it can be made with relative ease when the patient comes to therapy under duress, but willing to admit the problem and furnish a history. A patient who has been apprehended for a sex offense and denies it or refuses to give a history is very difficult to diagnose. Care should be taken in venturing an opinion in such cases. Suppose that one finds evidence of sexual conflict, aberrant impulses, and personality features compatible with the type of behavior of which the patient is accused. This in no way proves the patient guilty of the particular offense, or any other offense. There are many people with sexual conflicts and deviant impulses who do not put them into action. This is analogous to the fact that a normally heterosexual and happily married person has conscious or unconscious heterosexual impulses toward persons other than one's spouse, if not at other times, at least when the spouse is away, but not everyone puts them into action. Likewise, negative examination findings could scarcely establish that an offense did not occur. Medicolegal implications of sexual psychopath laws are discussed in Chapter 23.

In differential diagnosis of the Paraphilias, one should rule out Antisocial Personality, Schizophrenia, Obsessive Compulsive Disorder, Organic Mental Disorder, and Bipolar Affective Disorder.

Prevention

Prevention lies primarily in treating problems in psychosexual development and in the acquisition of the sex-appropriate role during childhood and preadolescence before aberrant behavior makes its appearance. Adequate sex education and the development of reasonable attitudes toward sexuality in the community are also of preventive value. Opportunities for healthy courtship activities during adolescence are important.

Treatment

In deciding whether and how to treat the Paraphiliac one should take into account any other symptoms and problems in living. Sometimes these are sufficient to warrant treatment on their own merits. One should also evaluate the patient's discomfort and dissatisfaction with the behavior and the motivation for change. Consideration should be given to the direct and indirect consequences of the behavior to the individual. A patient, for example, may engage infrequently in rather mildly deviant behavior that does little if any harm to others. However, if this behavior is likely to lead to arrests, loss of jobs, and disruptions of social life, it becomes clinically highly significant.

Most patients with minor Paraphilias can be treated on an outpatient basis. However, those whose behavior presents a real menace to others (e.g., the pedophilic patient; some sadomasochistic patients) must be hospitalized, not only to protect society but to protect them from the consequences of their acts. Possible treatment goal may be:

1. To help the patient accept the behavior and feel less guilty about it. This is sometimes appropriate in mildly disordered behavior between consenting adults (e.g., a member of a Sadomasochistic couple in which the behavior patterns are unlikely to lead to consequential injury to either party) and may also be appropriate in some other cases of deviant behavior which is highly chronic and apparently does not offer a good prognosis for change (e.g., some patients who have been fetishists for many years).

2. To help the patient control the behavior through the exercise of restraint, to behave more discreetly, or to meet deviant needs in a more socially acceptable manner. A suppressive therapy with the support of healthy defenses is likely to work only in a relatively mild case. Sometimes a patient who obtains sexual satisfaction through aberrant behavior outside of marriage can with the cooperation of the spouse find ways of meeting the needs in marriage. Before assuming that the social consequences of some types of deviant behavior could be eliminated or greatly reduced by greater discretion in the choice of time, place, and partner, one must be sure that the consequences are not part of the unconscious reason for the behavior.

3. Complete elimination of the symptom. This may be done in part through investigative psychotherapy. Support can be given to healthy sexual drives. Also, it is important to support the patient in his or her sex appropriate role. For example, when the woman with a Paraphilia is able to behave in an increasingly feminine way and to acquire a favorable image of herself as a woman she is less likely to feel deviant impulses.

Therapies based on learning theory or conditioning have also been used successfully with Paraphiliacs. They are indicated in those cases in which other symptoms and difficulties in living are either minimally present or are a consequence of the sexual behavior and do not require an investigative therapy themselves.

In the treatment of the married patient it is also helpful to involve the spouse. Sometimes this can be done in the form of family therapy. More often, separate therapy or case work for the spouse is recommended. In working with the spouse it is often desirable to remove first some of his or her feelings of guilt and responsibility for the disordered behavior even though these may not be consciously expressed. The mate is likely to feel that he or she is personally inadequate as a sexual partner and that this produces the disorder. This may lead only to less enjoyment of sexual activity and less comfortable participation in it; more often there is projection in the form of blaming the spouse. The constructive approach is not to try to fix responsibility, but to determine what can be done about the situation. The spouse can do much to help the deviant partner develop self-esteem and maintain a sex-appropriate role. In addition, the spouse can offer encouragement toward normal heterosexual behavior by making it more easily available and enjoyable. Finally, minor deviant needs can often be met effectively, and even sometimes major ones can be ameliorated (e.g., a man with fairly well-controlled pedophilic impulses was essentially freed of these feelings after his wife shaved her pubic hair).

Male Paraphiliacs have been treated with antiandrogen medications such as medroxyprogesterone acetate or cyproterone to reduce sexual drive and make it easier for the patient to control aberrant impulses. When a patient is seeking help voluntarily and can give informed consent without being under duress this is something that may be considered as part of a treatment program. When the patient is a sex offender and is ordered by or under pressure from the court to obtain treatment, the use of such medications may pose an ethical problem.

PSYCHOSEXUAL DYSFUNCTIONS

Before making a diagnosis of Psychosexual Dysfunction, the physician must determine that the condition is not secondary to another disease, psychiatric or otherwise, or the result of medication the patient is taking. Psychosexual Dysfunction
may be acute or chronic; complete or partial; partner-dependent or circumstance-
dependent. They include:

1. Inhibited Sexual Desire
2. Inhibited Sexual Excitement (frigidity; impotence)
3. Inhibited Female Orgasm
4. Inhibited Male Orgasm
5. Premature Ejaculation
6. Functional Dyspareunia (painful coitus)
7. Functional Vaginismus (vaginal spasms)
8. Atypical Psychosexual Dysfunction

   While many cases of sexual dysfunction are the result of emotional problems,
other sexual difficulties may represent endocrine or genitourinary system disorders, and a significant number are produced by toxins (including alcohol and some
commonly used medications). In marriage, or in any other specific relationship,
dysfunction may be secondary to some other interpersonal problem. Psychotherapy is indicated in some cases. Sex therapies, partially those employing behavioral
techniques, have an important role in the treatment of sexual dysfunction, but they
should not be undertaken until the problem has been thoroughly evaluated (and if
referral is made to a sex therapist, the referring physician should first carefully
investigate the therapist's qualifications and ethical standards).
   Sexual dysfunctions are quite common. In one study of patients in a medical
outpatient clinic a third of the men were found to be impotent (14 percent of these
cases were thought to be psychogenic). A history by systems should include questions about sexual behavior and function. Many patients do not make sexual complaints spontaneously, some because the subject is embarrassing to them, others
because they feel that nothing can be done to help them. Of course, not all patients with Sexual Dysfunction are sufficiently bothered by it to want complete
examination and treatment. Complete evaluation may require some specialized
techniques (such as the measurement of nocturnal penal tumescence in cases of
impotence), but once the cause of a dysfunction is understood, successful treatment
is often possible.

OTHER PSYCHOSEXUAL DISORDERS

1. Ego-Dystonic Homosexuality
2. Psychosexual Disorder Not Elsewhere Classified

Ego-Dystonic Homosexuality

A person's thoughts, feelings, and activities are described as ego-syntonic if he or
she finds them desirable, or at least acceptable. They are described as Ego-Dystonic (ego-alien) if the person regards them as inconsistent with his or her personality and finds them undesirable or distressing.
   For many homosexuals, homosexuality is ego-syntonic. A homosexual person
for whom homosexuality is ego-syntonic does not regard himself or herself as sick,
and does not seek treatment or change in sexual orientation.

On the other hand, if homosexuality is ego-dystonic either because the homosexual behavior is repugnant to the individual or because desired heterosexual capacity is lacking a diagnosis of Ego-Dystonic Homosexuality is made and treatment may be indicated.

Not all patients who come to the physician expressing concern about homosexuality are homosexual. A homosexual is one who habitually and by choice obtains sexual gratification from persons of the same sex. This definition excludes the occasional, more or less experimental, activity between persons of the same sex that is relatively common in preadolescence and adolescence and occasionally occurs in adult life. It also excludes "homosexual" (or isophilic) activity in situations in which access to the opposite sex is denied (e.g., prisons).

This definition is helpful when one encounters a patient who does not engage regularly in homosexual behavior, and clearly does not want to, but is afraid that he or she may be or may become homosexual. Fears of homosexuality are not uncommon among adolescents and young adults. They are frequently expressed by ones who are shy and introverted. They may stem from feelings of inadequacy as a man or woman or from difficulties in heterosexual relationships. They may also result from concern over isolated desires, impulses, or activities that occurred under unusual circumstances. Often they represent displacements from other sources of conflict.

Most such patients need little more than reassurance and information about sexual functions. However, the possibility that the patient has an Adjustment Disorder, a Neurosis, or a Personality Disorder must be considered.

The patient who believes that others think he or she is homosexual or accuse him or her of homosexuality presents a different problem in differential diagnosis. Something about the patient's behavior or life style may actually be giving rise to gossip. The patient may be insecure, feel inadequate as a man or woman, and project these feelings. The possibility of Schizophrenic or Paranoid Disorders must be considered.

Dynamically, the concept of latent homosexuality refers to strong impulses toward homosexual activity which are poorly controlled by the superego and which give rise to conflicts which may evoke more or less pathological defense mechanisms. In no sense should latent homosexuality be classed with the sexual deviations. In addition to the dynamic concept of latent homosexuality, it should be added that almost anyone has a capacity for facultative homosexuality. Latent homosexuality is not necessarily a factor in the fears expressed by some patients that they may be homosexual.

When homosexuality is actually present, in determining whether it is ego-dystonic one uses caution in evaluating the patient's initial comments about wanting, or not wanting, to change. Motivation for change may be superficial. On the other hand, the person who voluntarily seeks consultation about his or her sexuality (not about some other symptom) may be more dissatisfied with it than he or she is prepared to admit at first.

Though the patient's own feelings about his or her sexuality are more important, social pressure may be a factor in the desire to change sexual orientation. A patient who feels that being heterosexual would lead to better social adjustment or better acceptance by family and friends is not necessarily desirous of change, or diagnosable as having Ego-dystonic Homosexuality. On the other hand, this may be a greater motivating factor for the patient who is in a society, or subcultural group, that views homosexuality very negatively. This is analogous to the situation of a left-handed person in a culture that is prejudiced against left-handedness (e.g., certain Oriental groups). A person in a culture that accepts left-handedness as a normal variant may feel that life would be easier if she or he were right-handed, but is not likely to want to go to great lengths to change. A left-handed person encountering real prejudice would have reason to take this into account in weighing the possibility of trying to change hand preference.

The sexual and social behavior of homosexuals is as variable as that of heterosexuals. The homosexual man may or may not behave effeminately, and the homosexual woman may or may not copy masculine behavior. In sexual activity the homosexual may take a consistently active role, a passive one, or may vary his or her role. A homosexual may have a pattern of forming relatively lasting relationships or may be promiscuous. He or she may or may not affiliate with other homosexuals as part of the gay crowd.

There are multiple etiological factors in homosexuality. Constitutional endocrine abnormalities as such are rarely involved. Often the masculine-appearing woman homosexual or the feminine-appearing man gives this impression because of mode of dress, grooming, mannerisms, etc. However, the unfeminine-looking woman or the effeminate man may accept homosexual contacts more readily because of some relative inability to attract the opposite sex.

Though endocrine abnormalities as such are not a major factor as far as we know, there may be a biological precursor for some cases of homosexuality. This may be genetic, or it may be a result of biochemical influences during fetal growth.

Events during the phallic stage of development can contribute to homosexuality in some cases. Unsatisfactory resolution of the Oedipus situation may lead to fears of persons of the opposite sex, or in some cases, fears of competing with persons of the same sex. Sometimes a homosexual presents a history of growing up in a family who had wished for a child of the opposite sex and who were unwilling to accept the patient's actual sex. (Example: Parents had two older daughters and wanted a son badly. When a third daughter was born they gave her a boy's name, dressed her in boy's clothes, and until secondary sex characteristics developed in adolescence encouraged her to participate in masculine sports and activities. As an adult she was an Ego-Dystonic Homosexual, but she had no transsexual or transvestite tendencies.)

Undue restrictions of aim inhibited and partially sublimated heterosexual behavior in adolescence may contribute to homosexuality. Cases are found in religious groups that prohibit dating, dancing, attending motion pictures, mixed swimming, etc. It is not that these groups approve of homosexuality, but rather that they make such an issue of forbidding heterosexuality that homosexuality seems less prohibited.

There are other situations in which parents make youngsters so afraid or guilty about heterosexual impulses that they seek a different outlet for the sexual drive.

In treating the Ego-Dystonic Homosexual, as in treating the Paraphiliac, appropriate goals may be to make the patient more comfortable about his or her sexual behavior, to help the patient modify the behavior so as to prevent undesirable social consequences, or to help the patient change sexual preferences. For the latter, investigative psychotherapy is sometimes indicated. One looks for the reasons for rejecting heterosexuality as well as the reasons for accepting homosexuality. One does not focus on the sexual behavior alone, but works with the total personality. In the psychotherapy of homosexuality, supporting the self-esteem and the appropriate masculine or feminine qualities of the patient is important. Treatments based on conditioning have also been used.

Psychosexual Disorder Not Elsewhere Classified

There are a variety of other sexual problems and concerns that may be classified under the heading of Psychosexual Disorder Not Elsewhere Classified. Among these are nymphomania and the Don Juan syndrome.

Promiscuity implies frequent indiscriminate or casual affairs; not all premarital or extramarital sexual activity is properly described as promiscuous. A certain amount of promiscuity occurs in our culture. In addition to the individual and social problems created by venereal disease, unwanted pregnancies, and prostitution, premarital and extramarital sexual activity may become clinically important when it gives rise to feelings of guilt or anxiety, when individuals wish to restrain sexual impulses and are unable to do so, and when the behavior creates domestic or social problems. For some persons, superego values as such do not preclude relatively promiscuous sexual activity; however, if such a person has a spouse who has a different value system or lives in a social group whose values are different, the behavior may lead to stress-provoking situations. There are many factors other than a permissive superego which may produce promiscuity. The investigation of its possible clinical significance requires an understanding of what it means to the individual patient and its effects on his or her life. Promiscuity occurs in Antisocial, Histrionic, and some other Personality Disorders. In other cases, it may represent a form of compulsive behavior. Occasionally it is observed in mania, Schizophrenia, or Organic Mental Disorders.

Some persons who are promiscuous are motivated by a need to prove to themselves or others that they are attractive or that they possess masculine or feminine qualities. An inability to say No, a need to please others, may be a factor. Sometimes the behavior is aimed at punishing disapproving parents, a spouse, or one's self.

Each case must be studied on its own merits, without a premature negative value judgment on the one hand, and without a naive acceptance of the patient's rationalizations concerning the behavior on the other. At the beginning, the clinician wonders in what way the behavior proves a problem; does the patient enjoy it; is there guilt concerning it; does it appear to meet any needs other than ones primarily related to sex itself? If complications occur (e.g., pregnancy; discovery by a jealous spouse) are these coincidental or are they apparently an unconscious goal? Does the patient want to change the behavior; what has been tried; why has it failed?

Autoerotic practices often are not regarded as deviant, but they may be of clinical significance. Nearly all adolescent boys and many adolescent girls masturbate. Many single people continue this in adult life. Unfounded fears that masturbation will damage health, cause mental illness, or prevent adequate heterosexual functioning together with the guilt feeling of those who believe masturbation to be morally wrong bring some people to clinical attention. A more serious problem exists when masturbation and sexual fantasies are substituted for steps in the direction of adult heterosexuality. The adolescent who does not date and who does not make friends with members of the opposite sex and who masturbates frequently may need therapy. Often, fears of sexuality, fears of the opposite sex, or feelings of inadequacy or insecurity are involved. Also, the schizophrenic and the compulsive may have problems with masturbation. The married person who masturbates frequently may be showing hostility toward or fear of the spouse. Additional marriage problems, sexual and otherwise, may be involved.

REVIEW QUESTIONS

1. List and describe the major types of Psychosexual Disorders.
2. A woman complains that she is often bothered by peeping Toms; she has called the police on several occasions. She does not pull her shades before undressing, and explains, "If you pull your shades, people know you are

undressing. That would encourage sex perverts." What ego defense mechanisms may be involved in her behavior? If she were found to be mentally ill, what might her diagnosis be? What other possibilities are there? Could she be regarded as a Paraphilic?

3.   A woman patient usually does not reach orgasm during intercourse but has multiple orgasms while performing fellatio. How might you diagnose her case? What etiological factors may be involved? How would you treat her? What would be the goals of therapy?

4.   What changes have there been in prevailing attitudes toward sexual behavior in the United States in the past 25 years? Have there been corresponding changes in the incidence and prevalence of various types of sexual behavior? What data do you have to support your answer?

5.   Under what circumstances would you recommend a behavior therapy for Psychosexual Dysfunction? For other Psychosexual Disorders?

6.   A patient has been arrested three times for exhibitionism. A psychiatric examination following his third arrest revealed no positive findings other than his admitted urges toward exposing himself. Would you regard him as potentially dangerous? What elements in the history might lead you to modify your opinion?

SELECTED REFERENCES

1.   Berlin, Fred S., and Carl F. Meinecke: Treatment of sex offenders with anti-androgenic medication: Conceptualization, review of treatment modalities, and preliminary findings. *Am J Psychiatry* 138(5):601-607, 1981.

2.   Comfort, Alex: *Joy of Sex*. New York, Crown, 1972.

3.   Comfort, Alex: *More Joy*. New York, Crown, 1974.

4.   Cordoba, Oscar A., and James L. Chapel: Medroxyprogesterone acetate anti-androgen treatment of hypersexuality in a pedophiliac sex offender. *Am J Psychiatry* 140(8):1036-1039, 1983.

5.   Gagne, Pierre: Treatment of sex offenders with medroxyprogesterone acetate. *Am J Psychiatry* 138(5):644-646, 1981.

6.   Gallup, Gordon G., and Susan D. Suarez: Homosexuality as a by-product of selection for optimal heterosexual strategies. *Perspect Biol Med* 26(2):315-322, 1983.

7.   George, Linda K., and Stephen J. Weiler: Sexuality in middle and late life. *Arch Gen Psychiatry* 38(8):919-923, 1981.

8.   Karpman, B.: Perversions as neuroses (the paraphilic neuroses): Their curability by therapeutic means. *J Crim Psychopathol* 3(2):1-20, 1942.

9.   Kentsmith, David, and Merrill T. Eaton: *Treating Sexual Problems in Medical Practice*. New York, Arco, 1979.

10. Kinsey, A. C., W. B. Pomeroy, C. E. Martin, and P. H. Gebhard: *Sexual Behavior in the Human Female*. Philadelphia, Saunders, 1953.

11. Kinsey, A. C., W. B. Pomeroy, and C. E. Martin: *Sexual Behavior in the Human Male.* Philadelphia, Saunders, 1948.

12. Lothstein, Leslie M.: Sex Reassignment surgery: Historical, bioethical, and theoretical issues. *Am J Psychiatry* 139(4):417-426, 1982.

13. Masters, W. H., and V. E. Johnson: *Human Sexual Inadequacy.* Boston, Little, Brown, 1970.

14. Masters, W. H., and V. E. Johnson: *Human Sexual Response.* Boston, Little, Brown, 1966.

15. Schwartz, Mark F., and William H. Masters: The Masters and Johnson treatment program for dissatisfied homosexual men. *Am J Psychiatry* 141(2):173-218, 1984.

16. Moore, Stan L.: Satyriasis: A case study. *J Clin Psychiatry* 41(8):279-281, 1980.

17. Pattison, E. Mansell, and Myrna Loy Pattison: "Ex-gays": Religiously mediated change in homosexuals. *Am J Psychiatry* 137(12):1553-1562, 1980.

18. Slag, Michael F., John E. Morley, Michael K. Elson, Dace L. Trence, Carrie J. Nelson, Averial E. Nelson, William B. Kinlaw, H. Stephen Beyer, Frank Q. Nuttall, and Rex B. Shafer: Impotence in medical clinic outpatients. *JAMA* 249(13):1736-1740, 1983.

19. Wasserman, Marvin D., Charles P. Pollak, Arthur J. Spielman, and Elliot D. Weitzman: The differential diagnosis of impotence. *JAMA* 243(20):2038-2042, 1980.

20. Wise, Thomas N., Carol Dupkin, and Jon K. Meyer: Partners of distressed transvestites. *Am J Psychiatry* 138(9):1221-1224, 1981.

21. Zuger, Bernard: Early effeminate behavior in boys: Outcome and significance for homosexuality. *J Nerv Ment Dis* 172(2):90-97, 1984.

USE, MISUSE, AND DEPENDENCE

There are a number of chemical substances, naturally occurring and synthetic, which alter mood or state of consciousness and are spoken of as psychoactive. Many psychoactive drugs are used medically to treat mental and emotional disorders and to relieve symptoms accompanying other illnesses. Some of these, as well as other psychoactive substances which have no established medical uses, are used for purposes that are sometimes described as recreational. Caffeine-containing beverages, nicotine, alcohol, and marijuana are among the psychoactive substances most commonly used for nonmedical purposes.

Though psychoactive drugs have been used by some groups in connection with religious rituals and observances, other religious groups regard some or all recreational uses as unnatural or immoral apart from such demonstrable harm as the drug use may have for the person or for society as a whole. Varying viewpoints about the moral issues involved and inconsistent social attitudes toward the use of various substances create some confusion when one wishes to consider the clinical consequences of nonmedical drugs use objectively.

Many, perhaps all psychoactive drugs have a potential, often dependent upon the amount or frequency of use, for harming the user and for creating social problems. The harmful effects of an otherwise beneficial drug are sometimes spoken of as side effects. In medical use, one must weigh probable benefits against possible adverse consequences. A person using a psychoactive drug for nonmedical purposes must make similar value judgments. Unfortunately, such judgments are not always rational (cf. Chapter 1: Can a smoker honestly and rationally state that the pleasures associated with cigarette smoking are worth the added risk of lung cancer?).

The nonmedical use of a psychoactive drug, legal or otherwise, does not in itself merit a diagnosis. However, the possibility that the user has a Substance Use Disorder should be evaluated.

The diagnosis of Substance Use Disorder applies to the behavioral consequences of the substance use and not to Central Nervous System damage caused by the drug. If a patient develops an Organic Mental Disorder, including intoxication, while under the influence of the drug, the psychiatric syndrome is classified as a substance-induced Organic Mental Disorder. Furthermore, the Substance Use Disorders are separated into substance abuse and substance dependence categories. Substance abuse is defined as use of a drug for at least 1 month, with adverse social or occupational consequences, and either habituation or a pathological pattern of usage (behavioral abnormalities which can be directly attributed to the substance used, e.g., blackouts while alcohol intoxicated). Substance dependence requires the development of tolerance to the effects of the drug or a withdrawal syndrome. The course of the substance abuse or dependence is subclassified as: continuous, episodic, in remission, or unspecified.

Substance Use Disorders are classified as follows:

1. Alcohol abuse
2. Alcohol dependence (alcoholism)
3. Barbiturate or similarly-acting sedative or hypnotic abuse
4. Barbiturate or similarly-acting sedative or hypnotic dependence
5. Opioid abuse
6. Opioid dependence
7. Cocaine abuse
8. Amphetamine or similarly acting sympathomimetic abuse
9. Amphetamine or similarly acting sympathomimetic dependence
10. Phencyclidine (PCP) or similarly acting arylcyclohexylamine abuse
11. Hallucinogen abuse
12. Cannabis abuse
13. Cannabis dependence
14. Tobacco dependence
15. Other, mixed or unspecified substance abuse
16. Unspecified substance dependence
17. Dependence on combination of opioid and other nonalcoholic substance
18. Dependence on combination of substances, excluding opioids and alcohol

WHAT IS ALCOHOL ABUSE AND DEPENDENCE?

Alcohol abuse and dependence are defined using the general criteria listed above. Alcoholism is defined as a condition in which repeated use of alcoholic beverages has an adverse effect on the drinker's general health, vocational adjustment, or social adjustment.

If the alcohol-dependent person drinks daily, it is termed continuous alcohol dependence, while if there are sporadic periods of sobriety, it is labeled episodic alcohol dependence. In official nomenclature (see Chapter 4), alcohol dependence and alcoholism are synonymous.

The word "alcoholic" is likely to bring to mind first the skid row derelict, unemployed and unemployable, with a history of repeated arrests for drunkenness. However, this stereotype represents at most only an advanced stage of one type of Alcoholism. There are other drunks who do not reach skid row and who are unknown to the police, whose use of alcohol is gravely symptomatic. Examples: (1) A businessman each day drinks cocktails before lunch, a highball or two in the afternoon, several more cocktails before dinner, and additional drinks in the evening. He rarely misses a day of work and there are no complaints about his performance on the job. His social life is essentially normal. He never appears to be intoxicated. However, his intake of alcohol in relation to other nutrients leads to fatty infiltration of the liver and ultimately death from hepatic cirrhosis. (2) A housewife drinks each afternoon and evening. If callers arrive in the evening, they note that her speech is slurred and her gait unsteady. Often she sleeps late in the morning and neglects her housework. Her husband, tiring of the situation, spends increasingly more time away from home, becomes involved with another woman, and a divorce ensues. (3) A successful salesman never drinks during working hours, but each evening after dinner sits before the television with a glass and bottle and drinks until he drowsily staggers to bed. He and his family have essentially no social or recreational activities. (4) A rising young executive becomes extremely tense in stress situations. He keeps a bottle in his desk and has a drink or two when he feels anxious. This does not happen often, but it occurs frequently enough to give rise to rumors about his drinking habits. He is passed over for promotion. (5) A young woman rarely drinks, but when she does she takes one drink after another until someone takes her home or she passes out. At such times she loses a number of inhibitions. The consequences have included a break-up of an engagement, the loss of a job (after telling off her supervisor at an office party), the alienation of several friends, and unplanned pregnancy.

Though one can define and diagnose Alcohol Abuse or Dependence on the basis of descriptive criteria, such a definition does not address the nature and cause of alcohol problems. In the past, and to some extent today, intemperance was viewed as a moral problem rather than a medical one. Alcohol abuse was thought to be voluntary; dependence a result of repeated use of the substance itself. That is, drinking causes alcoholism. Currently, alcoholism is widely regarded as a disease, a single clinical entity. However, it is also possible that there are different kinds of alcoholism with different causes and that the abuse or dependence is more a symptom than a disease itself.

HOW MANY PEOPLE HAVE ALCOHOL PROBLEMS?

It is difficult to arrive at an accurate estimate of the incidence and prevalence of alcohol problems. Estimates based on the number of patients diagnosed or receiving treatment fail to include the problem drinkers who do not seek help and whose social behavior is not so aberrant as to require police intervention. The Jellinek formula, which is the basis of some estimates, relates the prevalence of Alcoholism to deaths from cirrhosis of the liver.

There are probably 10 million alcohol-dependent people in the United States. In the past it has been estimated that there are four times as many men with alcohol dependency as women. Certainly there are materially more men who are hospitalized for alcohol dependence, participate in alcohol treatment programs, or have alcohol-related arrests. Despite this, many clinicians believe that there are almost as many women with alcohol problems as men. It has been estimated that about one of every 13 alcohol users becomes a problem drinker, and in the United States there are about 120 million people who drink alcohol.

CAUSES OF ALCOHOL PROBLEMS

There are a number of factors which may play a part in the production of alcohol problems. These factors are discussed below.

Biological factors

There is an apparent familial predisposition to alcohol abuse and dependence. It has been reported that children raised separately from alcoholic parents have a fourfold greater frequency of alcoholic dependence than controls. Twin studies report 50 to 70 percent of identical twins to be concordant for alcoholism, but only about 25 percent of fraternal twins are concordant for this disorder. This may be the result of a genetically determined error in the metabolism of alcohol. A possibly related finding is that members of various ethnic groups react to and metabolize alcohol in different ways. Familial factors in alcoholism may be related to those contributing to Attention Deficit Disorders in childhood and to Affective Disorders. Children who have Attention Deficit Disorder are at risk for developing alcoholism as adults, and Affective Disorders frequently occur in alcoholics before as well as after the development of Alcohol Dependence. There are other hypotheses concerning biological factors. Some see the alcohol misuser as having a sensitivity, an allergy to alcohol. Others believe that the transition from social, controlled drinking to problem drinking occurs after long use of alcohol tends to damage an organ or system necessary for normal alcohol detoxication.

Social factors

By definition alone, social attitudes create some alcohol problems. A departure from established social ritual in the use of alcohol may lead to impaired social adjustment; drinking that is symptomatic in one social group may be "normal" in another. It is interesting and not altogether irrelevant that in a major study in social psychology in which an attempt was made to determine the prevalence of emotional disturbance in a population group, one of the signs sought was intoxication at an inappropriate hour. In our culture, even though some of us come closer to needing a drink in the morning than any other time, it is clearly more symptomatic to be inebriated at 8:00 AM than at 8:00 PM. On the other hand, a social group that is tolerant of alcohol intoxication, or even encourages it, may contribute to those alcohol problems manifested by impaired general health.

Another role of society in relation to alcohol use lies in its provision of facilities for recreational and social activities that do not include drinking, and in the provision of socially acceptable ways of relieving tension.

Poverty undoubtedly plays a role in the etiology of some alcohol problems. So does the general level of stress in the social environment. Though stress may be viewed as an individual, experiential, or psychological factor, social customs contribute to the total stresses experienced by the person.

Experiential factors

Experiential factors associated with alcohol problems include identifications with people who use alcohol symptomatically, use of alcohol to meet various emotional needs, and use of alcohol to relieve or narcotize unpleasant affective states.

The Effects of Alcohol

One approach to the question of why people develop alcohol problems lies in inspecting the effect of drink upon the individual. Alcohol has several effects which may lead certain individuals to use it repeatedly and at times to a symptomatic degree, some of which are discussed below.

Tranquilizing or Sedative Effect

Alcohol relieves anxiety and tension. It is "the people's tranquilizer." In moderate dosage this may be a desirable effect. Misuse of alcohol as a tranquilizer may relate to a limited ability to tolerate stress in some cases or to the magnitude of environmental stresses in others. The effects of stress in the etiology of alcohol use can be demonstrated in animal experiments. Laboratory animals generally reject beverages containing alcohol when they have a choice. However, if the animals are placed under stress (e.g., conditioned to perform certain operations to obtain rewards and then are given electric shocks or other unpleasant stimuli at times instead of rewards) they develop a preference for alcohol.

Increasing Aggressivity or Ability to Express Aggression

In the past, the idea that alcohol gave one strength and courage was accepted as common knowledge. During the American Revolution it was customary for troops to be provided with a rum ration before battles or forced marches, and contemporary historians attributed the loss of the Battle of Camden, perhaps America's greatest military defeat in that war, to the fact that rum was not available.

The belief that alcohol makes people braver (or not so frightened?) is less commonly held today, but many patients with alcohol problems refer directly or indirectly to feeling more aggressive or better able to assert themselves when asked what subjective changes occur when they drink.

Alteration of Mood

Some people become more cheerful when they drink; others become morose. People speak of "drowning their sorrow" in alcohol, but sorrow is a good swimmer. The apparent euphoriant effect which alcohol, basically a depressant, has is not fully understood. It may be due to sensorium clouding, though it is experienced with amounts too small to cause one to actually forget one's troubles; it may be a conditioned response related to the circumstances under which alcohol is usually consumed; or there may be a biochemical basis for it. The fact that any reduction of depression while drinking is more than offset by the feelings of the morning-after does not keep some depressed people from drinking or some relatively healthy people from wanting to drink at times of grief. Conversely, many manic patients increase alcohol use (sometimes with a deliberate intent to control symptoms).

Relaxation of Inhibitions

Alcohol is a superego solvent. It weakens cortical controls and permits more expression of id impulses. This may be a factor in increased expression of aggression. Some sexual impulses that are otherwise suppressed or repressed find expression under the influence of alcohol. Other conflicts may be resolved in favor of the id (e.g., a rather demure young woman who, despite strong exhibitionistic drives, usually does nothing that could be described as showing off sings, dances, and does imitations after having a few drinks at a party).

In some groups this effect of alcohol is reenforced by social attitudes which tend to excuse otherwise unacceptable behavior on the basis of intoxication ("He didn't mean anything by it, he was just a little high"). Instead of "in vino veritas," it is "Pay no attention to her, she's loaded."

Facilitating Social Contacts

Contrary to some popular opinion, most people with alcohol problems are not solitary drinkers. Many go to considerable effort to find a place to drink with other people. The tavern, the club, and the cocktail party are places where one may find others to talk with and where one may feel relatively free to strike up conversation with strangers. This opportunity, coupled with some relaxation of inhibitions, makes the drinking place especially comforting to the shy, lonely person.

Self-destructive Effect

The generally undesirable effects of alcohol dependence, the impairment of health, and the loss of social status may be unconsciously, or more or less consciously sought by the person with suicidal, masochistic, or other self-punishing and self-destroying impulses.

The Personality of the Alcohol Abuser

Another way of exploring the causes of alcohol problems is to study the personality types of problem drinkers. Many attempts have been made through psychological studies to predict alcohol dependence and to recognize an alcoholic personality without access to a history of problem drinking. A reason for failure of these studies to be conclusive and replicable lies in the fact that there are several common personality types among problem drinkers. These types are discussed below.

The Passive, Oral Dependent Type

Some patients with alcohol problems show a number of personality traits suggestive of fixation or regression to early oral stages of psychosexual development. They tend to be relatively helpless and inadequate and to depend on others. Smoking and eating habits together with other mouth activities may also suggest an oral character structure. It is more than a figure of speech to suggest that for them the liquor bottle symbolizes the nursing bottle or the breast. They drink to the extent of increased helplessness, increased need to be cared for by others.

The Compulsive Type

Some people who become alcohol dependent have primarily anal character structures. They are often hard-working and sometimes successful people. In some cases their use of alcohol seems to be a typical compulsion. They feel impelled to drink though they do not want to do it, nor do they enjoy the drinking as do the oral characters. Some need drinks daily; others maintain sobriety for periods of time, then after the first drink, they lose control and are unable to stop. In other relatively compulsive personalities, the alcohol problem is an indirect result of the character structure; these are people who do well at work but do not know how to relax. A feeling of being at a loss for something to do, coupled with fatigue, makes drinking a problem in their leisure hours.

The Sociopathic Drinker

The alcohol habits of Antisocial Personalities are discussed in Chapter 7 (Personality and Impulse Disorders).

The Symptomatic Drinker

There are patients whose drinking seems directly related to symptoms of emotional illness. Alcohol dependence may be symptomatic of psychiatric illness ranging from Adjustment Disorders to Schizophrenia. However, some problem drinkers do not have sufficient symptoms to justify another diagnosis, but nevertheless drink to relieve anxiety, depression, or loneliness. These often represent neurotic, cyclothymic, and schizoid personalities at what may otherwise be a subclinical level.

The Facultative Alcohol Abuser

A habit of drinking at a symptomatic level and some physiological dependence can develop in people who have no particular emotional need for alcohol. Bartenders, sales people working in settings in which it is customary to offer prospective customers a drink, and men and women whose social life involves almost daily attendance at functions at which liquor is served are likely to become facultative alcoholics. They differ from other people with alcohol problems in that when they become aware that their drinking is interfering with health, work, or social adjustment they are often able to modify it with relative ease.

Symptoms and Course

Since there are many types of alcohol problems, a description of symptoms and course cannot be expected to apply to all patients. The following stages are, however, observed in a number of patients.

Prodromal Phase

Though a few patients develop alcohol problems soon after they start to drink, most people have a period of 5, 10, or more years of controlled social drinking before alcohol use becomes symptomatic. During this period, some tolerance for alcohol appears. Larger amounts of alcohol are required to produce signs of intoxication, and alcohol is better tolerated by the gastrointestinal tract. The patient usually regards the effect of alcohol as pleasant, has no concern about drinking, and does not let drinking interfere with social life or work. There may not be any periods of marked intoxication. However, occasional drunkenness may occur in settings in which it is socially tolerated or encouraged (e.g., the college student who drinks a bucket of beer as part of his initiation into a fraternity).

Early Symptomatic Phase

At this time there is a definite dependence on alcohol. Drinking occurs daily. If alcohol is omitted, there is likely to be irritability, insomnia, and tremor. The patient may have a need for a morning drink. He or she tends to avoid social events at which alcohol is not served, or else takes alcohol along, or makes a point of drinking immediately before and immediately after.

In this stage the tolerance for alcohol may be maintained or may begin to decline. If it declines, the patient more frequently shows signs of intoxication. She or he becomes defensive about drinking, makes attempts to conceal the extent of alcohol use, and may worry about drinking and make attempts to control, ration, or stop drinking. A few patients in this stage enter therapy.

Family and social life are likely to be affected adversely. There is impaired efficiency at work. This is true whether there is drinking on the job or not. One does not work efficiently with a hangover. Absenteeism often increases. It has been estimated that employees with alcohol problems have about 22 days per year more absenteeism than the average employee.

Advanced Symptomatic Phase

Dependence on alcohol increases; tolerance decreases. Signs of intoxication are often observed. Periods of amnesia, "blackouts" while drinking, become frequent. Social, recreational, and occupational activities diminish as the patient's life becomes centered around drinking. Domestic crises occur. Jobs are lost. There may be arrests for public intoxication or drunken driving. Some patients continue to worry about drinking, attempt periods of abstinence, and may seek therapy. Others rationalize and/or project; they may blame their drinking on some person or circumstance. Physical changes include chronic gastritis and fatty infiltration of the liver. There may be some decrease in thyroid function.

Terminal Phase

Damage to the nervous system resulting in an Organic Mental Disorder is likely. Pancreatitis, cirrhosis of the liver, and nutritional deficiencies are usual. Untreated alcohol dependence is ultimately fatal.

Spontaneous Remissions

During the course of development of alcohol dependence, spontaneous remissions, temporary or lasting, may occur. Evidence of this is found in the biographies of patients seen for other reasons; there are some notable examples among historical personages. Remission is most likely in the early symptomatic phase but may occur at any stage of the disorder. Factors producing remission include the following.

Environmental Changes

Reductions in environmental stress or new ways of meeting emotional needs may contribute to remission.

Success in Voluntary Control of Drinking Habits

In early stages, patients who become aware of alcohol problems are sometimes able to reestablish controlled drinking. This possibility should not be overlooked in the management of early or borderline cases, but on the other hand, it should not be a basis for long delay of treatment.

A Decision to Quit Drinking

Some patients are able to implement such a decision without medical or other specific help. Sometimes this follows a particularly distressing episode resulting from alcohol use. It may come from a general awareness of the problem without a precipitating incident. It may be related to a decision to undertake some new activity; the patient stops drinking in order to achieve some other goal. Joining a religious group that forbids alcohol use was probably the commonest cause of remission of alcohol dependence until comparatively recent times.

Diagnosis

The prevalence of alcohol problems is such that the possibility of alcohol dependence should be considered in any complete psychiatric or general medical examination whatever the presenting complaint. Early diagnosis facilitates treatment
and prevents complications of the later phases.

A vague question about how much the patient drinks (generally answered and
recorded socially) is not likely to provide relevant information. The patient finds
the subject embarrassing and avoids furnishing details that are not requested. One
should ascertain what alcoholic beverages the patient uses, how frequently, and in
what quantity. If the quantity is sufficient to alert one to the possibility of an alcohol problem, further information concerning social and vocational adjustment is
necessary.

Patients may use mechanisms of rationalization, denial, projection, dissociation, and their conscious analogs to conceal from themselves the presence of alcohol problems. Direct questioning about alcohol problems may not elicit necessary
information even if the patient is really trying to be completely honest and candid.

Too often a patient is not told of the diagnosis or clinical suspicion of alcohol
dependence until the condition is far advanced. Fear of offending or frightening a
patient by raising the possibility of a potentially fatal disorder does not justify
withholding the diagnosis and recommendation for treatment.

Identification of problem drinking is inadequate for complete diagnosis. The
clinician must determine the type of alcohol problem and decide to what extent it
may be related to other emotional difficulties (e.g., anxiety, depression, dependency problems) before recommending appropriate treatment.

Patients who are concerned over their drinking habits when these are within
socially accepted limits and do not appear to interfere with health, occupation, or
social life, present another type of diagnostic problem. They may be healthy persons who need nothing more than reassurance; they may have other emotional problems, the concern about which is displaced to drinking, or they may be in the prodromal phase of alcohol abuse.

Prevention

Improvement of the Social Milieu

Elimination of poverty, reduction in the amount of stress in the environment, development of facilities for recreational and social activities that do not involve
drinking, and provision of socially acceptable ways of discharging tension can contribute to a reduction in the prevalence of alcohol problems.

Education

Young people should be instructed in the use of alcohol. They should recognize
the dangers of intemperance and risks of habituation. Risks involved in daily drinking should be emphasized. Adults should be taught to recognize the early signs of
alcohol problems in themselves and in members of their families. In industry, su-
pervisory personnel should learn to recognize alcohol problems and refer them for
treatment.

Identification of Early Potential or
Subclinical Alcohol Problems

Patients can modify potentially unhealthy drinking habits with relative ease before actual alcohol problems develop. If patients at times drink to relieve discomfort or to meet emotional needs, treatment of the underlying problems may prevent subsequent alcohol dependence.

Treatment

Patients with alcohol problems can be treated as outpatients if they present themselves during a period of sobriety. Also, some patients in the early symptomatic phase who are drinking daily can be treated without hospitalization. This can be considered if the patient is able to maintain employment and come to appointments regularly.

Motivation, recognition that alcohol has become a problem, and a wish to stop drinking are important, but these do not always need to be present at the beginning of therapy. If the patient still feels able to control drinking, one can encourage trying, but at the same time set a time limit on such efforts. In some cases it is desirable to have several appointments to establish a firm therapeutic relationship before attempting reduction or elimination of alcohol use.

In treating the alcohol abuser as a voluntary outpatient, the therapist's role in helping the patient stop drinking, not compelling it, must be clear to both physician and patient. The relationship should be such that the patient can feel comfortable and not afraid of criticism in reporting a relapse. Patients with alcohol problems have low self-esteem and require considerable support. They must feel that they are being treated with respect. Caution must be exercised in expressive or investigative psychotherapy. Any uncovering of conflictual material produces anxiety, and patients with alcohol problems can tolerate little anxiety without risk of increased alcohol use. Other features of the psychotherapy of the alcoholic depend upon the personality structure and the underlying causes of the drinking.

At the time when the patient decides to stop drinking, he or she is likely to experience some withdrawal effects and can benefit from tranquilizing medication. Use of medication beyond the withdrawal period is indicated only if free-floating anxiety contributes to the alcohol problems, or if there is another psychiatric disorder present which requires medication (e.g., Schizophrenia; Bipolar Affective Disorder).

Referral to Alcoholics Anonymous is frequently indicated. This self-help group meets many of the needs of persons with alcohol problems. Often, however, patients have tried AA before coming to psychiatric attention. Some patients are unable or unready to accept some of the features of AA, such as its "togetherness" or its quasireligious elements. Patients should not be referred to AA until thorough study rules out underlying psychiatric conditions in addition to alcohol dependence. If individual therapy is not used in addition to referral, follow-up appointments should be given to help evaluate progress and determine if other treatment is needed.

Disulfiram (Antabuse) is useful in some cases. This drug blocks the enzyme alcohol dehydrogenase (which converts alcohol to carbon dioxide and water) and causes the patient to become violently ill if she or he drinks alcoholic beverages. It helps prevent taking a drink on impulse. Patients must be well motivated and able to recognize the risks in taking disulfiram. If the patient does take a small amount of alcohol within 12 to 24 hours of taking disulfiram (in some cases the effects persist as long as 2 weeks), he or she will experience minor symptoms including headache, nausea, and palpitations; these are enough to keep one from drinking more. However, if a large quantity of alcohol is taken quickly, the result may be fatal. Disulfiram is contraindicated in cardiac decompensation and should be used with caution, if at all, in cases of any cardiac or hepatic disorder. Usually, it should not be started unless the patient has been abstinent from alcohol for several days; exceptions require a special treatment routine. Disulfiram must never be given without the patient's knowledge. Because of potentially dangerous drug interactions, disulfiram should not be given to patients taking antidepressants, dopamine-blocking agents such as phenothiazines, or drugs that affect the regulation of blood pressure.

Several other alcohol-sensitizing drugs have been studied, but none is widely used in the United States. In addition to alcohol-sensitizing drugs, a variety of other medications have been reported to reduce alcohol consumption, but their value lacks adequate confirmation. Lithium, which reduces alcohol consumption by animals, is of questionable value except for patients who have depression along with their alcoholism. Tricyclic antidepressants are also helpful in reducing alcohol consumption when depression is a feature of the disorder.

Aversive conditioning, once widely used, is still sometimes recommended. New techniques are under investigation. Other behavior therapies, including some which use positive reinforcement for modified drinking patterns have been tried, but follow-up studies indicate that these have not been successful.

Most patients in the advanced symptomatic phase require inpatient treatment. The initial phase of inpatient treatment includes detoxication, management of withdrawal symptoms, correction of nutritional deficiencies, and treatment of hepatic and gastrointestinal complications. Supplemental vitamins, including high doses of thiamine and folic acid, are usually given. Magnesium deficiency, due to urinary loss of the magnesium cation and a possible factor in the development of encephalopathies, should be corrected. Tranquilizing medicine, usually chlordiazepoxide, is required for the patient's comfort and may help prevent withdrawal delirium. After the first few days, tranquilizing medication is gradually reduced and should usually be discontinued within 2 weeks to avoid possible habituation. Dephenylhydantoin may be given to reduce the risk of convulsions during withdrawal.

Following the initial phase of treatment, best results are obtained with a comprehensive program of treatment and rehabilitation involving group living in a therapeutic milieu, group, and/or individual psychotherapy, education concerning alcohol problems, vocational counseling and vocational rehabilitation if needed, and ultimately follow-up outpatient care. A 6-month follow-up is adequate for most cases; however, some patients require lifelong professional attention.

Complete and permanent abstinence is the primary goal of alcoholism treatment. However, most reports of treatment results as well as giving the number of patients recovering list some others as improved. These are people who are drinking less, having less frequent drinking bouts, and/or having fewer alcohol-related problems in living. Even if the alcoholic does not recover, some benefit may result from treatment.

Recovering patients are advised never to take a drink of an alcoholic beverage under any circumstance. This is good advice; if one does not take the first drink, there will be no recurrence. However, one should not belabor the point to the extent that relapse after a single drink becomes a self-fulfilling prophecy. It takes up to 4 days to reestablish dependence on alcohol. The chief danger in taking the first drink lies in developing a false sense of security about drinking.

One advises permanent abstinence and advises against attempts to reestablish social drinking even after prolonged periods of abstinence. Rarely, one encounters a person who has had an alcohol problem but who has successfully resumed moderate drinking. However, the risk of recurrence is too great to make an attempt at social drinking advisable.

In treating people with alcohol problems one tries to avoid relapses. Patients are urged to seek help at times of stress or when an urge to drink becomes difficult to control. Nevertheless, one expects some relapses. Scolding the relapsing patient does not help; one simply resumes treatment and is glad if the patient seeks it promptly.

While abstinence, or at least reduced alcohol intake, is a sine qua non for recovery from an alcohol problem, it is not the sole measure of recovery. For the patient to be well, except for the facultative alcoholic, other personality changes must occur as a result of therapy. The overall emotional well-being of the individual must be considered in evaluating results.

Opioid Abuse and Dependence

Opiate addiction occurs in:

1.   Patients who develop dependence on drugs while they are being prescribed for the relief of pain.
2.   Persons who have relatively easy access to narcotics (e.g., physicians, nurses, pharmacists) and may be tempted to take them for the relief of minor discomforts.
3.   Individuals who begin the use of narcotics for psychological reasons under sociological and cultural influences. Among adolescents, curiosity, peer pressure, and hedonism rather than pain are among the reasons for beginning drug use. One the other hand, for some patients, environmental stresses, anxiety, and/or feelings of inferiority may be factors. Beliefs prevalent in some subcultures that drugs, especially heroin, produce bravery and sexual prowess (priapism is common in the early stages of opiate addiction; prolonged use causes a loss of sexual capacities) may contribute to some initial experimental use of drugs. The feeling of well-being accompanying drug use encourages repetition, and ultimately, dependence occurs.

As in the diagnosis of alcohol problems, the categorization of abuse and dependence upon opiates follows the general criteria for all substances.

The use of opiates produces some clouding of sensorium and impairment of intellectual function. As tolerance develops, these symptoms of intoxication are often less marked; however, a general loss of energy, ambition, and drive develops which interferes with work and other constructive activities. As the effects of each dose of the drug wear off, early withdrawal symptoms such as restlessness and discomfort cause the opiate dependent to seek medication. Since he or she requires steadily increasing doses, and since the drugs are difficult and/or expensive to obtain, the patient's life begins to revolve around efforts to maintain a supply of narcotics.

Diagnosis

Diagnosis of opiate dependence is usually made from a history furnished by the patient or by family members. The patient furnishes a history when:

1.   Genuinely seeking treatment for dependence (addiction).
2.   Deprived of the drug and needing treatment for withdrawal symptoms. This may occur when illegal supplies are cut off; it also occurs when the patient is hospitalized or incarcerated for any reason.

3. The habit gets too expensive. While many addicts regard their addictions as harmful, some do not. They hope to reduce physical dependence so as to obtain the results they feel are beneficial from smaller doses so as to be able to use narcotics for euphoria rather than to ward off withdrawal symptoms.
4. Trying to "cop a plea." The user in trouble with the law hopes that an apparent motivation for change will result in leniency.

In the absence of history, opiate dependence may be suspected when:

1. Patients appear to be malingering symptoms of painful illness so as to obtain a narcotics prescription.
2. Patients show signs of mild intoxication, lethargy, and a cyclic pattern of elation alternating with irritability.
3. Pupillary constriction (miosis) and scarring from hypodermic injections ("tracks") may occasionally be signs that arouse suspicion of addiction.
4. Diagnosis can also be made by hospitalizing the patient to remove easy access to drugs. However, patients entering a hospital may bring with them concealed supplies of drugs or may persuade visitors to supply them. Definite withdrawal symptoms begin between 8 and 48 hours after the last dose depending upon which narcotic is used. Withdrawal symptoms, more or less in the order of appearance, include:
    a. Anxiety and irritability together with a heightened desire (the yen) for narcotics
    b. Muscle cramps, chills, nasal stuffiness, watering eyes, nausea, and tremor
    c. Dilated pupils (mydriasis), piloerection ("goose flesh"), vomiting, marked insomnia, and agitation

Occasionally a test using a morphine antagonist, naloxone hydrochloride (Narcan), with caution, to precipitate withdrawal symptoms is justified. This test, of course, does not reveal meperidine (Demerol) addiction.

Prevention

In prescribing medication for relief of pain, physicians should be alert to risks of dependence. Special caution should be used in prescribing narcotics for relatively minor discomfort in patients who have dependent needs or experience noxious emotional states which might encourage the misuse of medication. The physician should evaluate the emotional state and personality of any patient for whom narcotics are prescribed. A casualness in prescribing mild narcotics (e.g., cough syrups containing opium for colds; codeine for menstrual cramps) based on the fact that these rarely are used by opiate dependents is unwarranted; the susceptible person who finds some relief from mild narcotics may be tempted to change to stronger ones (few alcoholics get drunk on crème de menthe or "pink ladies," but some were introduced to alcohol with such beverages).

If patients experiencing severe pain require medication over a protracted period, tolerance should be avoided by changing from one drug to another and, at times, omitting narcotics (other drugs which offer some relief of pain together with hypnotics can be used for a brief period). It is often suggested that patients not be told the names of opiate drugs they are receiving. In some instances it is appropriate to allow dependence to develop in terminal and/or incurable illnesses. If the source of pain is removed, patients who have developed an addiction in this way usually respond more favorably to treatment than do street addicts who take opioids primarily for their euphoric effect.

Instruction of medical and nursing students and others who have access to drugs should include warnings of the dangers, medical as well as legal, of taking drugs on one's own prescription.

Social action to eliminate poverty and some of the stresses of slum living can do much to reduce the prevalence of nonmedical dependencies. Enforcement of laws against the illegal sale of narcotics has been partially successful (certainly more successful than attempts at prohibition of alcohol); however, there are some who believe that if clinics could supply certain known addicts with regulated doses of drugs, the illegal narcotics traffic would be further discouraged by elimination of much of its profit.

Treatment

For all practical purposes, treatment of opiate dependence requires hospitalization. On admission, a thorough medical evaluation is done and treatment for illnesses other than the dependence itself is started. Infections, including hepatitis from the use of contaminated needles, are often present and there may be nutritional deficiencies. Other psychiatric disorders which may underlie the addiction must also be identified and treated.

The addict is observed until beginning withdrawal symptoms, at least pupillary dilatation, in presumed heroin addicts, are present. At that point, medication is started to control withdrawal symptoms. For heroin addicts, methadone hydrochloride (Dolphine) or its longer-acting derivative, methadyl acetate, is usually substituted for the drug the patient has been taking. The use of methadone is covered by federal regulations and methadone products can be dispensed only by authorized hospital pharmacies and by maintenance programs approved by the Food and Drug Administration and the designated state authority.

In selecting the dose of methadone, objective signs of withdrawal symptoms rather than the patient's history of the amount of drugs taken and the complaints of subjective discomfort are used. Patients may exaggerate amounts taken and discomfort experienced in the hope of getting more drugs, and even if an addict gives accurate information about the amount taken, the drugs that were used might have been adulterated. Overdosage is dangerous. A single dose of 15 to 20 mg of methadone may be sufficient to suppress withdrawal symptoms, but when patients are physically dependent on high doses of heroin or other opioids, repeated doses are often needed. Forty milligrams per day in divided oral doses usually constitutes an adequate stabilizing dosage level. After 2 or 3 days the dose of methadone can usually be decreased gradually (a 20 percent reduction at daily or 2-day intervals). A detoxication treatment course with methadone cannot legally exceed 21 days unless medical complications occur.

Instead of having methadone withdrawn, some patients are placed on a methadone maintenance program. The stabilizing dose may be continued indefinitely until the patient is physically and emotionally ready for withdrawal. This must be done in an approved methadone maintenance program.

A successful treatment program for narcotic addicts cannot be limited to detoxication and/or maintenance. It must include follow-up care and vocational rehabilitation. Individual and group psychotherapy are often indicated. In some areas there are self-help groups for addicts comparable to Alcoholics Anonymous. Other methods for treatment of dependence, including those using narcotic antagonists and various behavioral techniques, are still under study.

One of the risks associated with narcotic addiction and with methadone maintenance is overdosage (though some deaths attributed to overdosage are actually due to allergic phenomena). Naloxone (Narcan), a narcotic antagonist, is used to treat overdosage when respiration is compromised.

Minor Tranquilizers, Sedatives, and Hypnotics

The group comprising minor tranquilizers, sedatives, and hypnotics includes the drugs most commonly prescribed in the United States. As with alcohol, the two categories are those of abuse and dependence. All compounds in this group are associated with physiological addiction if large enough doses are used for a long enough time.

The addicting dose of chlordiazepoxide is about 300 mg, and diazepam about 100 mg daily for 2 to 4 weeks. The withdrawal syndrome is sometimes delayed with these two agents and may not occur for 1 to 2 weeks after the last dose. This is to be kept in mind in the differential diagnosis of an Organic Mental Disorder with delirium which develops in a patient hospitalized for another reason (e.g., a surgical procedure).

Withdrawal syndromes from minor tranquilizers and sedative-hypnotic agents are medical emergencies and require inpatient management. Tranquilizers should always be decreased slowly over time, since death occurs in about 15 percent of patients who cease them abruptly and do not receive treatment. For withdrawal purposes, one can use either the agent which the patient used, since all drugs in this category are prescription drugs, or one can convert the medication into an equivalent dose of phenobarbital and use it. Agents which lower seizure threshold, e.g., phenothiazines, should be used with caution, if at all.

Stimulant Abuse and Dependence

Cocaine is a short-acting stimulant which may be snorted into the nose or taken parenterally. The user experiences a feeling of euphoria or elation and becomes hyperactive. The drug is harmful to the general health of the user. Large doses over a period of time lead to psychotic reactions accompanied by hallucinations. Among the symptoms are haptic hallucinations (formication, tactile sensations, "the cocaine bug").

Amphetamine is another stimulant which produces euphoria, hyperactivity, and impaired judgment. Prolonged use of large doses invariably leads to the development of paranoid psychoses. Some addicts use massive doses (up to 200 times normal therapeutic doses) of amphetamine parenterally. Sometimes known as "speed freaks," these patients show sleeplessness, excitement, and irritability; they may develop toxic deliria or paranoid or schizophreniform psychoses.

Persons who have been habituated to stimulants for a prolonged period or who have been using high doses should be hospitalized for withdrawal. At the beginning of withdrawal the patient often falls into a deep sleep that lasts for 24 to 72 hours. On awakening, depression is present and there is an appreciable suicide risk. As in the case of other addictions, treatment cannot be limited to detoxication. Vocational rehabilitation and psychotherapy may be necessary. In planning treatment, one must identify the underlying problems which caused the need for stimulants in the first place.

Phencyclidine (PCP) and Hallucinogen Abuse

Drugs which produce hallucinations such as mescaline (peyote) and psylocibin (present in certain mushrooms) have been used ritualistically by subcultural groups and have occasionally been misused in the United States for many years, but only recently has the use of these drugs become a major problem.

Phencyclidine (Sernylan) is an animal tranquilizer which has hallucinogenic effects in humans. It is commonly called angel dust or hog. This hallucinogen became popular during the 1970s. The intoxication syndrome is that of an Organic Mental Disorder. Psychotic behavior with aggressive and paranoid features, as well as coma, can result from the use of phencyclidine. Some investigators feel that nystagmus is a prominent feature of overdose of this drug.

Experimentation with LSD-25 (lysergic acid diethylamide) became popular among young people in the 1960s, in part because psychedelic or mind expanding properties have been attributed to it. Aside from the experience sometimes being pleasurable and perhaps leading to some apparent insights into the user's personality, there is no evidence for mind expanding properties. At least there is no evidence of improved creativity or intellectual function. The drug causes a transitory toxic psychosis accompanied by hallucinations. Habituation probably occurs in some cases; frequent use tends to interfere with performance in other activities and with the user's overall adjustment. Isolated adverse reactions (bad trips) occur; patients seek hospitalization for persistent disagreeable hallucinations, panic, depression (sometimes with suicidal tendencies), or confusion. Recurring hallucinations after use of the drug has ceased (flashbacks) have been reported, as have been lasting psychotic reactions. The possibility of brain damage associated with misuse of this drug cannot be excluded.

Cannabis Abuse and Dependence

Cannabis, in large doses, acts as an hallucinogen; intoxication includes an early stimulant and later depressant effect. In small doses the drug is a mild euphoriant. Its possession is illegal throughout the United States, though in some states possession of small quantities is a misdemeanor rather than a felony.

The flowering heads of the plant *Cannabis sativa* (marijuana) are usually smoked in the form of cigarettes (joints; pot; tea; grass). Though this drug has long been used by millions of people in various parts of the world, little is known of its long-range effects. There are those who advocate legalization of marijuana in the belief that it is a generally harmless drug which gives pleasure and has fewer detrimental effects than alcohol or tobacco. Others cite reasons why the drug should be viewed as dangerous:

1. Habituation or at least frequent use over long periods of time does occur and may be accompanied by deterioration of personality functioning. How great the risk of habituation is to the occasional user is not known.
2. Acute adverse reactions occur and psychoses are sometimes precipitated.
3. As with any intoxicant, there is interference with judgment, unwise decisions may be made, risks may be taken, and accidents may occur.
4. Users may graduate to more dangerous drugs. We do not know how many marijuana users turned to "hard" drugs and there is an obvious fallacy in drawing a conclusion from the percentage of opiate addicts who have used marijuana. It may be that trying one drug tempts a person to experiment with others; it certainly is true that underworld suppliers try to convert customers to addictive drugs.
5. Physical harm may result from prolonged use. Cannabis can impair the T-cell component of the immune response, which may (or may not) have an important bearing on the total immune response and accordingly on susceptibility to disease. It can also reduce testosterone levels and can alter DNA synthesis, which suggests at least a possibility of danger to the human genetic process.

At present, most psychiatrists advise against Cannabis use, both because the drug is illegal and the user may get in trouble for possessing it, and because the degree of danger inherent in its use is not actually known. Short of advocating legalization of pot (in the sense that legalization would make it readily available to anyone desiring it), some psychiatrists advocate elimination or reduction of penalties for possession, feeling that these are disproportionate and that they interfere with the user's reporting experiences and seeking help when needed.

As with other drugs, not all users, or even all misusers, meet the criteria for a diagnosis of Abuse or Dependence. Cannabis Abuse is diagnosed in cases of more than a month's duration, manifested by almost daily use (or psychotic episodes) and showing impaired social or occupational functioning. For a diagnosis of Cannabis Dependence, tolerance must also be present.

Tobacco Dependence

Tobacco dependence is deemed worthy of attention because of the etiological role tobacco plays in various illnesses (e.g., chronic obstructive pulmonary disease, coronary artery disease, lung cancer). It is diagnosed when a smoker has made serious attempts to discontinue tobacco use, but he or she has been unsuccessful, when efforts to stop smoking have led to withdrawal symptoms, or when a person continues to use tobacco despite having a serious disease that he or she knows is made worse by using tobacco.

Supportive and behavioral psychotherapies have been used to treat Tobacco Dependence. Nicotine chewing gum or other nicotine preparations may prove to be useful during tobacco withdrawal.

Other drugs that are misused include a wide variety of volatile organic solvents found in glues and cements (glue sniffing), nail polish removers, cleaning fluids, paint thinners, etc. Of these intoxicants, some are hallucinogens and most are depressants. Some are productive of tolerance as well as psychological dependence. Brain, liver, and renal damage have occasionally been reported in connection with use of some of these agents, and sudden death sometimes occurs.

Primary prevention of hallucinogen, marijuana, and other drug misuse consists chiefly of educational programs aimed at making adolescents aware of the undesirable consequences and risks associated with drug misuse. Educational programs are also important in secondary prevention to the extent that users are persuaded to quit and, if necessary seek professional help. Programs should not overstate or overdramatize the dangers; to be of value they must be credible.

CRIME AND ADDICTION

Alcohol and Drug Dependence play a major role in the cause of crime. Though some alcohol abusers and some addicts have Antisocial Personalities, the majority do not. Nevertheless, intoxicants impair judgment, weaken cortical controls, and interfere with superego function. Indirectly, addictions contribute to crime, since they reduce employability and earning capacity, so that patients may turn to illegal activities to support themselves. This is accentuated by the dependence on alcohol or drugs and the cost of obtaining them. Hence, the prevention and treatment of alcohol and drug dependence is of intense social concern. However, patients with the conditions are not enemies of society or "fiends"; they are sick people in need of help, not punishment.

REVIEW QUESTIONS

1. Define Alcohol Abuse. Alcohol dependence. Alcoholism.
2. What is the difference between substance abuse and substance dependence?
3. How does one enquire tactfully about drinking habits when taking a medical history? Why?
4. Discuss the outpatient treatment of alcohol problems. Inpatient treatment.
5. What are the indications for using tranquilizing drugs in treatment of alcohol problems? Indications for antidepressants? Disulfiram?
6. Name some narcotic drugs that may produce dependence; some sedative or hypnotic drugs for which dependence occurs.
7. What do you know about methadone maintenance programs? What features make some methadone maintenance programs more successful than others?
8. A high school student who has been near the top of his class begins to do failing work. He smokes pot frequently. Indicate which of the following statements you think is most likely to be true and which least likely (explain): The two facts are unrelated. They result from a common underlying problem. Failure is a result of frequent intoxication (he cannot study when he is high or sleepy). The drug has caused cumulative brain damage. Preoccupation with the drug habit has caused failure (collecting stamps could interfere with school work too if he spent all his time doing it and thinking about it). He has adopted the life style of a social group that deemphasizes school performance.
9. Discuss the potential consequences, advantages, and disadvantages of legalizing marijuana. Of decriminalizing possession of it in small quantities.
10. What percentage of students in professional schools such as law schools and medical schools use marijuana? How do you account for this use among people who should be most likely to be aware of potential adverse medical and legal consequences associated with its use?

SELECTED REFERENCES

1. Brown, Barry S., Gloria J. Benn, and Donald R. Jansen: Methadone maintenance: Some client opinions. *Am J Psychiatry* 132(6):623-626, 1975.

2. Cohn, Sidney: Amphetamine abuse. *JAMA* 231(4):414-415, 1975.

3. Eckardt, Michael J., Ralph S. Ryback, Robert R. Rawlings, and Barry I. Graubard: Biochemical diagnosis of alcoholism: A test of the discriminating capabilities of γ-glutamyl transpeptidase and mean corpuscular volume. *JAMA* 246(23):2707-2710, 1981.

4. Goodwin, Donald W.: The genetics of alcoholism. *Hosp Community Psychiatry* 34(11):1031-1034, 1983.

5. Gottheil, Edward, Arthur I. Alterman, Thomas E. Skoloda, and Brendan F. Murphy: Alcoholics' pattern of controlled drinking. *Am J Psychiatry* 130(4):418-422, 1973.

6. Group for the Advancement of Psychiatry: *Drug Misuse: A Psychiatric View of a Modern Dilemma.* Report No. 80. June, 1971.

7. Kandel, Denise B.: Marijuana users in young adulthood. *Arch Gen Psychiatry* 41(2):200-209, 1984.

8. Ling, Walter, Walter Dorus, William A. Hargreaves, Richard Resnick, Edward Senay, Vicente B. Tuason, Elaine Holmes, C. James Klett, Manual Mejia, and Arthur Weinberg: Alternative induction and crossover schedules for methadyl acetate. *Arch Gen Psychiatry* 41(2):193-199, 1984.

9. McLellan, A. Thomas, Lester Luborsky, George E. Woody, Charles P. O'Brien, and Keith A. Druley: Predicting response to alcohol and drug abuse treatments. *Arch Gen Psychiatry* 40(6):620-625, 1983.

10. McLellan, A. Thomas, George E. Woody, and Charles P. O'Brien: Development of psychiatric illness in drug abusers: Possible role of drug preference. *New Engl J Med* 301(24):1310-1314, 1979.

11. Morse, Robert M., Mary A. Martin, Wendell M. Swenson, and Robert G. Niven: Prognosis of physicians treated for alcoholism and drug dependence. *JAMA* 251(6):743-746, 1984.

12. National Research Council Committee on Clinical Evaluation of Narcotic Antagonists: Clinical evaluation of naltrexone treatment of opiate-dependent individuals. *Arch Gen Psychiatry* 35:335-340, 1978.

13. Neubuerger, Otto W., Sheldon I. Miller, Robert E. Schmitz, Joseph D. Matarazozo, Herb Pratt, and Nancy Hasha: Replicable abstinence rates in an alcoholism treatment program. *JAMA* 248(8):960-963, 1982.

14. Sellers, Edward M., Claudio A. Naranjo, and John E. Peachey: Drugs to decrease alcohol consumption. *New Engl J Med* 305(21):1235-1262, 1981.

15. Snyder, Solomon H.: The opiate receptor and morphine-like peptides in the brain. *Am J Psychiatry* 135(6):645-652, 1978.

16. Vaillant, George E., and Eva S. Milofsky: Natural history of male alcoholism. *Arch Gen Psychiatry* 39(2):127-133, 1982.

17. Wood, David, Paul H. Wender, and Fred W. Reimherr: The prevalence of attention deficit disorder, residual type, or minimal brain dysfunction, in a population of male alcoholic patients. *Am J Psychiatry* 140(1):95-98, 1983.

18. Woody, George E., Lester Luborsky, A. Thomas McLellan, Charles P. O'Brien, Aaron T. Beck, Jack Blaine, Ira Herman, and Anita Hole: Psychotherapy for opiate addicts. *Arch Gen Psychiatry* 40(6):639-645, 1983.

Chapter 15

ORGANIC MENTAL DISORDERS

BRAIN SYNDROMES AND ORGANIC DISORDERS

Organic Brain Syndromes include Delirium, Dementia, Amnestic Syndrome, Organic Delusional Syndrome, Organic Hallucinations, Organic Affective Syndrome, Organic Personality Syndrome, and Atypical or Mixed Brain Syndrome. These are diagnosed independent of etiology on the basis of clinical signs and symptoms. The term Organic Mental Disorder is used to designate a brain syndrome for which the cause is known or presumed. Accordingly, the complete diagnosis for an organic mental illness includes the disorder (etiology) and the syndrome (manifestations). The brain plays a central role in all mental activity, and the use of the words organic and brain to describe these particular syndromes and the disorders of known etiology that contribute to them should not be understood to exclude brain malfunction as a feature of other psychiatric diseases, or to imply that the malfunction in those diseases is entirely the result of psychological or social factors.

SYMPTOMS OF BRAIN SYNDROMES

Each of the Organic Brain Syndromes has its own characteristic signs and symptoms, but there are some mental examination findings that are common to various of them. If any or all of these are present, one considers the possibility of an Organic Mental Disorder in arriving at a diagnosis. They include:

1. Sensorium Impairment
   a. Impaired orientation
   b. Loss of memory
   c. Disordered intellectual (cognitive) function
2. Faulty Judgment
3. Lability of Affect

Orientation

A disorder of orientation implies that the person to some extent has a lack of awareness of time, place, or person. If the time sense is distorted, the patient may not know the time of day or what week, month, or year it is. Some patients who are disoriented may not know where they are or how they came to the examination. Others will not recognize family or friends or may be unable to give familiar information about their own personal identity. Disorientation usually becomes more severe in twilight or darkness, when sensory stimulation is diminished, visual cues are limited, and fewer people are available to validate perceptions. Brain dysfunction results in impaired intellectual function and poor judgment which, coupled with the sensory deprivation, can markedly increase confusion. Confusion may increase in situations of overstimulation as well, such as a crowded emergency room. Some patients benefit from being taken to a quiet room where they are not bombarded by sensory input. Major difficulties in orientation are usually symptoms of advanced or severe brain dysfunction, but minor problems in orientation and transitory periods of disorientation may occur in milder cases.

Memory

Memory loss may be so mild as to be undetectable except with detailed questioning, or it may be severe. Memory for remote events is more likely to be retained than for recent events. Even a mild inability to recall recent events may be disturbing to some patients. Some will try to fill in the gaps in their memory with confabulation. Hiding the memory loss by confabulation is characteristic of Korsakoff's syndrome, the Amnesic-Confabulatory Syndrome.

Intellectual Function

As with the other findings in the Organic Brain Syndromes, intellectual impairment may vary from mild to severe. A subjective feeling of not being able to think clearly, difficulty in concentration, or inability to recall familiar names might be present in mild impairment. In a coma, which would represent a severe impairment, intellectual functions are inoperative. Perceptual loss, slowed thought processes, some degree of inability to plan ahead or carry out instructions, and difficulty formulating abstractions indicate impairment of intellectual function.

In assessing the intellectual function of a person suspected of having an organic deficit, it is helpful to know something about previous performance level. If a person were capable of above average intellectual functioning prior to an illness or injury, and an average level afterward, this represents an impairment in function even though he or she can still perform at a normal or average level.

Judgment

One of the earliest signs of the Organic Mental Disorder may be deterioration of judgment. This coupled with lability of affect may produce much of the character change described in many people who have Organic Mental Disorders. Impaired judgment may become evident in a decreased ability to make sound business decisions (i.e., investing heavily in speculative or manifestly unprofitable businesses; making grandiose plans for sweeping changes in a well-functioning organization) or in tendencies to commit social errors and indiscretions.

Affective Changes

Lability of affect may be an outstanding feature. Patients may react excessively, laughing or crying in response to trivial events or minor stimuli. Others may appear dull, shallow, or unresponsive. Affective lability also occurs in some Personality Disorders (e.g., Histrionic Personality Disorder) and in some cases of Dysthymic Disorder.

Personality Changes

Personality alterations in the form of an exaggeration or caricature of the previous personality may occur. Whereas the common findings of disorientation, memory loss, intellectual deficit, defective judgment, and lability of affect are related to the severity of the cerebral pathology, some of the personality changes which appear in the course of the illness are related to the premorbid personality. Any of the various psychiatric disorders can occur concomitantly with the Organic Mental Disorders. Past experiences, including other illnesses and injuries, emotional conflicts, interpersonal factors from the past or current environment, and personal reactivity to stress may contribute to the amount and form of the person's response to illness or injury.

Psychotic manifestations may include illusions, delusions, and hallucinations. Reality may be perceived and interpreted incorrectly. Hallucinations in the Organic Brain Syndromes are more often visual than auditory, although both may be present. The combination of impaired intellectual function, defective judgment, and threatening hallucinations can result in injury if the patient is not prevented from attempting to flee from the threat.

In any Organic Mental Disorder, neurotic symptoms such as depression, anxiety, obsessions, compulsions, and phobias may become apparent. Depression may result in part from the systemic effects of the illness or an awareness of its gravity. Compulsive ritualistic behavior is not uncommon in brain-damaged individuals as part of their attempts to compensate for their disabilities. Behavior disorders including excessive drinking, promiscuity, and aggressive or impulsive acts may occur. Disordered behavior may result from diminished cortical control and impaired judgment.

The psychotic, neurotic, and behavioral disturbances which accompany the Organic Mental Disorders may masquerade as any other psychiatric illness.

CLASSIFICATION OF ORGANIC MENTAL DISORDERS

The Organic Mental Disorders are classified in three main groups (see Chapter 4):

1. Senile and Presenile Dementias
2. Substance-induced Disorders
3. Organic Brain Syndromes resulting from another disease which is classified separately

When diagnosing a disorder in any of these main groups, one also identifies the type of brain syndrome present. The syndrome, dementia, is included in the names of the disorders in the first group (Primary Degenerative Dementia, Senile Onset; Primary Degenerative Dementia, Presenile Onset; Multi-infarct Dementia), but patients with these disorders can also have other brain syndromes in addition to it.

The second group, Substance-Induced Organic Mental Disorders includes:

1.   Alcohol
     a. Intoxication
     b. Idiosyncratic intoxication
     c. Withdrawal
     d. Withdrawal delirium
     e. Hallucinosis
     f. Amnestic disorder
     g. Dementia associated with alcoholism
2.   Barbiturate or similarly acting sedative or hypnotic
     a. Intoxication
     b. Withdrawal
     c. Withdrawal delirium
     d. Amnestic disorder
3.   Opioid
     a. Intoxication
     b. Withdrawal
4.   Cocaine
     a. Intoxication
5.   Amphetamine or similarly acting sympathomimetic
     a. Intoxication
     b. Delirium
     c. Delusional disorder
     d. Withdrawal
6.   Phencyclidine (PCP) or similarly acting arylcyclohexylamine
     a. Intoxication
     b. Delirium
     c. Mixed organic mental disorder
7.   Hallucinogen
     a. Hallucinosis
     b. Delusional disorder
     c. Affective disorder
8.   Cannabis
     a. Intoxication
     b. Delusional disorder
9.   Tobacco
     a. Withdrawal
10. Caffeine
     a. Intoxication
11. Other or unspecified substance
     a. Intoxication
     b. Withdrawal
     c. Delirium
     d. Dementia
     e. Amnestic disorder
     f. Delusional disorder
     g. Hallucinosis
     h. Affective disorder
     i. Personality disorder
     j. Atypical or mixed organic mental disorder

Note that the classification includes, in addition to Delirium, Dementia, Organic Hallucinosis, and several other brain syndromes previously mentioned, intoxication and withdrawal. The definition of these two syndromes differs from those of the other brain syndromes in that etiology is implied.

When one makes a diagnosis in the third main group, one lists the causative condition as an Axis III Diagnosis and the type of brain syndrome (Dementia, Delirium, Amnestic Syndrome, Organic Delusional Syndrome, Organic Hallucinosis, Organic Affective Syndrome, Organic Personality Syndrome, Atypical or Mixed Organic Brain Syndrome) on Axis I.

Delirium, a word that from its derivation literally means off the track, is used to designate an acute brain syndrome that has a rapid onset over a few hours or days and a short duration (1 to 4 weeks). Delirium may be superimposed on another brain syndrome, e.g., Dementia, or it may occur in a person who has had no previous signs of mental illness. Depending on cause and treatment, it may end in recovery, in the appearance of another type of brain syndrome, or in death. The main clinical feature of delirium is clouding of consciousness. The delirious patient is confused, bewildered, and disoriented. The patient has difficulty in understanding environmental stimuli and in maintaining attention. Hyperactivity and restlessness may be present and may alternate with periods of preoccupation, daytime drowsiness, or coma. The sleep cycle is disturbed. Memory is impaired. Illusions and hallucinations frequently occur. Delusions, if present, are likely to be transitory and unsystematized.

While delirium usually has an acute onset, dementia often develops gradually. It is manifested by intellectual deterioration and memory loss without clouding of sensorium. The amnestic syndrome (the word amnesia is derived from a Greek word meaning forgetfulness and describes both memory loss and gaps in memory) is manifested by short-term (recent) and/or long-term (remote) memory impairment without either clouding of sensorium or generalized intellectual deterioration.

For Brain Syndromes in which delusions, hallucinations, or emotional disturbances are the main symptoms and occur in the absence of marked clouding of consciousness or significant intellectual impairment, the diagnoses of Organic Delusional Syndrome, Organic Hallucinosis, or Organic Affective Syndrome can be used.

When the main symptoms of an Organic Brain Syndrome are behavioral and reflect personality changes without marked clouding of consciousness, intellectual deterioration, or memory loss, the diagnosis of Organic Personality Syndrome is applied.

ORGANIC MENTAL DISORDER:
PRIMARY DEGENERATIVE DEMENTIA

In the classification system, a distinction is made between Primary Degenerative Dementia of Senile Onset (over age 65) and those of Presenile Onset (under age 65). The distinction is arbitrary, as there is no clinical or pathological difference between cases having early and late onset and there is no bimodal grouping. The vast majority of these Dementias are associated with Alzheimer's disease. On postmortem examination the brains of people with Alzheimer's disease show characteristic placques and neurofibrillary tangles resulting from loss of neurons, often accompanied by cortical atrophy. In clinical practice the diagnosis must be made by excluding other causes of progressive Dementia with insidious onset in persons over 50 years of age (Alzheimer's disease rarely occurs in patients under 50 except in association with Down's syndrome).

Alzheimer's disease is common. It is the fourth leading cause of death in the United States. It affects nearly 5 percent of people over 65 and, debatably, up to 20 percent of people over 80.

The cause of Alzheimer's disease is unknown. There are undoubtedly genetic factors involved.

The course is steadily progressive with death occurring in 2 to 5 years. First signs often are of memory impairment, making mistakes in doing familiar tasks, and getting lost in familiar places. As the disease progresses, aphasia, agnosia, apraxia, and amnesia may appear.

Possible early Alzheimer's disease must be distinguished from normal aging. Older people are often concerned about mild forgetfulness. Sometimes the concern is totally unrealistic and the examples are ones that might normally occur for a healthy person of any age. Sometimes there is some actual memory loss accompanying normal aging. In normal aging one loses some cortical neurons; some brain atrophy may occur. Atrophy, incidentally, does not correlate well with measurable intellectual changes. As any teacher knows, people are endowed with far more brain cells than they ever use. One can have a lot of atrophy without having intellectual impairment (or can have intellectual impairment without having atrophy). A constriction of interests in the aging may be more responsible for apparent mild intellectual dysfunction than are changes in the brain.

In differential diagnosis in cases where there is actual dementia, one must rule out chronic toxic and metabolic encephalopathies. These are common in the aging. One also rules out normal pressure hydrocephalus. One must also rule out depression (depressive pseudodementia), and in cases of reasonable doubt, a trial of antidepressant medication is certainly warranted. It must, of course, be remembered that patients often have both dementia and depression.

MULTI-INFARCT DEMENTIA

Persons who have multiple cerebral infarctions become intellectually impaired and develop dementia. Multi-infarct Dementia is usually associated with cerebral arteriosclerosis, generalized arteriosclerosis, and hypertension, but these conditions are not usually direct causes of dementia. They are indirect causes, since they predispose to thrombotic or embolic cerebral infarctions. Various cardiac and inflammatory disorders can also cause Multi-infarct Dementia.

Multi-infarct Dementia usually has a sudden onset, though the onset may appear gradual if early mild episodes are overlooked. The course is intermittent or step-wise, in contrast to the steadily progressive dementia of Alzheimer's disease. The deterioration is patchy; some intellectual functions are preserved. Focal neurological signs can usually be found. Prodromal or early episodes may include transitory periods of confusion, clouding of consciousness, or alterations in behavior. After repeated episodes, complaints, in addition to those related to memory loss and intellectual impairment, may include dizziness, headache, and sometimes feelings of fatigue or weakness. Confusion becomes troublesome, especially at night. Patients may have periods of delirium or excitement. Affective symptoms and/or delusions may appear. The progress of the disorder can usually be halted if the underlying cause can be treated successfully.

SUBSTANCE-INDUCED ORGANIC MENTAL DISORDERS

Substance-Induced Organic Mental Disorders are classified under the heading of the substance that is the causative agent by indicating the type of brain syndrome present.

Alcoholic Psychoses

Syndromes associated with alcohol ingestion include:

1.   Acute Alcohol Intoxication
2.   Idiosyncratic Intoxication (pathological intoxication)
3.   Withdrawal
4.   Alcohol Withdrawal Delirium (Delirium Tremens)
5.   Amnestic Disorder (Korsakoff's psychosis)
6.   Hallucinosis
7.   Dementia Associated with Alcoholism (Alcoholic Deterioration)

Simple intoxication is a good paradigm for an Organic Brain Syndrome. This state usually exists when a person's blood alcohol level exceeds 10 mg% (0.10 on breath analyzer). Most people in our society are familiar with this syndrome either by observation or from personal experience. The intoxicated individual has some sensorium clouding and impaired intellectual functioning, faulty judgment, and sometimes lability of affect. Personality changes, often representing desires or behavior patterns that are suppressed or repressed most of the time, but sometimes revealing otherwise compensated psychiatric disorders, may be observed.

In Idiosyncratic Intoxication, small quantities of alcohol produce severe symptoms, including disorientation, hyperactivity, aggressive behavior, and amnesia. This syndrome occurs almost exclusively in people who have a history of previous brain damage.

Alcohol Withdrawal is the diagnosis used for a clinically significant hangover. Ordinary hangovers are uncomfortable, reduce efficiency, and increase accident risk, but the diagnosis is restricted to episodes following cessation of heavy drinking that has been going on for several days. Symptoms develop a few hours after drinking stops. Tremors are always present and malaise is usually a complaint. Anxiety, irritability, or depression may be present, as may be insomnia, nightmares, illusions, and even transitory hallucinations. However, the diagnosis is not made if the criteria for Alcohol Withdrawal Delirium are met.

Withdrawal Delirium (Delirium tremens) commonly occurs in persons over 30 years of age who have been drinking heavily for at least 3 to 4 years. Opinion is still somewhat divided as to the cause of Withdrawal Delirium, but it is thought to be primarily an abstinence syndrome beginning when someone accustomed to drinking heavily either stops suddenly or cuts his or her intake sharply. Other factors which play a part in its onset may include metabolic disturbances, liver malfunction, vitamin B and other nutritional deficiencies, and disturbed water balance. Early signs of impending delirium may be restlessness, irritability, and loss of appetite. Nightmares and restless sleep may precede the onset of hallucinations of terrifying small creatures or fantastic animals. Tactile and olfactory hallucinations as well as frightening visual ones may be present. The person having Withdrawal Delirium is confused, disoriented, and terrified. Because of fear and apprehension the patient becomes agitated and may become aggressive and destructive.

Hyperactivity and efforts to escape from the hallucinations may be exhausting. Gross tremors of the face, tongue, and hands are common. Convulsions may occur. The acute stage of Withdrawal Delirium lasts approximately 3 to 10 days. The death rate in untreated cases is relatively high, 15 to 20 percent.

Amnestic Disorder (Korsakoff's disease) may appear following Withdrawal Delirium or Wernicke's encephalopathy, or may arise separately. In this disorder, because of disturbed memory and attention, the person suffers from memory gaps which are filled by confabulation. This Amnestic-Confabulatory Syndrome is often accompanied by polyneuritis. Though a result of alcoholism, the direct cause is thiamine deficiency.

In Alcoholic Hallucinosis the sensorium is clear, in contrast to other Brain Syndromes associated with alcohol ingestion. Vivid accusatory or threatening auditory hallucinations occur and may be terrifying to the patient. Some clinicians believe Hallucinosis is actually a type of Schizophrenia.

Dementia Associated with Alcoholism follows several years of heavy drinking. It differs from the Amnestic syndrome in that cognitive functions are impaired in addition to memory loss. Dementia is often relatively mild and is reversible if abstinence can be achieved. Sometimes, however, one encounters severe dementias of the Alzheimer type in persons with a history of chronic alcoholism. There is some question as to whether these cases are actually caused by alcoholism, or they are simply cases of concurrent Alzheimer's disease. It is possible, though by no means proven, that alcoholism predisposes to Alzheimer's disease.

In addition to the syndromes specifically listed in current nosology, some chronic alcoholics develop a condition difficult to distinguish from a paranoid psychosis, characterized by jealousy and delusions of infidelity.

Other Substances

Organic Mental Disorders can be caused by narcotics, sedative hypnotics, psychostimulants, hallucinogens, cannabis products, and a variety of other substances. It would be redundant to discuss in detail each of the possible brain syndromes produced by each substance.

Narcotic intoxication is sometimes called being on the nod. The sensorium is clouded and the person is not very attentive to surroundings. Apathy has a prominent and impressive association with narcotic intoxication. During intoxication with the sedative-hypnotic drugs and minor tranquilizers such as the barbiturates, chlordiazepoxide, and diazepam a triad of symptoms is present: slurred speech, ataxia (motor incoordination), and nystagmus. Sensorium is markedly impaired and disorientation is the rule. All of these medications suppress respiration and can be toxic to the kidneys. In withdrawal, the addicted patient runs the risk of convulsions and cardiovascular collapse. On occasion these patients develop withdrawal deliriums. (Example: A 45-year-old man was admitted to the hospital for a hemorrhoidectomy. His mental status examination was normal on admission. On the sixth day postoperatively he became markedly disoriented, paranoid, and had visual hallucinations. His wife told the surgeon that her husband had been taking diazepam four to eight times a day and barbiturates at bedtime for the past 2 years. The patient responded to treatment with diazepam by returning to his preoperative mental status.)

The psychostimulants, amphetamine, cocaine, and methylphenidate can all produce Organic Mental Disorders. Amphetamine use may result in intoxication or delirium. With massive doses and sometimes following prolonged use of smaller amounts (at or above the upper limits of recommended clinical use) one sees a delusional disorder with auditory and visual hallucinations and paranoid delusions among its features. It is similar to Paranoid Schizophrenia. An Amphetaminelike Psychosis can also be produced by methylphenidate. Chronic cocaine use can lead to an Organic Mental Disorder. These patients often have haptic hallucinations (the sensation that bugs are crawling under their skin). Users refer to this as the "cocaine bug." It is also called formication.

Acute intoxication occurs with hallucinogens such as lysergic acid diethylamide (LSD). Chronic use has been associated with flashbacks, repeated druglike experiences without taking the hallucinogen. Flashbacks seem to be made worse by cannabis, repetitive boring visual stimuli (highway posts, TV test patterns), stress, and anticholinergic medications.

Recently, phencyclidine (PCP; angel dust) has become a very popular hallucinogen. Use of this drug may result in intoxication, delirium, a mixed Organic Mental Disorder, or coma. Intoxicated patients are frequently combative and paranoid.

Cannabis products including marijuana, hashish, and hash oil can produce an Organic Mental Disorder very similar to LSD intoxication if the dose taken is high enough. The active hallucinogen is Δ^9-tetrahydrocannabinol (THC). Many drug users who think they have been taking TCH have actually been sold a combination of drugs including LSD and/or phenylcyclidine (Sernylan).

Bromide intoxication, usually from proprietary medications, can produce an Organic Mental Disorder. The sensorium is clouded and neurological disturbances such as ataxia, tremor, and decreased deep tendon reflexes are usually present. Patients may have delusions and hallucinations.

The sniffing of glue, gasoline, paint thinner, enamel reducer, hair spray, and related compounds have produced Organic Mental Disorders, including severe Amnestic Syndrome.

Among the poisons commonly implicated in Organic Mental Disorders are lead, mercury, manganese, organic phosphorus, and carbon monoxide.

Adults may be exposed to lead inhalation in the course of an occupation such as paint spraying. Children are more likely to be poisoned by chewing objects coated with lead-based paint. Lead poisoning may be characterized by an acute delirium of sudden onset, or it may appear as a progressive deterioration. In addition to the cerebral signs, patients with lead poisoning may complain of gastrointestinal distress or of muscle weakness which has led to a wrist- or footdrop. Adults may have a dark lead line deposited at the gum margins. Examination of the blood will reveal a hypochromic anemia and basophilic stippling of cells. In children, x-rays of the long bones will show increased density from lead deposition at the ends of the growing bones. Children who have suffered from lead encephalopathy may develop permanent brain damage manifested by learning defects or behavior disorders.

Carbon monoxide poisoning may result in mild to severe symptoms, depending on the concentration of carbon monoxide and the exposure time. Permanent mental changes are most likely to occur following severe intoxication or a long period of unconsciousness. Chronic exposure to small amounts of carbon monoxide gas can produce mild clinical symptoms.

OTHER CONDITIONS CAUSING
ORGANIC MENTAL DISORDERS

In addition to Senile, Presenile, and substance-induced conditions, psychotic or nonpsychotic Organic Brain Syndrome can occur in the following conditions:

1. Intracranial or systemic infection
2. Brain trauma
3. Circulatory disturbance
4. Epilepsy
5. Disturbance of metabolism, growth, or nutrition
6. Intracranial neoplasm
7. Degenerative disease of the Central Nervous System

Intracranial Infection

Intracranial infections such as encephalitis, meningitis, or brain abscess commonly produce Organic Brain Syndromes of varying severity. For example, in meningo-coccal meningitis, with delirium paralleling the seriousness of the illness, along with cerebral signs, the patient will have characteristic systemic signs, rash, fever, and neurological changes. In recent years these conditions are on the increase, since so many patients are taking immunosuppressive agents which lower resistance to infection, especially to viral and fungal diseases.

Systemic Infection

With severe systemic infections, particularly with high fever, manifestations of an acute Organic Brain Syndrome are likely to appear. Personality changes may appear before definitive evidence of the underlying disorder can be found. Sometimes delirium appears after the onset of fever and may accompany illnesses such as pneumonia and typhoid fever. Occasionally, a delirium may persist after the fever has subsided or may begin in the postfebrile period.

Central Nervous System Syphilis

Neurosyphilis, meningoencephalitic (paresis; general paresis) or meningovascular, used to be one of the commonest causes of Organic Brain Syndromes. Since the introduction of antibiotics, successful treatment of primary and secondary syphilis has made symptomatic neurosyphilis a relatively rare condition. Nevertheless, it is a possibility one must think of in evaluating an Organic Brain Syndrome of otherwise unknown cause.

Brain Trauma

The amount of actual tissue damage may be difficult to assess in head injuries, and many of the symptoms which arise after head injury are not related to the degree of apparent tissue destruction. Minor temporary damage may result from a concussion in which there is no evidence of external injury. The patient may be dazed or unconscious, may suffer from varying degrees of retrograde amnesia, and may exhibit psychotic or behavioral disturbances. Trauma of greater magnitude such as a penetrating wound, skull fracture, or the pressure of a large hematoma may produce irreversible tissue damage with concomitant loss of mental functions.

Following a head injury, patients may complain of irritability, diminished ambition, decreased tolerance to stress, lability of affect, tendencies toward irresponsibility, easy fatigue, dizziness, slowed thinking or decreased concentration, headache aggravated by effort or stooping, intolerance to alcohol, and memory deficits. The importance that mental facility has had to the person prior to the injury may to some extent influence the emotional and behavioral reactions to injury. Depression with feelings of anxiety, despair, helplessness, and hopelessness may be prominent in a person whose profession seems threatened by the injury and the subsequent memory deficits, impaired judgment, or slower thought processes. Some patients may become withdrawn, avoiding the stress of new people and new situations. Others will attempt to compensate for their disability by an increased orderliness. Some will attempt to deny to themselves and others that there has been any loss of function even though it may be painfully obvious that their judgment or their ability to solve problems has declined.

Often unrelated to the severity of the head injury is a group of symptoms sometimes labeled Post-Traumatic Neurosis. This condition is not to be confused with the Post-Traumatic Stress Disorders discussed in Chapter 8, though a Post-Traumatic Stress Disorder can occur following head injury. A post-traumatic neurosis usually does not appear immediately after the injury, but begins about the time the person is returning to work. Though an increase in activity may re-activate head injury symptoms, and some disability may not be apparent until a person actually tries to return to work, secondary gain is an important factor in many cases. If the injury has resulted in the patient's getting attention and consideration that is lacking in his or her daily life, and if it removes him or her from a trying home situation or an unsatisfactory job, there may be an unconscious rebellion against a return to everyday life. The headache, vertigo, and anxiety resulting from this are not to be confused with conscious malingering for purposes of compensation.

Positive attitudes in the people who care for a person who suffers a head injury help prevent post-traumatic disability. The injured person should, of course, have good physical care. In addition, one should be encouraged to begin to engage in suitable activities as soon as one is able and to make plans for an early return to work.

Epilepsy

In idiopathic epilepsy and other cerebral dysrhythmias, Organic Brain Syndromes may occur. There is nearly always a confused period lasting from several minutes up to several hours after a grand mal (tonic and clonic) seizure. Occasionally, confusion occurs before a seizure as a prodromal symptom or as part of the aura. Sometimes an epileptic patient may have a clouded and confused period without actually having a seizure. In psychomotor, temporal lobe, or diencephalic epilepsy a behavioral disorder or a transient psychotic state may be a seizure equivalent. In cases of unexplained temper outbursts, for example, one must consider cerebral dysrhythmia as a possible cause. Patients with epilepsy may have a variety of emotional disturbances secondary to the social problems and limitations on activity resulting from the disease (or from overconservative management in which the patient is overprotected). In some epileptic patients whose disorder has been poorly controlled, Organic Mental Disorder develops after a number of years. This is an insidious dementia with narrowing of interests, slowing of mentation, and apathy. This chronic state is more likely to occur in patients who have been institutionalized and who have had frequent prolonged seizures. Finally, in evaluating psychiatric symptoms in epileptic patients one must remember the possibility of toxic psychoses resulting from anticonvulsant medications.

Disturbance of Metabolism, Growth, and Nutrition

The syndromes associated with nutritional, metabolic, or endocrine disturbances such as uremia, thyrotoxicosis, diabetes, etc. are often transient but may have permanent residuals. Hypoglycemia may produce apathy, disorientation, confusion, stupor, and other manifestations of an Organic Brain Syndrome. Repeated or prolonged hypoglycemic comas may produce permanent damage. Hyperthyroidism and myxedema, hepatolenticular degeneration (Wilson's disease), and porphyria all have associated mental symptoms, some of which may appear before other demonstrable evidence of disease.

Metabolic changes may have an important role in the development of some postoperative confusional states. Anxiety, possible dehydration, disturbances in the nutritional state, medications, and anesthesia may all contribute to the development of delirium in the postoperative period. The onset of other psychoses appearing postoperatively may be delayed for several days and they are more likely to occur after operations involving emotionally important organs such as the eyes, genitals, and heart.

The vitamin deficiencies usually do not result in an acute Organic Brain Syndrome, but are frequently involved in the development of chronic ones. Deficiencies in the B complex vitamins are implicated in Organic Brain Syndromes, including those associated with Korsakoff's psychosis, Wernicke's syndrome, pellagra, etc. Wernicke's syndrome, consisting of ophthalmoplegia, confabulation, ataxia, and progressive dementia results from thiamine deficiency. The triad of diarrhea (and other gastrointestinal disturbances), dermatitis, and dementia is characteristic of pellagra. Pernicious anemia may be accompanied by delirium, paranoid ideation, depression or agitation, and deterioration. The reversibility of mental symptoms in many of the nutritional disturbances depends to some extent upon the promptness with which treatment is begun.

Intracranial Neoplasm

Subtler personality changes representing intensifications of the premorbid personality are often the first signs of brain tumor. The degree to which other mental symptoms develop depends in part upon the nature and location of the tumor and on the development of increased intracranial pressure. Frontal and temporal lobe tumors are particularly likely to produce psychosis. Emotional lability, apathy, irritability, euphoria, and silliness may occur along with visual, auditory, or olfactory hallucinations. Rapidly increasing intracranial pressure may precipitate an acute delirium.

Metastatic carcinoma from breast, lung, etc., can present as an Organic Brain Syndrome, as can leukemia and lymphoma, Hodgkin's disease, and the collagen vascular diseases. Carcinoma of the pancreas often presents with signs of depression and sometimes a mild Organic Brain Syndrome.

Postoperative mental symptoms are determined by the location of the tumor, the degree of tissue damage resulting from the tumor and its removal, and, as with head trauma, the patient's individual reactions to the disability.

Degenerative Disease of the
Central Nervous System

Huntington's Chorea is an inherited disorder transmitted by a single non-sex-linked dominant gene with good penetrance. Although some cases have been diagnosed in younger persons, in the majority this disorder begins after the age of 30. Choreoathetosis and mental deterioration have an insidious onset and progressive deterioration is inevitable.

Multiple Sclerosis is the most common of the demyelinating diseases. In Multiple Sclerosis, multiple scattered patchy areas of demyelination appear and are followed by gliosis. Neurological manifestations such as involuntary movements, dysarthria, and ataxia occur in a variable pattern of remissions and relapses. Emotional lability, euphoria, depression, or irritability are common, and Dementia sometimes occurs in the terminal stages. Dementia also occurs during the later stages of amyotrophic lateral sclerosis. Mild dementia sometimes accompanies Parkinsonism.

TREATMENT

Treatment of Organic Mental Disorders is directed to both the underlying cause, if known and treatable, and to the Brain Syndrome itself. When the underlying cause is a physical disorder, curing or arresting that disorder is one's first goal. In treating Multi-infarct Dementia one seeks to eliminate any specific cause for the infarctions, and in any case to control hypertension, and one may use anticoagulants. In Substance-Induced Disorders one seeks to eliminate the use or exposure to the causative substance. With some substances gradual withdrawal or substitution of an appropriate drug is necessary to prevent causing a Withdrawal Delirium.

A person suffering from an acute delirium must be provided with safeguards against injury. The patient may need someone in the room at all times, not only to observe and prevent accidental injury, but also to provide a feeling of security and some contact with reality. Having familiar people near and keeping the same people in attendance rather than changing nurses may have a calming effect on a fearful, agitated patient. Since disorientation is often more troublesome in relative darkness, leaving a light on in the patient's room may diminish agitation. When not contraindicated by other factors, tranquilizers and mild sedatives may prevent exhaustion and make the patient more comfortable.

During the early phases of treatment of a person who has suffered a brain injury or a cerebrovascular accident in which the extent of permanent residual damage is uncertain, a positive attitude on the part of those caring for the patient is essential, so that all possible physical functions are retained and attitudes of hopelessness do not develop. Planning a flexible program for rehabilitation, and whenever possible, focusing on a return to work can often prevent unnecessary disability. Some people who have suffered brain damage profit from psychotherapy, especially those who are depressed. A very active and enthusiastic rehabilitation program is essential for a good long-term prognosis.

Even the treatment of Dementia need not be discouraging. Some Dementias are reversible. Many, especially those of the Alzheimer type, are not. Often, one does not know whether a Dementia is reversible, whether its progress can be halted, or even if the patient can be made more comfortable and given a better quality of life until one has tried treatment.

Treatment requires intellectual stimulation. Efforts are made to get the patient to use the cognitive capacities he or she has, and to make positive efforts to retain remote and recent memory. Social interactions are encouraged. Disturbing behavioral symptoms accompanying Dementia sometimes respond to behavior modification techniques. Sometimes symptomatic medication may be needed (e.g., for aggressive outbursts), but large doses of sedatives or tranquilizers are best avoided.

General supportive measures are often helpful. Intercurrent diseases, even though they do not directly contribute to the Dementia, should be treated. Unnecessary medications should be discontinued. Nutritional disorders are to be corrected. Visual and hearing disorders should not be neglected.

Psychotherapy helps some patients deal with feelings that they have about their disorders. Anxiety or depression accompanying Dementia requires appropriate treatment.

The two most important things in the successful treatment of most patients with Organic Brain Disorders are:

1.   Maintaining therapeutic optimism
2.   Keeping the patient intellectually stimulated

Certainly not all patients can be cured, but if one keeps trying, improved functioning is possible for many patients. Intellectual stimulation helps improve the functioning of portions of the brain that are still intact. Of course, placing too many demands on the patient can be frustrating and detrimental, but providing things that the patient can do to keep the brain active and to awaken interest in the environment does not need to exceed the patient's capacity.

REVIEW QUESTIONS

1. How do you evaluate sensorium impairment? Judgment? Affect?
2. Define Delirium. Dementia. Organic Personality Syndrome.
3. Name six substances which can produce an Organic Mental Disorder. Discuss the types of disorder produced by each.
4. Discuss the clinical features and prognosis of each of the seven psychiatric syndromes associated with alcohol misuse.
5. A 50-year-old man presents with postprandial epigastric fullness, vague abdominal pain, and an atypical depression with some mental confusion. If you were the physician, what would your differential diagnosis be and how would you work up this patient?
6. What are the differences in the symptoms and course of Alzheimer's disease and Multi-infarct Dementia?
7. A 48-year-old woman presents with recent memory loss, mental confusion, and a labile affect. What is the differential diagnosis? How would you proceed in evaluating this patient?
8. Look up current literature and give treatment recommendations for a patient with each of the following conditions: Alcohol Withdrawal Delirium; Alzheimer's disease; caffeine intoxication; phencyclidine intoxication.
9. An 80-year-old patient clearly has an Alzheimer-type Dementia. Other causes of Brain Syndrome have been ruled out to your satisfaction. You do not suspect that drug toxicity is a primary cause of the Dementia. However, the patient is taking 12 different medications, prescribed and proprietary, for various nonpsychiatric disorders and symptoms. Insofar as possible, would you try to reduce the amount of medication being taken? Why? Might this be helpful in the management of the Dementia? If so, why?

SELECTED REFERENCES

1. Brandt, Jason, Nelson Butters, Christopher Ryan, and Roger Bayog: Cognitive loss and recovery in long-term alcohol abusers. *Arch Gen Psychiatry* 40(4): 435–442, 1983.

2. Caine, Eric D., Robert D. Hunt, Herbert Weingartner, and Michael H. Ebert: Huntington's dementia. *Arch Gen Psychiatry* 35:377–384, 1978.

3. Cummings, Jeffrey L.: Dementia: Definition, classification, and differential diagnosis. *Psychiatr Ann* 14(2):85–89, 1984.

4. Comfort, Alex: Alzheimer's disease or "Alzheimerism"? *Psychiatr Ann* 14(2):130–132, 1984.

5. Hammeke, Thomas A., Charles J. Golden, and Arnold D. Purisch: A standardized short, and comprehensive neuropsychological test battery based on the Luria neuropsychological evaluation. *Int J Neurosci* 8:135-141, 1978.

6. Heston, Leonard L., Angeline R. Mastri, V. Elving Anderson, and June White: Dementia of the Alzheimer type: Clinical genetics, natural history, and associated conditions. *Arch Gen Psychiatry* 38(10):1085-1090, 1981.

7. Larson, Eric B., Burton V. Reifler, Harvey J. Featherstone, and Dallas R. English: Dementia in elderly outpatients: A prospective study. *Ann Intern Med* 100(3):417-423, 1984.

8. Lipowski, Z. J.: Transient cognitive disorders (delirium, acute confusional states) in the elderly. *Am J Psychiatry* 140(11):1426-1436, 1983.

9. McAllister, Thomas W.: Overview: Pseudodementia. *Am J Psychiatry* 140(5):528-533, 1983.

10. Pierson, Eric W., John R. Thompson, and George J. Wolcott: Normal pressure hydrocephalus: A treatable cause of dementia. *Neb Med J* 67(1):6, 1982.

11. Rabiner, Charles, Allen Willner, and Jirina Fishman: Psychiatric complications following coronary bypass surgery. *J Nerv Men Dis* 160(5):342-348, 1975.

12. Read, Stephen L., and Lissy F. Jarvik: Cerebrovascular disease in the differential diagnosis of dementia. *Psychiatr Ann* 14(2):100-108, 1984.

13. Reifler, Burton V., Eric Larson, and Ray Hanley: Coexistence of cognitive impairment and depression in geriatric outpatients. *Am J Psychiatry* 139(5): 623-626, 1982.

14. Schneck, Michael K., Barry Reisberg, and Steven H. Ferris: An overview of current concepts of Alzheimer's disease. *Am J Psychiatry* 139(2):165-173, 1982.

15. Spar, James E.: Psychopharmacology of Alzheimer's disease. *Psychiatr Ann* 14(3):186-189, 1984.

16. Stephens, Louise P.: *Reality Orientation, A Technique to Rehabilitate Elderly and Brain Damaged Patients with a Moderate to Severe Degree of Disorientation.* Washington, D.C., American Psychiatric Association Hospital and Community Psychiatry Service, 1969.

17. Stillner, Verner, Michael K. Popkin, and Chester M. Pierce: Caffeine-induced delirium during prolonged competitive stress. *Am J Psychiatry* 135(7):855-856, 1978.

18. Yesavage, Jerome A., Jared R. Tinklenberg, Leo E. Hollister, and Philip A. Berger: Vasodilators in senile dementias. *Arch Gen Psychiatry* 36:220-223, 1979.

19. Yudofsky, Stuart, Daniel Williams, and Jack Gorman: Propranolol in the treatment of rage and violent behavior in patients with chronic brain syndromes. *Am J Psychiatry* 138(2):218-220, 1981.

Chapter 16

MENTAL RETARDATION

CHANGING CONCEPTS OF
MENTAL RETARDATION

The Mentally Retarded as a group were not differentiated from the "insane" until John Locke suggested the separation in 1689. In 1801 the Wild Boy of Aveyron was treated by Itard, and hopes of reversing environmental deprivation were raised. Guggenbühl promised treatment success through education in the mid 1800s. He failed because his promises could not be entirely fulfilled. In 1848 Séguin wrote the first textbook on Mental Retardation, *The Physiological and Moral Instructions of Idiots.*

The Mentally Retarded were thought of as constitutionally deficient or degenerate and were often neglected or rejected throughout the last half of the nineteenth century and the early part of this century. In 1930 Garrod developed the concept of inborn errors of metabolism which was followed in 1934 by Föllings' discovery of phenylketonuria. With the advent of penicillin in the 1940s, which offered an effective treatment for syphilis, the discovery of Rh incompatibility, and improved obstetrical care, the possibility of preventing some cases of Mental Retardation directed more attention to the field. In the early 1960s President John F. Kennedy's interest in Retardation helped stimulate federally financed programs for the Retarded. In the mid 1960s, Potter labeled the field of Mental Retardation the Cinderella of psychiatry.

More recently the development of amniocentesis has added significantly to the accuracy of prenatal diagnosis. Appropriate use of cesarean section and improved techniques of fetal monitoring have reduced some risks of mental retardation. Advances in neonatology are currently reducing some risks, but at the same time making it possible to keep many more potentially retarded infants alive.

MAGNITUDE OF THE PROBLEM

Over 200 conditions may be associated with Mental Retardation, and the resulting deficits in adaptational ability may vary from incapacitatingly severe to so mild as to be almost undetectable in the adult. Mental Retardation (or mental deficiency) is a symptom as well as a diagnostic entity. It can be defined as a state of arrested, imperfect, or subnormal intellectual functioning which appears during the developmental period and which is manifested by impaired ability in learning, adaptive behavior, and social adjustment.

Although an estimated 3 percent of babies born each year can be expected to be diagnosed as Mentally Retarded some time in their lives, the number and types of recognized retarded persons in the community may vary in each age group. In infancy, babies with obvious malformations such as microcephaly, or with congenital disorders such as Down's Syndrome, are more likely to be diagnosed early. This group, with readily apparent abnormalities, constitutes a relatively small percentage of the Retarded, but includes many of the cases with relatively serious impairment. Milder degrees of Retardation are not usually detected during the first year. In the years prior to entering school, children who have marked delays in maturation, those who do not develop speech or language skills, or those with incoordination or other motor deficits may arouse suspicions of Retardation. Mild Retardation, if unaccompanied by other handicaps, may not become evident until after the child has begun school, where the lack of academic success may be complicated by behavior problems, aggression, or negative attitudes. After leaving school, many mildly retarded people obtain suitable employment and again become indistinguishable from others in their environment. The majority of mentally retarded persons are in the Mildly Retarded group, and these are most apparent during their years in school. Because of a somewhat higher mortality rate among the severely Retarded, and the blending of the least Retarded into the general population, the number of people in a community who can be identified as Retarded at a given time is probably only about 1 percent.

CLASSIFICATION OF MENTAL RETARDATION

Mental Retardation is subclassified according to its severity. This is usually measured by the Intelligence Quotient, because the IQ is known to correlate closely with adaptive behavior. Nevertheless, even though they are hard to measure, social and adaptive capacities must be taken into account before making a diagnosis of Mental Retardation or deciding about its severity. In using arbitrary IQ values one is most likely to err in the mild and borderline ranges and in dealing with members of socially disadvantaged groups.

Mental Retardation is subclassified as follows:

1. Mild Mental Retardation (IQ 50-70)
2. Moderate Mental Retardation (IQ 35-49)
3. Severe Mental Retardation (IQ 20-34)
4. Profound Mental Retardation (IQ Below 20)
5. Unspecified Mental Retardation

A sixth category, Borderline Intellectual Functioning (IQ 71-84) is not regarded as a disorder, but it is classified among Conditions Not Attributable to a Mental Disorder That Are a Focus of Attention or Treatment.

The classification of Unspecified Mental Retardation is used when Mental Retardation can be readily diagnosed on the basis of adaptive and social behavior but the patient is untestable by standard intelligence tests.

The IQ ranges need not be applied rigidly. Test results are not totally reliable and retesting or the use of another test may show a variation of as much as five points. In determining the presence and degree of Mental Retardation, clinical judgment must be used.

The diagnosis of Mental Retardation is made only when the onset is before age 18. It requires, in addition to an Intelligence Quotient in the retarded range, evidence of concurrent deficits in adaptive behavior.

The Mildly Retarded is by far the largest category, comprising almost 80 percent of the total. People in this category can attain educational skills to about the sixth grade level (which is sometimes called functionally literate) and are usually able to function in society normally except at times of heavy stress.

The Moderately Retarded comprise about 12 percent of the population of retarded and can attain skills to about the second grade level. With sheltered conditions and assistance, they can function within society.

The Severely Retarded category contains about 7 percent of the retarded. Under complete supervision they can attain some self-help skills.

The Profoundly Retarded make up less than 1 percent of the total. They require continuous nursing care.

In the assessment of functioning, the degree of Retardation is modified, ameliorated, or intensified by other elements. Retarded individuals may have significant physical handicaps such as visual or hearing losses, paralysis, spasticity, incoordination, etc., which increase the problems in adaptation. Rejection or overprotection by the family can contribute to emotional disturbances. Interpersonal relationships in the school and community can influence the performance level. Many Mildly Retarded and some Moderately Retarded persons are keenly aware of the diagnosis and its social implications. Their feelings about this influence adaptation. Social isolation and cultural deprivation can compound the problems inherent in Retardation.

CAUSES OF MENTAL RETARDATION

Although many conditions are known to carry a high risk of Retardation, in about three-fourths of mentally retarded persons a definite cause for the Retardation cannot be determined. Factors usually implicated in the development of Mental Retardation can be primarily biological, that is, within the individual, or experiential and environmental. The biological elements leading to Retardation can be present prior to birth (prenatal), as in the genetically determined disorders, and in conditions resulting from complications during pregnancy; may begin at birth as with birth trauma or anoxia (perinatal); or may have their onset in the postnatal period (i.e., infections and trauma). Experiential factors include abnormalities in the mother-child interaction, lack of stimulation in the early months of life such as might occur in an institution, and cultural deprivation because of social or economic status.

The causes of Mental Retardation include:

1.   Infection
2.   Intoxication
3.   Trauma or Physical Agent

4. Disorders of Metabolism, Growth, or Nutrition
   a. Proteins
   b. Lipids
   c. Carbohydrates
   d. Other
5. New Growth
6. Unknown Prenatal Influence
7. Chromosomal Abnormalities
8. Prematurity
9. Unknown Postnatal Causes
10. Psychosocial (Environmental) Deprivation

Infection

Viral infection in the mother during pregnancy, especially rubella in the first trimester and cytomegalic inclusion virus infection, carry a risk of Retardation and
congenital malformations. Acute viral and bacterial infections in the last trimester of pregnancy may precipitate a premature labor with the resultant increased likelihood of Retardation associated with prematurity. Congenital syphilis can be prevented by adequate therapy for the mother during pregnancy. When
it occurs congenital syphilis may result in the meningovascular type of neurosyphilis or it may produce a diffuse encephalopathy leading to juvenile paresis. Toxo-
plasmosis, a protozoan infection which can be transmitted from the mother to the
fetus, can cause microcephaly, hydrocephaly, convulsions, choreoretinitis, and Mental Retardation. In the postnatal period, permanent neurological sequelae, including Retardation, may follow infectious meningitis or encephalitis.

Intoxication

Toxemia in the mother may increase the risk of Retardation directly or as a result of premature labor. In any condition in which there is a high serum bilirubin,
bilirubin encephalopathy (kernicterus) and severe Retardation can occur if the infant's blood is not exchanged promptly. Rh and ABO blood incompatibilities are
probably the most common causes of kernicterus, but prematurity and neonatal
sepsis may also be associated with an elevated serum bilirubin. The effects on the
fetus of medications taken by the mother during her pregnancy are difficult to
assess or predict. Drugs often have an increased toxicity in the newborn, and especially in prematures. Some antibacterial agents and tranquilizers may predispose the infant to hyperbilirubinemia. The antimetabolites are likely to cause
anomalies or spontaneous abortion.

A few children will develop a chronic encephalopathy after some childhood infections with a prolonged high fever. Other encephalopathies implicated in Retardation include carbon monoxide and lead poisoning.

The fetal alcohol syndrome, which includes developmental and neurological
abnormalities, is a toxic syndrome which can contribute to Mental Retardation.
Though not every child of an alcoholic mother develops the fetal alcohol syndrome,
there is no doubt that the woman who drinks heavily (daily use of 4 oz or more of
100-proof alcohol or its equivalent) during pregnancy places her child at risk for
birth defects and mental retardation. The risks associated with moderate drinking are not known and research has not established a safe level for maternal alcohol use. The mechanism for the development of fetal alcohol syndrome is unknown. A possible association with zinc deficiency has been suggested.

Trauma or Physical Agent

Anesthetic agents used during delivery, especially in premature infants, may depress respiration, or interference with placental circulation may result in anoxia at birth. Intracerebral bleeding, subarachnoid or subdural hemorrhage, may occur with precipitate or difficult deliveries, especially when forceps are used. The site of the bleeding determines the nature of the damage, and muscular dysfunction, perceptual impairments, or convulsions may occur along with Retardation. As in the infant, brain injury in a young child may result in Retardation.

Disorders of Metabolism, Growth, or Nutrition

Mental Retardation may be associated with the congenital inability to metabolize certain proteins, lipids, and carbohydrates. With early recognition of some of these inborn errors of metabolism, Retardation may be avoided or minimized by altering the diet, as in phenylketonuria and galactosemia, or by supplying the deficient substance, as in hypothyroidism. In those disorders known to have a genetic basis, early detection allows for genetic counseling regarding future pregnancies.

Disorders of Protein Metabolism

Some of the disorders of protein metabolism often with associated aminoaciduria are Hartnup disorder, oasthouse urine disease, homocystinuria, phenylketonuria, maple syrup urine disease, argininosuccinicaciduria, histidinemia, cystathioninuria, and citrullinuria. All of these disorders may be associated with brain damage, Retardation, or neurological symptoms.

Phenylketonuria results from a defect in the enzyme phenylalanine hydroxylase which prevents the metabolism of phenylalanine to tyrosine. Genetic transmission is by a simple autosomal recessive gene. The disorder can be detected by testing the infant's urine with ferric chloride, by the Guthrie bacterial inhibition assay on blood, and by determination of the serum phenylalanine. Marked reduction in the amount of phenylalanine in the diet as early as possible may prevent Retardation.

The branched chain amino acids, valine, leucine, and isoleucine, have been implicated in maple syrup urine disease. Infants with this enzymatic defect fail to thrive, are severely Retarded, and have multiple neurological dysfunctions. A diet low in these branched chain amino acids may prevent the profound Retardation and early death in infancy which otherwise would result.

Defective tryptophan transport is thought to be involved in Hartnup disorder. In the child with this condition, irritability and mental deficiency follow the development of a pellagralike skin rash on the exposed parts of the body. Neurological signs such as ataxia, nystagmus, and tremor of the hands and tongue are associated with this disorder.

Although aminoacidemia is present in Wilson's hepatolenticular degeneration, mental and neurological symptoms occur usually in adolescence or early adult life so that deterioration of mental function rather than Retardation usually occurs.

Disorders of Lipid Metabolism

Progressive mental and motor deterioration occur with the disorders involving faulty lipid metabolism. Like the aminoacidurias, these disorders, the cerebral lipoidoses, are genetically transmitted.

In Amaurotic Family (or Familial) Idiocy, the most frequently seen form is the early infantile type, or Tay-Sachs disease. After developing normally for a few months, the infant gradually deteriorates physically and mentally. Spasticity, convulsions, and blindness ultimately appear. A typical cherry-red spot is present in the macular area of the retina. In the juvenile type, Spielmeyer-Vogt disease, the onset is later, and degeneration occurs more slowly. Although there is macular degeneration, the cherry-red spot is not present. The early juvenile type, Bielschowsky-Jansky disease, and the late juvenile type, Kufs' disease, occur later and progress somewhat more slowly, but in all forms of the disorder degeneration and death result.

Niemann-Pick disease resembles Tay-Sachs disease in its onset and course. They differ in that in Niemann-Pick disease the liver and spleen are greatly enlarged due to the deposition of sphingomyelins in the reticuloendothelial system.

Gaucher's disease, lipid histiocytosis of the kerasin type, occurs in two forms, the acute infantile type which is likely to be accompanied by Mental Retardation and early death, and the chronic form which is usually slowly progressive but without Retardation. In this disorder, kerasin is deposited in the cells of the reticuloendothelial system. Usually, central nervous system involvement is present only when the onset of the disease is during infancy, usually at 4 to 6 months of age.

Disorders of Carbohydrate Metabolism

Children with galactosemia have an enzymatic defect which interferes with metabolizing galactose to glucose. They lose weight and develop jaundice, liver enlargement, and cataracts along with Mental Retardation if they continue to ingest galactose. Early elimination of milk and substitution of a diet free of galactose is necessary for the child with this disorder.

A high protein diet may be useful in glycogenosis, Von Gierke's glycogen storage disease. Liver enlargement, hypoglycemia, and sometimes convulsions because of the defect in conversion of glycogen to glucose, abnormal responses to testing with epinephrine and glucagon injection, ketosis, and an abnormal glucose tolerance test are characteristic of the disorder. The associated Mental Retardation is often relatively mild.

Other Metabolic Disorders

Hypothyroidism may be present at birth or may become apparent in the first few months of life. Retarded growth; lethargy and irritability; anemia; constipation with abdominal distention and sometimes an umbilical hernia; dry, puffy, cold skin; thick lips and protruding tongue; thin hair; and neurological signs such as ataxia, tremor, or rigidity may be found in children with congenital or acquired cretinism. Early replacement of the missing thyroid hormone may eliminate or minimize the degree of Mental Retardation.

Accumulation of mucopolysaccharides in all tissues is characteristic of gargoylism. In this disorder, also known as lipochondrodystrophy or Hurler-Pfaundler's disease, varying degrees of Mental Retardation from mild to severe may be associated with the multiple deformities present in this syndrome. Children with gargoylism are dwarfed and have kyphosis and other skeletal deformities. Their skulls are enlarged and deformed with characteristic coarse facial features, saddle nose, bushy eyebrows, and thick lips. They develop corneal opacities and an enlarged spleen, liver, and heart.

New Growths

In several conditions frequently associated with Mental Retardation growths within the cerebrum account for the symptoms. These are intracranial neoplasm, neurofibromatosis, trigeminal cerebral angiomatosis, and tuberous sclerosis.

With neurofibromatosis, von Recklinghausen's disease, the intelligence level may vary from severely Retarded to normal. This is a hereditary disorder in which there are light brown patches of pigmented skin and sometimes pedunculated soft tumors of the skin. Mental symptoms are probably related to the presence of neurofibromatous tumors within the cranial cavity.

Tuberous sclerosis, epiloia, is also transmitted genetically. In this disorder, sebaceous adenomas are distributed in a butterfly-shaped rash over the face. Tumors of the eye, brain, and other organs, convulsions, psychosis, and varying degrees of Mental Retardation are also found.

In trigeminal cerebral angiomatosis, Sturge-Weber-Dimitri disease, vascular malformations over the meninges of the parietal and occipital lobes and maldevelopment of the cortex are associated with a cutaneous angioma of the face in the trigeminal region.

Unknown Prenatal Influences

Congenital cerebral defects may result in early death or they may be associated with severe Retardation. These congenital defects of undetermined etiology include anencephaly, hemianencephaly, malformations of the gyri (agyria, microgyria, and macrogyria), porencephaly, and multiple congenital anomalies of the brain. Porencephaly, in which there are cavities communicating from the ventricles to the surface of the brain, may also result from known causes such as postnatal trauma or asphyxia at birth.

Mental Retardation does not always occur with the primary cranial anomalies, acrocephaly, scaphocephaly, and hydrocephaly. When present, Retardation probably results from brain damage secondary to pressure. Premature closure of the coronal suture produces the tower skull characteristic of acrocephaly or oxycephaly. Acrocephaly is sometimes accompanied by syndactyly in the Apert-Park syndrome. Premature closure of the sagittal suture results in the typical boat-shaped head of scaphocephaly. Hydrocephalus may be congenital, resulting from prenatal factors, or it may be secondary to other conditions such as meningitis or hemorrhage. The severity of the handicap in hydrocephalus can vary from complete helplessness to nearly normal activity. Surgical procedures have been devised in an attempt to alleviate all of these conditions, and they should be carried out as early as possible to minimize damage to the brain.

Severe Retardation is associated with macrocephaly, as are headaches, visual disturbances, and convulsions. The skull and brain are both enlarged.

Primary microcephaly is thought to be transmitted genetically by a single recessive gene. The head is small, less than 17 in (43.5 cm) in circumference, and the face is of normal size. Moderate to severe Retardation occurs with this disorder and other defects, deafness, cataracts, etc., may be present.

In the Laurence-Moon-Biedl syndrome, obesity, Retardation, polydactyly (often with syndactyly), skull deformities, and retinitis pigmentosa are accompanied by neurological disturbances such as ataxia, nystagmus, and facial palsies.

Harelip, cleft palate, and congenital abnormalities of the teeth, hands, feet, and heart are often associated with hypertelorism. In this disorder there is an abnormal development of the sphenoid bone which results in a separation of the nasal bones and an increased distance between the eyes.

Chromosomal Abnormalities

Of the chromosomal disorders, which account for about 5 percent of cases of mental retardation, Down's Syndrome, formerly called mongolism, is clinically the most important because of its frequent occurrence and the consequent need for genetic counseling. Most patients have trisomy of chromosome 21 with the result that they have 47 chromosomes instead of the normal 46. This form of Down's Syndrome is more likely to occur when the mother is older, with the risk increasing with increased maternal age. A small percentage have double trisomy with 48 chromosomes, mosaicism in which some cells have 46 and some have 47 chromosomes, and translocations in which there are 46 chromosomes with segments of chromosomes exchanged. When a translocation is present the disorder is more likely to be transmitted genetically and is unrelated to maternal age.

Because of their obliquely set eyes with narrow palpebral fissures and characteristic epicanthal fold, the short stubby nose, and a somewhat flattened face and occiput these children seem to resemble each other. They may have palatal deformities and their protruding tongues are usually large and fissured. Their abdomens may be large and their genitalia underdeveloped. They are of relatively short stature with a generalized muscular hypotonia and moderate incoordination. The fifth finger is usually short and curved. Instead of two creases across the palm there may be only one, the simian line. The skin may be dry, circulation poor, and the hair thin and fine.

Trisomy 18 and trisomy 13-15 are associated with characteristic multiple congenital anomalies. Recurrence risk is thought to be low in these conditions.

In Kleinfelter's syndrome (XXY) and Turner's syndrome (XO) the chromosomal abnormalities are in the sex chromosomes. These disorders may or may not be associated with Retardation. The patients are always sterile in these two conditions.

Prematurity

One of the most important of the known causes of Mental Retardation is prematurity, which is defined as a birth weight of less than 2500 gm (5 lb, 8 oz), assuming a single birth. The premature infant is more vulnerable to central nervous system insult than the full-term child. Seizures, motor disturbances of other types, neurological deficits, and hyaline membrane disease may, singly or in combination, complicate prematurity. Although all premature children do not develop Mental Retardation, their risk is much greater because of lack of development.

Unknown Postnatal Causes

Several conditions of unknown etiology appear to involve demyelinization and diffuse sclerosis. Among these are Krabbe's disease, Merzbacher–Pelizaeus disease, infantile metachromatic leukodystrophy, and Schilder's disease. These disorders are considered to be familial and all of them have mental deterioration with other symptoms, such as convulsions and motor disturbances.

Psychosocial (Environmental) Deprivation

Overall, Retardation associated with psychosocial (environmental) deprivation probably accounts for 75 percent of the Mentally Retarded. Only 25 percent of the Mentally Retarded can be accounted for with known biological causes. The more severe forms of Mental Retardation are found in similar proportions throughout all socioeconomic groups, but cultural-familial Retardation is more common in the lower socioeconomic groups. This Retardation is usually mild and several members of the family may be affected. The relationship of genetic and environmental factors is difficult to assess. Parents who are limited both in intelligence and financial resources may be unable to provide intellectual stimulation to the child. Mental or physical illness in the mother may deprive the child of experiences necessary for normal intellectual development. Severe deprivation such as would occur in a child with a sensory handicap such as blindness or deafness may result in mild mental deficiency. Similarly, children who have spent long periods in an institution where they had few opportunities for close physical and emotional contact may show evidence of this deprivation with mild retardation in learning and adaptive behavior.

Infantile Autism and childhood Schizophrenia may be associated with or confused with Retardation. Retarded children have the same needs and the same emotional disorders as other children, but they may have an additional stress load imposed by their Retardation. The retarded child is likely to experience frequent frustration and may be anxious when too much is expected of him or her. This anxiety may then interfere with learning. Social skills can to some extent compensate for slowness or deficiencies in thought processes, but acquisition and utilization of these skills may be hampered by emotional problems.

PREVENTION

The physician who is aware of the conditions which predispose to Retardation is in a more favorable position to prevent or correct these conditions and in this way to decrease the incidence of Retardation.

Better maternal care during pregnancy can decrease the incidence of severe toxemia, bleeding, and premature delivery with their risk of Retardation. Women of the lower socioeconomic groups are particularly prone to complications of pregnancy because of a lack of adequate facilities for their care or because prenatal care is not considered essential by their cultural group. Very young mothers may be ignorant of their need for care and of the increased incidence of complications in younger mothers. During the prenatal period, mothers with endocrine disorders such as diabetes and hyperthyroidism need special attention to avoid complications in the infant. The toxic and teratogenic effects of medications on the fetus are often difficult to evaluate, making it necessary for the physician to use extreme caution in prescribing medication for pregnant women; it is also essential that self-medication during pregnancy be discouraged.

Warnings should be given about the use of alcohol and recreational drugs during pregnancy. Since the safe level of alcohol consumption is not known, the best advice is not to use alcohol at all. However, if the patient is unable or unwilling to follow that advice, one should at least try to reduce alcohol consumption. On the other hand, one should not frighten the patient by overstating the risks associated with alcohol consumption prior to the diagnosis of pregnancy. One can be reassuring to the patient who is concerned because conception occurred while under the influence of alcohol. One can be somewhat reassuring concerning subsequent drinking before the recognition of pregnancy, especially if drinking has been moderate and pregnancy is recognized promptly.

Because of possible damage to the fetus the mother should be protected from exposure to irradiation. Elective diagnostic x-ray studies should not be performed when a woman is pregnant or during the last half of the menstrual cycle when there is the possibility of pregnancy.

A woman planning to become pregnant who is not already immune to rubella should be vaccinated. Influenza vaccination is also desirable. Vaccination for cytomegalovirus is also possible. Syphilis and other chronic infectious diseases in prospective mothers should be diagnosed and treated. The treatment of an infectious disease acquired early in pregnancy, especially during the first trimester, must take into consideration not only the risk that disease creates for the mother and the risk to the fetus from it, but also the possible effects of medication on the fetus. Effective treatment of infections arising later in pregnancy, since they may cause premature delivery and in some cases may be transmitted to the fetus, may help prevent Retardation.

Amniocentesis is recommended when genetic, enzymatic, chromosomal, or metabolic defects are suspected. It should be recommended, despite the slight (about 1 percent) risk of inducing abortion, if the mother is over 35, if she has had a previous child with a disorder that can be detected in this way, or if either parent is a known carrier of a chromosomal abnormality. Selective abortion is recommended when a condition causing Mental Retardation is found unless the prospective parents reject therapeutic abortion on moral or religious grounds.

Hyperbilirubinemia can result from many factors. It is common in ABO and Rh blood incompatibilities, may occur with other conditions, and is particularly dangerous in the premature infant. To avoid damage, hyperbilirubinemia must be corrected promptly. The infant's blood can be exchanged repeatedly if necessary. Rh-negative mothers can be immunized against developing Rh antibodies by administration of Rh-immune globulin after each incompatible but nonsensitized pregnancy.

Anoxia at the time of birth may be associated with excessive sedation of the mother or with any condition which lowers the mother's blood pressure. Infants who breathe poorly at birth have a high incidence of Retardation, cerebral palsy, and neurological dysfunction. When the newborn infant's breathing, color, or condition is poor at birth, the physician and the family must be sensitive to the possibility of neurological damage. A careful record of developmental progress is desirable on all infants, but in those with a known risk of Retardation, such a record becomes essential so that any problems which develop can be recognized early and remedial steps instituted as soon as possible.

Prolonged high fever in an infant or a series of prolonged febrile seizures with asphyxia may result in brain damage. Prompt treatment of febrile disorders and, if necessary, anticonvulsive medication for febrile seizures may prevent some cases of retardation.

Early identification of the inborn errors of metabolism such as phenylketonuria and galactosemia is necessary if Retardation is to be avoided. The physician should be alert to the signs of these disorders and aware of any family history suggestive of them. For example, phenylketonuria (PKU) must be suspected in siblings of children known to have the disorder. Routine testing of newborn infants for PKU is recommended (and is required by law in some states). However, routine screening misses some cases and reevaluation is necessary if family history or clinical findings arouse suspicion.

There are more than a dozen other genetic disorders that cause retardation and can be detected with urine tests. While infants with chromosomal disorders have characteristic appearances, including abnormal facies, at birth, those with metabolic disorders do not. One must be alert to possible abnormalities in early development or for acidosis, and be ready to search for metabolic disorders so as to be able to start treatment promptly.

Screening for hypothyroidism also reduces the incidence of Retardation.

When one child in the family is born with a defect the parents may wish counseling about their chances for having another child with a similar disorder. Sometimes the family doctor can reassure them that the disorder is not genetically determined. However, in case of doubt, the family may be referred to a genetic
counseling center where chromosome studies can be done, if indicated, to determine whether or not the couple may be carriers of a genetically determined defect.

The number of children who suffer brain damage from accidents and poisoning
can be reduced through education of the parents and other adults in the community.

Many factors are implicated in cultural-familial Retardation. Any condition
which interferes with the mother's healthy interaction with her baby may interfere
with adaptive capacity. If the mother is physically or emotionally ill, or if she has
too many other responsibilities to be able to devote time to her new infant, the
child is likely to suffer from lack of stimulation. Arrangements for additional mothering for the child or help for the mother can sometimes be made. In some families, lack of time, money, or inclination to encourage the child to learn may result in the child's entering school deficient in experiences which would facilitate
progress in school. Exposure to more varied opportunities for learning will sometimes remedy the apparent defect in a mildly retarded child (often referred to as
culturally deprived). When there is a lack of intellectual stimulation in the family
setting nursery school, when it is available, may be helpful. In those families
where it is impossible for the child to receive proper care, foster home placement
may be necessary and is a more satisfactory arrangement than institutionalization
because of the additional stimulation likely to be available in a family setting.

DIAGNOSIS

The diagnosis of Mental Retardation is usually made in childhood, but it can be
made during adult life if history indicates an onset before the age of 18. An onset
after the age of 18 calls for a diagnosis of Dementia.

As may be evident from reviewing the causes of Mental Retardation, certain
children are more likely to become Retarded than others. For example, children
with congenital abnormalities (either genetically determined or resulting from prenatal influences), premature infants, infants with a history of hyperbilirubinemia,
or those who were anoxic at birth constitute an at risk group. The family physician
or pediatrician who keeps a careful record of the progress of these children through
the developmental stages will be in a position to suspect Retardation if the child
begins to lag behind other children of the same age. There might be concern about
Retardation in the child who is too good, too placid, or apathetic, or in the irritable hyperactive child who may show signs of minimal brain damage. When there
is a suspicion of Retardation, the doctor's first task is to establish a diagnosis.
The family physician may examine the child and make arrangements for the other
examinations necessary for a thorough evaluation of the child's potential. The initial examination usually includes a careful physical and neurological examination,
searching for minimal (so-called "soft") signs of neurological dysfunction, for defects in vision or hearing, for discrepancies between the child's performances and
the developmental norms applicable to his or her age, and for evidence of metabolic or genetic disorders. Additional studies such as an electroencephalogram,
x-rays of the skull and extremities, and appropriate blood and urine examinations
may be included.

An accurate measure of intelligence is essential for the diagnosis of Mental
Retardation. Standardized intelligence tests are most reliable for children over
age 6, but can be used for children as young as 2. In evaluating infants, one must
rely on clinical judgment.

One uses caution in accepting parental reports of previous IQ measurements, and verifies conditions under which testing was done, tests used, and the qualifications of the person doing the testing. One usually needs to use more than one test and test on more than one occasion.

The Stanford Binet Intelligence Scale and the Wechsler Scales are the most widely used and reliable intelligence tests. However, when a nonverbal test is needed (e.g., for a patient with a language problem) the Columbia Maturity Scale is probably the most satisfactory.

Retardation is not diagnosed on the basis of intelligence testing alone; there must be impairments in adaptive behavior. Though the clinician can usually assess these from history and observation, testing is also available. The Adaptive Behavioral Scale measures 28 areas of functioning. The Vineland Social Maturity Scale yields a Social Quotient.

If the physician is unable to determine the cause or the extent of the child's deficiencies, and feels that the services of several specialists are necessary, the family may be referred to a clinic where speech and hearing specialists, psychologists, psychiatrists, cytogeneticists, neurologists, and other specialists are available. The age of the child and the nature of any associated problems such as convulsions, spasticity, or blindness to some extent determines what additional services would be necessary in making a complete assessment of the child's capabilities and limitations. As previously noted, severe Retardation with associated neurological deficits is more likely to be recognized in infants, and the evaluation procedures in these infants differ somewhat from those used in evaluating a mildly retarded child referred because of behavioral problems at school.

INTERPRETATION

As important as making the diagnosis is the interpretation of the results of the examinations to the parents. If the parents are to help the child achieve his or her potential, they must know both the limitations and the assets. In addition, they will want to know what changes in the child they may reasonably expect as he grows older.

The physician should inform the parents of available facilities in the community. They need to know about support groups and organizations that may help them and the child. They need to know what the community offers in training and special education for the retarded, what options there are, if any, and the advantages of each. If the child cannot be cared for at home, is hospital care, residential schooling, or placement in a group home feasible? If there are options, what are the advantages and disadvantages of them?

The parents need help in explaining the problem to the child's siblings and handling the siblings' feelings about the retarded child. They are likely to need counseling or psychotherapy to help deal with their own feelings about the child.

MANAGEMENT OF PROBLEMS COMMON TO RETARDED PEOPLE AND THEIR FAMILIES

Although the treatment and recommendations pertinent for any one retarded patient and the family would be specific to the underlying cause of the disorder and would be unsuitable for another, some common problems are likely to develop, particularly at crucial points in the retarded person's life.

Nearly all families will need support and understanding during the process of diagnosis and in accepting the diagnosis of Retardation when it has been made. Some will not accept the fact that the child is Retarded and will go from clinic to clinic hoping to find someone who will rescind the diagnosis. Whether the first suspicion of deficiency comes from the family doctor's appraisal of the child's condition, or from the family's noticing that something seems wrong, some degree of distress is usually evident in the family. The impact of having a retarded child may be greater in one family than in another and may depend to some extent upon the aspirations for that child. Many parents will deny that the child is Retarded. Others will feel angry and try to find someone or some event to blame. Still others will feel guilty about having produced a handicapped child. Often the doctor will need to encourage the parents to explore their feelings about the child. Then the physician can help them accept the child, with the strengths and the limitations, and can help the family see that although there are problems associated with rearing a retarded child, there are challenges and rewards also.

Parents of a retarded child may become overprotective and thus deprive the child of experiences which would help integration into society. They may become rejecting and expect performances beyond the child's capabilities. As with normal children, either overprotection or rejection can result in emotional problems which may become evident in behavior such as hyperactivity, aggressiveness, or withdrawal. Parents may need support and guidance in their efforts to train the child in the fundamentals of self-care and the rules of social living. Acquisition of social skills is important for any child and may to some extent help the retarded child compensate for deficiencies in other areas.

Unless encouraged to look for areas of aptitude the parents may not become aware of the child's abilities. They may need support in helping the child learn to do those things which he or she is capable of learning. For example, the child may have aptitudes in art or music, or she or he may be able to develop skill in handicrafts, and can gain self-esteem and confidence from becoming proficient in these areas. The parents can teach good work habits; they can praise the child when he or she performs well when doing household tasks or learning skills which may help later when looking for work. The physician may have to help the family shift their focus from the child's disabilities to abilities so that these can be developed.

The family physician may need to help the family obtain special diets, braces, medications to control convulsions, and special schooling and other services for the handicapped child. The doctor should introduce them to organizations such as the National Association for Retarded Children. The physician may help the family arrange for additional group contacts such as a preschool enrichment program or nursery school. If necessary, he or she may advise the family about placement in an institution or foster home when the family is unable to provide care.

In considering institutional placement, the family should know the indications for placing the child away from their own care. Only a very small percentage of the Retarded are institutionalized at any time in their life. Placement is more likely to be required for those with severe physical handicaps which make constant nursing care necessary. Most families are unable to provide constant care to one member of the family without neglecting the needs of other family members. Institutional placement may be the only solution when the parents of a severely retarded person become unable to care for the child because of their own illness or when one parent dies unless community programs can provide considerable assistance within the home. Temporary placement may be possible for less severely retarded people while they are learning elements of self-care, or while they are participating in rehabilitation programs designed to prepare them for working and handling their own affairs. If permanent or temporary institutional care seems indicated, delay in placement until the child has had an opportunity to gain experience in family living is desirable. A period of living in a home setting seems to help the child develop emotionally and often makes adjustment to the institution easier when placement becomes essential. Families may need help in choosing between a private or state-supported facility, weighing the difference in cost between them and the suitability of the institutions for meeting their child's needs.

Starting in public school may be difficult for the retarded child and the family. For the mildly retarded youngster, it may be the first time that anyone has noticed his or her inability to compete on equal terms with the other children. Frustration may lead to behavior problems or withdrawal from competition and contacts with other children. In the past, these problems sometimes led to institutionalization, as this was the only way that these children could get special education. However, with the development of community programs other options are available, including special learning centers that the child may attend while living at home, special classes for the handicapped within the public school system, and mainstreaming (being kept in regular classes but having supplemental instruction and supervision by teachers trained in special education), which is often best for the mildly retarded.

Public school systems are required by law to provide appropriate education for the handicapped. School systems usually provide some special educational services and may contract for others. In addition, when a particular student needs services not routinely provided, payment for these may be authorized. School systems have different procedures for handling these situations, and the physician needs to be familiar with them so as to advise parents about the methods for obtaining help from the school system and he or she also needs to be prepared to interpret the child's special needs to school officials.

The family's attitude toward the child and his or her accomplishments can help during the school years. If they can encourage the child without making demands beyond his or her capabilities and can give support without being overprotective, they can help the child to develop a realistic sense of confidence in his or her abilities as well as an acceptance of limitations. This together with practical experience and exposure to people of different age groups and to a variety of social and vocational situations maximizes the opportunity for emotional and intellectual growth.

When a retarded child reaches adolescence the parents often become concerned about sexual behavior. Some retarded children are impulsive and show poor judgment in their interpersonal relationships; others will exhibit more social awareness and control. The mildly retarded adolescent usually will not differ in sexual development and inclinations from others in the age group. The severely Retarded are often not sexually active. As with training in other areas of social interaction, parents will find that being patient, firm, and consistent in limit setting will result in acceptable behavior. Simple explanations of what is considered proper behavior, encouragement in activities which are not sexually stimulating, and adequate parental supervision while the youth is learning how to cope with his or her newly developing urges may prevent problems from arising.

Some parents will ask advice about contraception or sterilization at this time. However, most families need the opportunity to explore their fears and concerns about the patient's sexuality more than they need specific advice. Contraceptive advice, taking into account the patient's possible difficulties in understanding and following procedures should certainly be given, if the patient is sexually active or seems about to become so. Before advising sterilization one needs to explore the feelings of the patient and family thoroughly, and take into account the moral and legal requirements for informed consent.

Except in communities where the child would be passed from grade to grade without regard for having profited from the previous one, the retarded youth may not attend high school, as such. Vocational training should be begun early and will occupy the time usually devoted to academic training at the high school level. In choosing the line of work best suited for the individual retarded youth, all capabilities, social, physical and mental, must be weighed. Some will be able to learn semiskilled trades, others may need a sheltered workshop, and others may be able to do only simple repetitive tasks under supervision. Since learning rates as well as abilities vary, the training period may extend beyond the usual high school years.

It is in the years after completion of schooling or training that the number of recognized retarded persons decreases. The severely Retarded have a somewhat increased susceptibility to illness and a higher death rate, so that there are proportionately fewer of them in this age group. Many of the more mildly Retarded are able to marry and become an indistinguishable part of the community. Those who are slightly more handicapped may still be able to support themselves but cannot maintain a family. Others may be only intermittently employed and may need some support from public funds. Still others, who could live in the community without needing institutional care, may be unable to provide for any of their own support and are therefore dependent upon family or public funds. For the last group, provision for their care and for management of their financial and legal affairs is essential. Especially after their parents are no longer available to care for them, they may need to have a guardian appointed or possibly be placed in a nursing home or private family.

Mildly and Moderately Retarded patients often need counseling or psychotherapy to help them with their feelings about being retarded and about the social attitudes they encounter. They also need help with problems in interpersonal relationships and with a variety of problems in living. However, they are, like everyone else, subject to other psychiatric disorders and these must be correctly diagnosed, not merely attributed to retardation, and treated on their own merits.

Management is a continuing process throughout the retarded person's life, and the amount and kind of help needed or required will differ with each stage of life.

REVIEW QUESTIONS

1. Discuss the prevalence of recognizably mentally retarded people in the population in each age group.
2. What examinations should be carried out in the diagnosis of Mental Retardation in a child of school age?
3. Give at least one example of each of the major categories of inborn errors of metabolism which may be associated with Retardation.
4. In making a diagnosis of Down's Syndrome, what physical characteristics would you look for? What is the chromosomal abnormality usually associated with this disorder? In what way is the maternal age a factor in the incidence of this syndrome?
5. In classifying the degree of Mental Retardation, the IQ range or a descriptive term may be used. What is the IQ range for Mild Mental Retardation? Moderate? Severe? Profound?
6. How is Borderline Intellectual Functioning classified? Under what circumstances is it important to recognize and diagnose this condition?
7. If you were a primary care specialist, what would you do to help reduce the incidence and prevalence of the fetal alcohol syndrome?

8. Suppose you have a pregnant patient who is drinking heavily and is unwilling to stop drinking or even to attempt to modify her drinking habits. Is there anything you might do that could possibly reduce the chance of her child's having fetal alcohol syndrome?

SELECTED REFERENCES

1. American Medical Association, Council on Scientific Affairs: Fetal effects of maternal alcohol use. *JAMA* 249(18):2517-2521, 1983.

2. David, Oliver J., Gary Grad, Barbara McGann, and Arnold Koltun: Mental retardation and "nontoxic" lead levels. *Am J Psychiatry* 139(6):806-809, 1982.

3. Eaton, Louise F., and Frank J. Menolascino: Psychiatric disorders in the mentally retarded: Types, problems, and challenges. *Am J Psychiatry* 139(10): 1297-1303, 1982.

4. Efron, M. L., and M. G. Ampola: The aminoacidurias. *Pediatr Clin North Am* 14:881-903, 1967.

5. Jakab, Irene (Ed.): *Mental Retardation.* Vol. 2, Karger Continuing Education Series. New York, Karger, 1982.

6. Menolascino, Frank: *Psychiatric Approaches to Mental Retardation.* New York, Basic Books, 1970.

7. Menolascino, Frank: *Psychiatric Aspects of the Diagnosis and Treatment of Mental Retardation.* Seattle, Special Child Publications, 1971.

8. Menolascino, Frank, and Michael L. Egger: *Medical Dimensions of Mental Retardation.* Lincoln, Nebraska, University of Nebraska Press, 1978.

9. Menolascino, Frank J., Ronald Neman, and Jack A. Stark: *Curative Aspects of Mental Retardation: Biomedical and Behavioral Advances.* Baltimore, Brookes, 1983.

10. Reiss, Steven, and Betsey A. Benson: Awareness of negative social conditions among mentally retarded, emotionally disturbed outpatients. *Am J Psychiatry* 141(1):88-90, 1984.

11. Saunders, Edward J.: The mental health professional, the mentally retarded, and sex. *Hosp Community Psychiatry* 32(10):717-721, 1981.

12. Sovner, Robert, and Anne DesNoyers Hurley: Do the mentally retarded suffer from affective illness? *Arch Gen Psychiatry* 40(1):61-67, 1983.

13. Tarjan, George: Mental retardation. *Psychiatr Ann* 4(2):5-44, 1974.

14. Review: The role of zinc deficiency in fetal alcohol syndrome. *Nutr Rev* 40(2):43-45, 1982.

Chapter 17

PSYCHIATRIC DISORDERS OF CHILDREN AND ADOLESCENTS

INTERACTIONS BETWEEN PARENTS AND THE CHILD

The prevention and treatment of mental disorders in childhood is particularly important, not only because of the immediate problems created by the illnesses, but also because of the importance of childhood experiences in the etiology of adult disorders. Although there are child psychiatrists accessible to most communities and general psychiatrists see some children and adolescents, most of the treatment of the psychiatric disorders of children is done by primary physicians in Pediatrics and Family Practice.

Anyone who has observed newborn infants in the hospital nursery is aware that each infant shows individual characteristics. The babies vary in size, physical appearance, and response to stimulation even at this early age. Some are awake, hungry, and crying loudly before scheduled feeding times; others may sleep intermittently, even while being fed. Some appear irritable and others placid. On being taken home from the hospital, some will sleep through the night but most will awaken at least once to be fed. As each child is different, so are the family reactions to him or her.

Important factors in the interaction with the parents may be present before the infant is born; whether the child was wanted and planned strongly affects parental reaction. An infant born prematurely, spending weeks in the hospital before going home, or a baby with a physical deformity may experience a different set of early parental attitudes than a normal, full-term baby without obvious handicaps. Example: The difficulties in feeding an infant with a cleft palate may add to the mother's feelings of guilt or disappointment over having had a disfigured baby, and she may then react with rejection or be oversolicitous.

Constitutional factors influence the child's reaction to the family atmosphere into which he or she has been born. An irritable child and a phlegmatic one experience their environments in different ways and evoke different responses from their parents. A mother who would accept the responsibilities of caring for a placid, cheerful baby may be uncomfortable and covertly rejecting of an impatient, demanding infant who cries frequently.

Seemingly unrelated events and circumstances may influence the way a child is accepted. A move or job change, or a family crisis such as divorce, illness, or death can alter the emotional climate of a family. A mother who is left without the support of significant family members may not welcome a child's dependence on her. If these crises occur when the children are older, she may be unaware of the effect on them of parental absences, serious illness, or death, or of separation and divorce, and therefore may not offer explanation, reassurance, or comfort.

The child's position in the family may to some extent determine how he or she is received. New mothers with a first-born child often feel inadequate to deal with unfamiliar tasks of caring for the child and communicate their anxiety to the child. A mother who already has more children than she feels she can care for may regard another new one as, at best, a mixed blessing. For the children in a large family, each newcomer may mean less attention for the older children.

Parental rejection and overprotection are often cited as the most important sources of later maladaptive behavior in children, and parental attitudes are considered to be the most important factors in a pathological parent-child interaction. The rejection or overprotection is often unconscious, and not within the parents' awareness, but may occasionally be overt and recognized. For the most part, pathological attitudes of the parents are inadvertent, the product of their own immaturity and conflict, and are not a deliberate attempt to handicap the child. Parents of a disturbed child may be perplexed by his or her behavior and oblivious to their part in it.

Family, usually maternal, rejection of a child can be expressed in many forms and varying degrees. Outright hostility, cruelty, abandonment, or neglect are obvious manifestations, but the mother who cares only for her infant's physical needs and does not provide emotional warmth may be evidencing her unwillingness or inability to accept the child. As the child grows a little older, the mother may expect performance in excess of the child's ability and may complain of failures to conform to her unreasonably high standards. The child then learns to feel that acceptance in the family depends upon achieving perfect performance. Example: A mother calls her 2-year-old son bad and destructive when he will not willingly share toys with another toddler. In an effort to convince herself that she is not rejecting, a mother may bend over backward to avoid overt rejection and may become overprotective.

Overprotection may arise from an effort to conceal rejection, but it may have other roots as well. A mother to whom the child is especially precious because of being the only surviving infant, or the last baby prior to a hysterectomy, may tend to stand between the child and real or imagined dangers more than necessary, as will some mothers of handicapped children. Overprotection does protect the child from danger, but its restrictions prevent one from growing self-reliant and having confidence in his or her ability to solve life's problems. As part of either the pattern of covert rejection or of overprotection, the mother may become overindulgent with the child. Example: The mother may give the child everything he or she wants and permit any behavior. Excessive permissiveness and indulgence in every whim prepare a child poorly for the realities of living in a society where one is certain to experience some deprivations, restrictions, and frustrations. Overindulgence, like all overprotection, tends to promote infantile behavior patterns, as the child is deprived of experiences necessary for maturity and self-esteem.

Although rejection and overprotection are most easily seen in mothers, because of their greater closeness to the child, especially in the early years, others may exhibit these attitudes. A father who is never home or one who is brutal to the child may be showing his rejection not only of the child, but also of the mother and of the marriage as well. Grandparents and other relatives may contribute to overprotection and/or rejection in cooperation with the mother or despite her efforts to prevent their interference. When parents show favoritism or preference for one child, jealousy among siblings may become a source of rejection. Occasionally, an older child will become overprotective of a younger one as a reaction formation against hostile impulses toward the sibling.

Exposure to other attitudes outside the home may modify the effect of pathological home attitudes, and the child may show disturbances only when confronted with a particularly distressing situation. A child who is belligerent or cries a great deal at home may seem different in nursery school or with a warm, responsive babysitter. Alternately, exposure to the outside world can be a difficult experience if the child has a physical or mental difficulty or if there is a large discrepancy between the home and the environment, e.g., racial, religious, socioeconomic.

Marital difficulties can influence parental attitudes toward the child. For example, a parent who feels that responsibilities to the child prevent dissolving an unsatisfactory marriage may show resentment. A child is sometimes encouraged, overtly or covertly, by one or both parents to take sides in their disputes. This may generate feelings of insecurity, fear, and/or guilt.

When separation or divorce does occur, the child may feel abandoned by the noncustodial parent. At the very least, new adjustments are required by the changed relationship. If the custodial parent remarries, as happens in the majority of cases, the child encounters new relationships and attitudes.

Interaction with other significant people (e.g., siblings; other relatives or nonrelatives living in the home; the persons who take care of the child while the mother works) in addition to the parents help shape the child's personality and may be factors in his or her problems.

To understand the child, one must understand the family, know what is happening in it, and appreciate the interaction between the child and its members.

ENTRY OF THE CHILD INTO A PSYCHIATRIC SETTING

A child is usually brought to a psychiatrist on the complaint of someone else, not by choice. The parents, grandparents, neighbors, school, or court are the ones who most often feel that there is something wrong with the child. Because they are disturbed by a behavior and because the child is often unable to express concern about what is happening in his or her life, information about the child is usually obtained from others. Behavior which is normal at one age may be an indication of trouble in another, and the symptoms for which the child is brought to treatment will vary with the age of the child.

In the infant, feeding problems, sleep disturbances, apathy or hyperactivity, breath-holding spells, excessive crying, or vomiting may alarm the mother. In the preschool child, she may be concerned about toilet problems, masturbation, thumbsucking, or temper tantrums. In older children, the presenting complaints may be school problems, fighting, enuresis, or sleepwalking. Sometimes the child will have regressed, that is, returned to behavior patterns normal for an earlier age. Children often do this under the stress of illness or when a sibling is born.

Whatever the symptoms are, they provide a reason for the parents to bring the child for help. They are the ticket of admission. They may represent the child's inept way of coping with a situation beyond one's capabilities. They may herald the beginning of a major illness or indicate only that the family needs to make minor adjustments in their relationships. They may be satisfactory modes of behavior to the child, but they may be a source of annoyance to the family. Sometimes there has been no change in the child's behavior, but a new family crisis has called attention to the distress of the child and within the family.

The child may exhibit disturbing behavior only in certain restricted situations, such as when asked to share with siblings, when in the presence of certain relatives, or while dining in a public place. The youth may act in an acceptable manner when not confronted with what for him or her may be excessive stress. One may react to coercion by a parent, especially by the mother with rebellion, but conform readily under other circumstances which do not involve a power struggle. In some instances, careful investigation of the complaints and observations of the child over an adequate length of time will reveal no abnormalities, and the problem will be found not within the child and her or his reactions, but in the parents' expectations of the child.

A youth may develop symptoms in the effort of trying to solve conflicts. One may respond to parental dissension with symptomatic behavior. Children sense when parents are in disagreement even if there is no outright fighting, and the child may react appropriately for the age with crying, thumb-sucking, temper tantrums, or demands for increased attention. If the stress is overwhelming, for example, if one becomes convinced that one's parents are going to separate and one will be abandoned, one may begin to exhibit regressive behavior, with patterns appropriate to an earlier age.

When a child is brought to a clinical setting depends on many elements, but the parents' tolerance for deviant behavior is often a determining factor. The nuisance value of the symptoms is important in the parents' (and later, the teachers') reactions to the child's behavior, but parental tolerance of this irritation may vary (e.g., to a perfectionist mother, any evidence of normally aggressive behavior may be cause for alarm). Stealing change from mother's purse may be viewed with amusement in one home and with horror in another.

EXAMINATION OF THE CHILD

Since the child is not a miniature adult, some modifications in examination techniques must be made. The age of the child to some extent determines how much he or she can participate actively in the examination. An infant can be observed under various circumstances and simple neurological tests performed. As motor skills develop, spontaneous activities and responses to the examiner may be included in the evaluation. The older child who can talk and play with toys can cooperate in both examination and treatment. The adolescent may be able to participate on an adult level.

Playrooms are often used in the examination of children. A child may reveal feelings and attitudes through play activities. A playroom setting provides the child with materials for self-expression and also may ease the tension of trying to communicate with a strange adult. Interviewers often introduce the child to the playroom with the indication that it is a room which has toys to play with while they talk together and in this way sets the scene both for playing and talking. The playroom is often viewed as a sort of projective test area in which the child, who is provided with more or less standard toys, equipment, paper, paints, blocks, dart guns, dollhouse and doll family, etc., reveals attitudes and conflicts through play. The child who draws a picture can often be induced to tell about it as he or she may tell a story in response to the CAT cards used in psychological testing. Children often set up the doll family to mirror their own family and may show important family behavior patterns in the make-believe adventures of the dolls. How the patient approaches the play materials, whether cautiously, aggressively, or methodically may reveal some of the habitual ways of reacting to new situations. Since many children find talking with adults difficult at best, the toys and opportunities for activity can diminish the child's restlessness and anxiety while becoming acquainted with the interviewer. Even older children may welcome the diversion of some toys or games during the initial stages of the interview, and some adolescents are more comfortable in any setting which allows them to channel some of their anxiety into activity. When an adolescent is interviewed in an office, a piece of modeling clay or a puzzle may satisfy the need to doodle.

Information from other sources is usually more necessary in the evaluation of children than with adults. The child may be unaware of why she or he is being examined and may not have been told of the appointment until the hour of the examination. Even a patient aware of a disturbing life situation may have difficulty expressing this in words, especially to an adult. Parents are the most frequent informants and the story from the mother may differ from that given by the father, or from information elicited in a joint interview between the parents. If the child is the scapegoat for other family problems, each parent may blame the other for the child's behavior or may wish to attribute the problem to "bad heredity," from the spouse's family, of course. The child may be unfortunately similar in appearance to a relative who is disliked or feared, or may be exhibiting behavior acceptable to one parent but not the other. Because she is more likely to be available to accompany the child the mother is more likely to be seen in the initial interview and give her version of the symptoms. However, whenever possible, the father and other significant members of the household should be interviewed. Grandparents or aunts and uncles who live in the home, full-time domestic employees who care for the child, or even a regular, frequent babysitter may be able to provide data about the child and her or his habits. Not only can they provide useful information, but by their interaction with each other and with the child they may give the observer a picture of the family attitudes which may be provoking the child to symptomatic behavior. The manner in which the information is given may reveal some basic feelings toward the child. The mother who looks daggers at her husband while she recounts a list of the shortcomings of *his* son may be suspected of displacing some of her disappointment in her husband onto the child. Overt rejection may be obvious. Perfectionist expectations and subsequent disappointments with the child's performance may be cataloged in detail. Sometimes acceptance of the youth, but puzzled consternation about the symptoms, may be the parents' prevailing attitude.

Still other sources may provide information or register complaints about the child. The school will often suggest that the child needs psychiatric evaluation because of poor scholastic performance, inattention, aggressiveness, or poor socialization. The child who conforms, no matter how personally uncomfortable, is not likely to be regarded as a school problem. Even when it is not involved in the referral, the school may report observations of the child's interactions with other children and with teachers and the child's academic performance and intelligence level. The school and family may not see the child in the same light unless the parents have attempted to alert the teachers to the child's "bad" behavior and have inadvertently promoted the same behavior in school that appears at home. If the juvenile court has a part in the referral, that is, if the child's behavior takes the form often labeled delinquent, information may be available from this source. Social agencies such as the county welfare office or the Visiting Nurses Association may occasionally be able to supply information about the family and home conditions.

Information about the child from community sources, from the parents, from the family, and from the child, the interviewer's observations of the child, and the interactions between the family members are the raw materials from which the differential diagnosis is formulated.

As with the adult, physical and neurological examination and indicated laboratory tests should be done when they appear warranted, such as for a child with significant somatic complaints, or with evidence of possible brain damage, endocrine disorder, or toxicity. Psychological testing may be needed to establish the child's intellectual level or to obtain additional projective material.

CLINICAL SYNDROMES IN CHILDREN

Children are remarkably plastic and adaptable, changing their reactions in response to the circumstances in which they find themselves. Therefore, the clinical syndromes are often not as clearly definable in children as in adults and may be more closely related to the interaction which provokes the symptoms. A child who is rebellious and defiant with a rigid, critical teacher may become cooperative in a classroom where the teacher is warm, accepting, and free with praise. The youth who resumes bedwetting after the birth of a sibling may become dry again when he learns through experience that his place in the family has not been usurped. The child may exhibit different symptoms under different conditions and at different ages.

Many of the psychiatric illnesses of adults may also occur during childhood or adolescence, and if they do, the same diagnostic terms are used as would be used for adult patients. However, some childhood disorders are classified separately, as they are ones that are usually first evident in infancy, childhood, or adolescence (see Chapter 4). These may be divided into five groups depending on whether the main symptoms and findings are:

1. Intellectual
2. Behavioral
3. Emotional
4. Physical
5. Developmental

The Intellectual group, used for Mental Retardation, includes mild, moderate, severe, profound, and unspecified subtypes. The Behavioral group is divided into Attention Deficit Disorders (with hyperactivity, without hyperactivity, and residual) and Conduct Disorders (undersocialized, aggressive; undersocialized, nonaggressive; socialized, aggressive; socialized, nonaggressive; atypical). The third division, Emotional, is subdivided into Anxiety Disorders (Separation Anxiety Disorder; Avoidant Disorder; Overanxious Disorder) and Other Disorders of Infancy, Childhood, or Adolescence (Reactive Attachment Disorder of Infancy; Schizoid Disorder; Elective Mutism; Oppositional Disorder; Identity Disorder). Those in which the main symptoms and findings are physical include the Eating Disorders (Anorexia Nervosa; Bulimia; Pica; Rumination Disorder of Infancy; Atypical Eating Disorder), the Stereotyped Movement Disorders (Transient Tic Disorder; Chronic Motor Tic Disorder; Tourette's Disorder; Atypical Tic Disorder; Atypical Stereotyped Movement Disorder) and Other Disorders with Physical Manifestations (Stuttering; Functional Enuresis; Functional Encopresis; Sleepwalking Disorder; Sleep Terror Disorder). The last group is Developmental, which includes Pervasive Developmental Disorders (Infantile Autism; Childhood Onset Pervasive Developmental Disorder;

Atypical Developmental Disorder) and Specific Developmental Disorders (Developmental Reading Disorder; Developmental Arithmetic Disorder; Developmental Language Disorder; Developmental Articulation Disorder; Mixed Specific Developmental Disorder; and Atypical Specific Developmental Disorder).

INTELLECTUAL DISORDERS

Mental Retardation is discussed in Chapter 16. An estimate of intelligence should be made as a part of the evaluation of any child or adolescent patient. Remember that Mental Retardation is a separate and additional diagnosis when it is present along with another psychiatric disorder.

BEHAVIORAL DISORDERS

The Behavioral Disorders include Attention Deficit Disorders and Conduct Disorders.

Attention Deficit Disorders of Childhood and Adolescence

This disorder has been called the hyperactive child syndrome, minimal cerebral dysfunction, and hyperkinetic reaction. The term Attention Deficit Disorder is probably more specific and appropriate. There is some evidence to suggest that this syndrome may be a genetically transmitted disorder of the catecholamine system. Characteristic features of the Attention Deficit Disorder include: (1) increased activity; (2) impulsivity; (3) low frustration tolerance; (4) short attention span; (5) distractibility; and (6) increased aggression. "Soft" neurological signs may or may not be present. There is an increased incidence of Somatization Disorder, Alcohol Dependence, Antisocial Personality, and "hyperactivity" in parents of children with Attention Deficit Disorder. Attention Deficit Disorders are subclassified into those with hyperactivity and those without. A subclassification of residual type is used for those patients who initially showed hyperactivity but no longer have that symptom. These patients are impulsive and continue to have difficulty in sustaining attention.

Though other treatment may be effective in some cases, many patients with this syndrome respond best to the psychostimulants including amphetamine, methylphenidate, and pemoline. Before using these medications (even a brief clinical trial may be misleading because of a transitory placebo effect) one must be certain that the diagnosis is correct, and the medications must be used conservatively because large doses may lead to interference with growth and development, and long-term side effects are possible. Chemical dependence is very rare in later life among persons treated for this condition, but casual use in inappropriate cases would increase the risk.

The critical factor in the Attention Deficit Disorder is to differentiate those cases which have another etiology from the pattern described above. Other causes of increased activity include: (1) Organic Mental Disorder; (2) Schizophrenia; (3) Anxiety Disorders, and (4) Mental Retardation. In the Organic Mental Disorder cases there is a history suggestive of cerebral insult and usually "hard" neurological signs. Memory and new learning are impaired regardless of whether the attention span is short or not. The schizophrenic child has a short attention span because of overutilization of fantasy and autistic thinking. This child has a thought disorder as the primary problem. In an Anxiety Disorder, one finds the physiological signs and symptoms of anxiety which are not present in the true Attention

Deficit Disorder. Intelligence testing is helpful in differentiating the Attention Deficit Disorder from Mental Retardation. Though Retarded children can have Attention Deficit Disorder, most children with this condition are of normal intelligence. The mildly mentally retarded child in the classroom may be disruptive and hyperactive because of frustration or boredom. For that matter, teachers, school nurses, and sometimes parents suspect some perfectly normal and healthy children of being hyperkinetic. An apparent overactivity with disruptive behavior in group situations can result not only from boredom, but also from normal curiosity, and from a lack of readiness for group experience. This condition tends to improve as children get older, and if the child is on medication this should be discontinued from time to time to determine whether it is still needed. Though improvement and apparent remission usually take place before or during adolescence, about a third of children with Attention Deficit Disorder have residual symptoms in late adolescence and adult life. In addition, persons who have had this disorder show a significantly higher incidence of delinquency and of other psychiatric disorders in adolescence and as adults.

The nonhyperactive Attention Deficit Disorder is manifested by an inability to concentrate and sustain productive activity, although the child is able to sit quietly. Impulsivity and noncooperative behavior are seen in both conditions.

Conduct Disorders

The Conduct Disorders are termed undersocialized or socialized, and further defined as either aggressive or nonaggressive. The diagnosis of Atypical Conduct Disorder is used for those cases of Conduct Disorder which do not fall into any one of the four specific types. Undersocialized Aggressive Conduct Disorder is the diagnosis utilized for children with aggressive antisocial behavior, poor interpersonal relationships, and behavioral problems at school. In the Nonaggressive Undersocialized Conduct Disorder, the same triad of symptoms is seen (i.e., poor interpersonal relationships, antisocial behavior, and difficulties at school), although aggression is absent. There are two patterns apparent in this Conduct Disorder: one is seen in shy, timid, compliant behavior, and the other in overingratiating, manipulative behavior with superficial friendliness.

In the Socialized Conduct Disorders one observes antisocial behavior, either aggressive or nonaggressive, with difficulties at school, but with unimpaired interpersonal peer relationships, e.g., friendships are established and loyalties expressed.

EMOTIONAL DISORDERS

The disorders primarily manifested by emotional symptoms include the Anxiety Disorders of Childhood or Adolescence, including Separation Anxiety Disorder, Avoidant Disorder, Overanxious Disorder, and another group of disorders which appear in the classification as Other Disorders of Infancy, Childhood, or Adolescence, and include Reactive Attachment Disorder of Infancy, Schizoid Disorder, Elective Mutism, Oppositional Disorder, and Identity Disorder.

Separation Anxiety Disorder is to be distinguished from the normal reactions of infants and children to parental absences. Up to about the age of 8 months the infant, if well cared for in the parent's absence, tolerates separation well. At about 8 months, the baby shows greater ability to discriminate between strangers and familiar persons, tends to be frightened by strangers, and will often seem distressed when the mother, or the person who usually cares for it, is away even for brief periods. As the baby gets older the fear of strangers lessens and the child, secure that the parent will return again, tolerates brief absences comfortably. Sometimes, instead of this normal developmental pattern, perhaps as the result of prolonged parental absences or events associated with them, a Separation Anxiety Disorder appears in the infant or very young child. This may be manifested by panic upon being separated from the parent. Older preschool children express fears of abandonment, or of getting lost, or vague fears of something bad happening. Still older children have more specific fears, sometimes partially reality based, of things that might happen when the parent is away, and these fears may reach phobic proportions.

Another reaction to prolonged separations from the parent is the development of depressive symptoms which are sometimes severe (when this occurs, the condition is sometimes described as an anaclitic depression; the word anaclitic, derived from a Greek word meaning to lean, refers in this context to depression caused by a failure to have dependent needs met). Infants with this condition fail to thrive.

Another manifestation of Separation Anxiety Disorder which occurs in older children is school refusal (school phobia). This is not a true phobia even though the child may indicate fear of a teacher, classmates, or the school room. It is usually a manifestation of the interaction between the mutual anxiety the child and the mother feel when separated (sometimes due to their hostile dependence on each other), and the child's fear of failure. The mother may wish, consciously or unconsciously, to have the child stay home and may covertly encourage him or her not to go to school. The condition is a self-perpetuating one in which it becomes more difficult for the child to resume attendance after being allowed to remain at home (hence, in treating the condition, one encourages parents to take the child to school despite his or her expressed fears without waiting for the underlying problems to be resolved in therapy). Elements of repressed aggression toward the parent who forces the dependence are important. Any event which threatens to separate the parent and the child may precipitate symptoms. In an older child who begins to complain of fears of school, there is often a history of earlier, less marked difficulties in separating from the mother on entering kindergarten or when a sibling was born. Note: In truancy, the child avoids home as well as school, while in school phobia, as a form of Separation Anxiety Disorder, the child is invariably found at home. Of course, before assuming that fear of going to school is symptomatic of a disorder, one must be sure that there is no real basis for it.

In the Avoidant Disorder, the primary feature is shyness. The child has a clinging, whiny, frightened appearance, especially when exposed to new or unfamiliar people or events. When in the presence of parents or familiar surroundings the child warms up and participates actively without symptoms.

The Overanxious Disorder of Childhood involves excessive worry, obsessive thinking, overt anxiety, and is not focused on a situational event or psychosocial stressor. Also present is initial sleep disturbance with frequent nightmares.

The diagnosis of Reactive Attachment Disorder is utilized for those cases where there is failure to thrive in the absence of any organic etiology or any other diagnosable psychiatric condition that might account for it. It results from neglect, from failure to meet the infant's emotional needs. With adequate mothering it can be reversed. In managing infants with this condition one wants to be sure that the child is receiving attention and physical contact (being held).

In the Schizoid Disorder, shy, introverted behavior is seen as well as a constricted or blunted affect. There is little or no expression of aggressive feelings; age-appropriate interpersonal relationships are sorely lacking. Elective Mutism is the diagnostic term for the child who uses silence as the way to interact with his or her environment.

Oppositional Disorder is the diagnosis for the child who is argumentative and directly obstructionistic toward authority, especially that of parents and/or teachers. Peculiar to this condition is its persistence even in the face of obviously negative consequences, e.g., school suspension. Antisocial behavior does not occur in this disorder. Oppositional behavior is a relative matter. The normal 2-year-old goes through a stage of being quite oppositional. Normal older children are oppositional to an appreciable number of parental demands; the oppositional child simply exceeds the usual frequency of negativistic behaviors (is oppositional about twice as often). Mothers of such children are frequently described as "depressed" or "controlling" (even before the syndrome appears). They tend to give vague instructions to the child and get angry or upset when the child's behavior does not meet their expectations.

Reasoning with healthy children works fairly well, if the children can understand the reasons. With oppositional children it only serves to generate arguments. Attempts at positive reenforcement of desired behaviors lead to patients rejecting the reenforcers. Conventional psychotherapy and behavior therapy (with time out as an aversive measure) are sometimes used in treatment, but teaching parents to give fewer and clearer instructions and commands and to know when and how to ignore oppositional behavior may make treatment unnecessary.

The diagnostic term Identity Disorder is used to describe the childhood or adolescent behavior of a person who as an adult would be called Borderline Personality Disorder. The key feature of these behaviors is very stormy interpersonal relationships.

PHYSICAL DISORDERS

Among the disorders manifested by physical symptoms are five eating disorders: Anorexia Nervosa, Bulimia, Pica, Rumination Disorder of Infancy, and Atypical Eating Disorder. In Anorexia Nervosa, the patients starve themselves. The typical history is of an early adolescent girl who was slightly overweight (10-15 lb). She was also a straight A student, hypersensitive, and compulsive. She decides to diet following an object loss such as a friend moving away. Ideal weight is rapidly attained, but she continues to starve herself. Bizarre eating habits and induced vomiting become part of the syndrome. Most patients view themselves as fat even though they are obviously very thin. Secondary amenorrhea occurs. Numerous physiological abnormalities result from the starvation, especially in those functions regulated by the hypothalamus. The condition may be fatal if untreated.

Anorexia literally means a lack of appetite, but that is not the real problem in Anorexia Nervosa. The problem is one of self-image, of feeling that one is too heavy despite what the scales and mirror show, and what amounts to a phobic dread of gaining weight. Underlying this disorder, which is at least 10 times more common in girls than in boys, is a maturational conflict, a rejection of growing up, a retreat from puberty. Dependency needs and conflicts, fears of adult sexuality, and occasionally fantasies of oral impregnation may be present. There are frequent conflicts with parents who may be overcontrolling and demanding. One should not assume that the condition is purely an eating disorder. One often finds other emotional problems and/or behavioral manifestations.

Early treatment is desirable and a long-term treatment relationship is an important factor in successful management. The latter is sometimes difficult to achieve, as families of patients with Anorexia Nervosa tend to become dissatisfied and shop around for quick cures. With treatment, about two-thirds of patients ultimately regain normal weight. About half of the patients continue to have eating difficulties and/or other psychiatric symptoms. Psychotherapy, behavior therapy, or a combination of behavior modification with individual and/or family therapy can be used in treating these patients. Medications, including tricyclic antidepressants and lithium carbonate, have also been used, and they should be considered if the patient is not responding to other treatment or if depressive features are present. It should be remembered that suicide, other than by starvation, is one of the causes of death among these patients.

Bulimia is manifested by binges of high calorie foods, purging with cathartics and/or self-induced vomiting, and depression. The person is often consciously aware of the problem, unlike those with the anorexias who perceive themselves as fat regardless of how thin they get. However, some patients have combinations of Anorexia Nervosa and Bulimia.

In Pica, the child eats things which have no caloric or food value — such as wood, paint, carpet, etc. He or she also eats "people food" at meals. It is a disorder primarily of preschool children and is sometimes seen as a feature of Infantile Autism or Schizophrenia.

Rumination Disorder of Infancy is the term used to describe a syndrome in which the child regurgitates his or her food. Nausea is absent. Weight loss can be severe, as can failure to thrive.

The diagnosis of Atypical Eating Disorder is used for any other eating disorder than the four just described.

There are five *Stereotyped Movement Disorders:* Transient Tic Disorder, Chronic Motor Tic Disorder, Tourette's Disorder, Atypical Tic Disorder, and Atypical Stereotyped Movement Disorder.

A tic is an involuntary, purposeless motor movement which is made worse by stress or anxiety. If such a tic has been present for at least a month but less than 1 year, the diagnosis of Transient Tic Disorder may be applied.

A diagnosis of Chronic Tic Disorder is made in cases where the tic persists for more than 1 year. Tourette's Disorder (formerly called Gilles de la Tourette's Syndrome) is a condition characterized by multiple tics, movement disorders, and verbal obscenities. It is important to distinguish the early symptoms of Tourette's Disorder from Attention Deficit Disorder, since stimulants used for the latter make Tourette's Disorder worse. The diagnosis of Atypical Tic Disorder is used for tics which do not seem to fit the other tic categories.

Atypical Stereotyped Movement Disorders (characterized by head-banging or rocking) differ from tics in that the movements are voluntary and the patient seems to enjoy the activity.

Other disorders primarily manifested by physical symptoms include: Stuttering, Functional Enuresis, Functional Encopresis, Sleepwalking Disorder, and Sleep Terror Disorder.

Stuttering is a disorder of speech in which there are repetitions of sounds and interruptions of the normal flow of speech. It affects about one of every hundred children, is four times more common in males than females, and remits spontaneously at least half of the time. This type of speech disorder nearly always begins before the age of 12.

Functional Enuresis is the diagnostic term for involuntary urination by a person who is old enough to control it and who has no organic disease that would explain the behavior. Bedwetting is symptomatic after the age of 5. There are two forms: primary enuresis (80 percent) in which the patient never was dry, and secondary (20 percent) in which there is regression after a period of dryness. Most enuresis occurs during deep sleep. Except in cases of secondary enuresis for which the cause of regression is clearly apparent, an evaluation of sleep pattern and a thorough medical examination to uncover nonpsychiatric conditions is required. In evaluation of the family, one often finds a greater than expected dependency upon the opposite sexed parent. Before treating the enuretic child, one must determine whether the child or a significant adult in the family needs psychotherapy. If individual or family therapy is not required, behavioral techniques or tricyclic antidepressants may be effective. These can also be used along with psychotherapy when it is indicated. While more elaborate behavioral techniques may be needed, as simple a device as the "star chart," used by Leo Kanner long before contemporary techniques of behavior modification were developed, which rewards the child with a silver star for a dry night and a gold star for a dry week may be helpful. Aversive conditioning is to be avoided, though devices which simply awaken the child when urination begins are acceptable.

Functional Encopresis is involuntary defecation without another disease (e.g., anal fissure; aganglionic megacolon) to explain it. This condition, just like Enuresis, is more common in male children. Intrafamilial stress is often high in patients with Encopresis. The mother of the child is usually punitive and controlling. The father is aloof and passive. Encopresis is much less frequent than enuresis and the patients tend to have more psychopathology. The patients use much denial and usually are poorly socially integrated. Despite this, they are usually friendly and well-liked by adults. The disorder tends to improve with age, which is fortunate because treatment is seldom effective over a short term.

Sleepwalking Disorder (Somnambulism) is 10 times more prevalent in children than in adults. Most patients recover spontaneously by the end of adolescence or early in adult life. Those who do not or who have a recurrence during adult life are likely to have other psychiatric symptoms. Some have Somatoform Disorders.

Sleep Terror Disorder (Pavor Nocturnus) is a behavior in which the child awakens screaming, the parent finds the child in an altered state of consciousness, and he or she appears disoriented even with eyes open. This disorder occurs primarily before age 4 and usually responds to reassurances by the parents. The child seldom remembers the incident the following day.

DEVELOPMENTAL DISORDERS

Developmental Disorders include Pervasive and Specific categories. The Pervasive Developmental Disorders are divided into: Infantile Autism, Childhood Onset Pervasive Developmental Disorder, and Atypical Pervasive Developmental Disorder.

Infantile Autism

In 1943 Leo Kanner described a syndrome he called Primary Infantile Autism, which he believed to be different from Childhood Schizophrenia. Autistic children are described as unable to make affective contact with people very early in their lives. They are unresponsive to mothering. They resist cuddling and do not display the usual anticipatory responses and postures for being picked up. Mothers become worried, since the children do not cry to get attention and do not seem to care whether they are there or not. Autistic children relate more to objects than to people. Their play is solitary, stereotyped, and repetitive. They have an extreme need for "sameness," insisting on their environment remaining precisely the same. There is little or no language. Many autistic children are mentally retarded, but about a fourth have IQs above 70 and some have superior intelligence. The lack of crying and speech development occurs even in patients with normal intelligence and causes numerous difficulties for these children and their families.

The parents of autistic children are often both highly educated. The child is frequently the first-born to a mother in her 30s. Both parents seem to overutilize isolation of affect as an ego defense mechanism. However, since autism can occur virtually at birth and is not diagnosed unless symptoms are present by the age of 30 months, there is some question as to the relative importance of environmental factors in this disorder.

It has been reported that some autistic children have fragile X chromosomes and respond to treatment with folic acid. A substantial number of Autistic children develop seizures; unless one has ruled out fragile X chromosome disorder, one should avoid giving phenytoin (Dilantin) to these children, as it suppresses folic acid.

Treatment of Infantile Autism should be started early. One should employ multiple treatment modalities. At best, the prognosis is poor and if verbal communication is not established by age 5, it is very poor. However, at least a third of patients benefit from treatment.

Childhood Onset Pervasive Developmental Disorder

Originally described by Loretta Bender as Childhood Schizophrenia, Childhood Onset Pervasive Developmental Disorder occurs at a later age than does Infantile Autism, usually beginning after age 30 months. The onset of illness commonly follows a traumatic family situation or an event which the child may experience as traumatic such as the birth of a sibling. The child then begins to regress. Speech which has been acquired may be lost and those words that are retained may be distorted or used in such a manner as to negate their communication value. Behavior is predominantly autistic with retreat into fantasy, bizarre gestures, and mannerisms. The child is distressed by changes in the environment. Twirling or rocking repetitive movements are found. There may be a family history of Schizophrenia.

The diagnosis of *Atypical Pervasive Developmental Disorder* is used for conditions which do not fit the two mentioned above.

Specific Developmental Disorders

Specific Developmental Disorders are learning disabilities and are not regarded as diseases, but they are included as diagnoses (Axis II), since the physician must evaluate them for diagnostic purposes and is often involved in their management. In the Developmental Reading Disorder, one finds difficulty with reading which cannot be explained by age or education. It is more common in boys and tends to be a familial trait. Developmental Arithmetic Disorder also cannot be accounted for by age or educational deficit; it, too, is more common in boys.

Developmental Language Disorders are divided into expressive and receptive groups. In the former, one understands language but cannot produce it; in the latter, one cannot comprehend the language. In making a diagnosis, the physician must rule out neurological causes.

In the Developmental Articulation Disorders, the patient finds difficulty in the pronunciation of language, although there is no physical reason for this.

The diagnosis of Mixed Specific Developmental Disorder is used to describe multiple developmental problems in the same patient. If one disorder predominates, it should be listed separately.

The category of Atypical Specific Developmental Disorder is used for patients who do not fit the preceding five diagnoses.

THE BATTERED CHILD SYNDROME

Child abuse is not truly a psychiatric disorder of children. If a diagnosis is used, the classification of Parent-Child Problem which is included among the Conditions Not Attributed to a Mental Disorder that are a Focus of Attention or Treatment would be the one chosen. It may be a cause of psychiatric disturbance (if the child survives). The possibility of child abuse should be kept in mind when one sees unexplained injuries in children. Laws in most states require reporting suspected child abuse.

The child that becomes a victim is often one who has been scapegoated because of special difficulties, e.g., "hyperactivity," Retardation, prematurity, etc. The battering parent may be Schizophrenic, Mentally Retarded, Alcoholic, or may have had very punitive parenting modeled at home while a child. Child abuse is an offense, but most courts recognize the possibility that the parent who abuses a child is more a sick person than a criminal, and psychiatric consultation is likely to be requested in such cases. When it is possible to treat the offender, and perhaps other members of the family, this is preferable to punishment. Long-term follow-up is necessary and sometimes placement outside of the home is indicated for the child.

TREATMENT

Treatment of emotional disturbances in children must take into account the many differences between adults and children. The greater malleability of children and their normal maturational processes are assets in the treatment program. Although past experiences are important in shaping current behavior, behavior patterns are not yet fixed. The young child is especially likely to react to people in terms of the real emotions being expressed rather than in terms of expectations from past experiences.

Therapy with children attempts to promote their learning to accept and express their emotions in the presence of an understanding, relatively permissive adult. In play therapy, or with interviews in a playroom, the child can express some feelings and try out solutions to problems using the play materials. Hostile, aggressive feelings can often be worked out in pummeling a dummy or shooting enemy soldiers with a dart gun. Competition can be expressed with a friendly adversary, the therapist. Family situations which are distressing or puzzling to the child may be experimentally resolved in the dollhouse family play. Important in the playroom approach is the presence of the therapist, his or her attitudes, and the relationship which develops between therapist and child as they attempt to explore and remedy the difficulties which have been causing the child to react with symptoms. The primary physician who wishes to use play therapy and does not have access to an elaborate playroom may use simple materials. Even a few crayons and some paper may work nicely (some child psychiatrists prefer this sort of material to the use of the playroom for many cases).

Where the therapy of the child takes place depends upon several factors. If the family lives in an area served by a child guidance clinic, they may contact the clinic personally, be referred by a school or court, or be referred by the family physician. In a child guidance clinic, the child and family are usually evaluated and treated by a team consisting of a psychiatrist, psychologist, and social worker. These clinics are often the major service agency for helping with behavior problems of children. Children may be treated as outpatients in private offices or clinic settings if their disorders are such that they can carry on with most of their daily activities. If the child's symptoms are grossly disabling or if the family setting is unusually noxious, there may be a need for hospitalization. Removing the child from a stressful or hostile environment may be the first step in effective treatment.

Because of the importance of the parent-child interaction, simultaneous treatment of the child and parents is usually attempted, with the focus on the problems of the child as they relate to the family. Such interviews can help the family adapt to the changes in the child as these come about in therapy, and their participation can modify attitudes in the home which have been detrimental to the child. With infants or very young children the therapeutic efforts are, of necessity, directed almost entirely toward helping the parents. Most therapists prefer to treat families of adolescents whenever possible, but they are more likely to accept an older adolescent without the parents being in treatment if the parents are unwilling and the youth wishes to be treated.

Adolescents are particularly likely to be concerned about confidentiality. Accordingly, many therapists restrict talking with parents to those situations in which the patient can also be present. When the parents are willing but the adolescent is not, interviews with the parents may be indicated and a realistic discussion of the adolescent's alternatives to therapy are presented.

An adolescent who feels he does not need psychiatric help may come for interviews to satisfy his parole officer, to keep his parents from nagging, or to ensure that his parents will attempt to modify their behavior toward him. If he has no real choice about seeing the therapist, he may need to be encouraged to use the time to work on problems so that he does not spend his own and the therapist's time unnecessarily.

The parents and child are usually treated individually, or the child may have one therapist and both parents another. In conjoint family therapy all members of the family are seen together and problems in family interaction are explored cooperatively in the presence of one or more therapists.

Consultation with the school may be important to the child's well-being. Placement in another school room or in a class more suited to one's abilities may relieve some of the pressure. A change of teachers may decrease the objectionable behavior or improve performance. A cooperative principal and teachers can be helpful in the therapeutic program for the child.

Social agencies may be utilized for family counseling, for help with family financial problems, or when placement of the child outside the home is necessary. Families known to family service agencies can often be referred back to the agencies for supportive follow-up visits after they leave psychiatric treatment. Social agencies perform a major service in their selection of foster homes for children who have lost their families through death, illness, desertion, separation, or other major family disruptions. By choosing the foster home wisely the social agency can minimize some of the emotional turmoil associated with acquiring a new family and thus prevent the child's having to be placed in a succession of homes. Foster home placement may be necessary for children with emotional problems when their parents' inability to modify cruel, hostile, and rejecting attitudes would make their staying in or returning to the family home disastrous. Careful choice of the foster home, then, becomes one of the therapeutic measures in the child's treatment program.

An equally important service of the social agencies is in the attempted prevention of emotional disorders by careful selection of couples to be adoptive parents. Because of the careful preadoption investigations, both of the prospective parents and the adoptive child, child and parents are usually well matched, and the child is more likely to become part of a family which can offer affection and security.

PREVENTION

For emotional growth to occur, a child needs a family which can give affection, security, and respect to him or her as an individual; one which can provide the guidance and consistent discipline necessary to help one learn the rules of living in society, yet allow freedom to develop individual characteristics; one which can impart the feeling of importance and the object of love; a family which can be tolerant of failures, develop strengths, and be stimulated by successes. Any measure which improves the quality of the care of the child gives him or her a better chance to become a healthy adult. Attempts to prevent disorders in children can be made in essentially three spheres: within the child, through the family, and in the community.

Contact with an individual child is likely to come about after there are signs of disturbance. Early treatment lessens the likelihood of the symptoms becoming more serious and helps the patient to learn techniques for coping more effectively with the environment. Since disturbed children grow into adults who marry and have more children, treating the disturbed child can often break the chain of anxious parents having anxious children, etc. Parents who were themselves rejected often have difficulty in relating warmly to their children.

Counseling with the parents of a disturbed child may be helpful, not only in the life of the child brought for treatment, but also in preventing difficulties with other children in the family. Helping the parents work out the personal conflicts which provoke rejection or overprotection of their children can benefit all of the family. Education of the parents before they begin to have children, even before they marry, can help prevent many interpersonal problems within the family.

In preparation for parenthood, numerous practical considerations are made. Children are expensive; the couple has to budget money differently. Housing arrangements will need to take into consideration the addition of another person. The parents, if lacking personal experience, will need to read about parenting, or at least ask questions of those with more experience. The emotional preparation varies from individual to individual and couple to couple. The addition of a child can be a stressful period for either or both parents. If nothing else, the helplessness and complete dependency of the infant will require some adjustment. For example, who feeds the child? When? Who changes diapers? Where does father get his dependency needs met? Where does mother get hers met?

Many community agencies are involved in activities which help prevent emotional illness in children. Nursery school can ease a young child into socialization and learning situations. Organizations such as the Boy Scouts, Campfire Girls, and 4-H can begin to teach children skills appropriate to their age. Recreational facilities provide opportunities for children to relate to people outside the family. Community centers can offer supervised activities to help youth learn community customs. Centers for recreation and other supervised activities are often helpful when both parents work.

Prenatal instructions for pregnant women can ease some of their anxieties about childbearing and their qualifications as mothers. Well-baby clinics and, in some instances, instructions from the visiting nurses can all play their part in helping mothers learn how to care for their children. School courses can provide basic information for dealing with marriage problems, economic planning, or home management. Child guidance clinics or other family service agencies can offer support for families in crisis. Welfare agencies often can relieve overwhelming financial hardship, or through Aid to Dependent Children can provide funds to allow a mother to stay home to take care of her children.

An increasingly large number of mothers work outside the home and must find care for their children in their absence. The important factor in this circumstance is the quality of maternal care both while the mother is at work and when she is home.

In those instances where adequate individual mother substitutes are not available, day nurseries staffed with people trained in child care can provide supervision for children. As with community recreation centers, day nurseries are most needed in urban areas.

In addition to those factors which affect the children and their families directly, general community conditions have an influence. As noted in Chapters 7 and 11, both major mental illness and antisocial behavior are more common in areas characterized by poverty and crowded living conditions. Community efforts to raise living standards, encourage education, or expand vocational opportunities may be reflected in improved mental health.

REVIEW QUESTIONS

1. What symptoms of Separation Anxiety Disorder are seen in infants? Small children? Contrast these to the normal reactions of children at various ages to brief parental absence.

2. How may parents show their rejection before a child is born? During infancy, childhood, or adolescence?

3. Discuss the problems which would be likely to arise when a child who has been overprotected goes to school for the first time.

4. When his mother returns from the hospital with a new baby, a 3-year-old begins to suck his thumb, demands to be fed, and although previously toilet trained, occasionally wets or soils. What conditions would you include in your differential diagnosis? What recommendations would you make to the mother?

5. Discuss the differential diagnosis of a child with what appears to be a Conduct Disorder. How are Conduct Disorders subclassified?

6. An adolescent girl has had a significant weight loss in recent weeks. Physical examination does not reveal a possible cause. She complains of poor appetite, is worried about her weight loss, and appears mildly depressed. Discuss differential diagnosis. What do you think is the most likely diagnosis? Why?

7. What community resources may be helpful in the treatment of a disturbed child?

8. A 9-year-old boy does not seem to pay attention in school, has trouble concentrating, and is easily distracted. He is impulsive and overactive. What is the most likely diagnosis? If this diagnosis proves to be correct, how would you treat him?

9. A mother complains that her child always says "No" when asked to do anything. What would your initial impression be if the child is $2\frac{1}{2}$ years old? Ten years old?

SELECTED REFERENCES

1. Agras, W. Stewart, and Helena C. Kraemer: The treatment of anorexia nervosa: Do different treatments have different outcomes? *Psychiatr Ann* 13(12): 918-928, 929, 932-935, 1983.

2. Barkley, Russell A., and Charles E. Cunningham: The effects of methylphenidate on the mother-child interactions of hyperactive children. *Arch Gen Psychiatry* 36:201-208, 1979.

3. Bindelglas, Paul M., and George Dee: Enuresis treatment with imipramine hydrochloride: A 10-year follow-up study. *Am J Psychiatry* 135(12):1549-1552, 1978.

4. Bowlby, John: *Grief and Mourning in Infancy and Early Childhood, Psychoanalytic Study of the Child.* Vol. 15. New York, International Universities Press, 1960, pp. 9-53.

5. Bruch, Hilde: Anorexia nervosa: Therapy and theory. *Am J Psychiatry* 139(12):1531-1538, 1982.

6. Crisp, A. H.: Anorexia nervosa: Getting the "heat" out of the system. *Psychiatr Ann* 13(12):936-941, 945, 949, 952, 1983.

7. Duffy, John: *Child Psychiatry. Medical Outline Series.* 2nd ed. New Hyde Park, New York, Medical Examination Publishing Co., 1977.

8. Gittelman, Rachel, and Brenda Eskenazi: Lead and hyperactivity revisited. *Arch Gen Psychiatry* 40(8):827-833, 1983.

9. Goodwin, Jean, Catherine G. Cauthorne, and Richard T. Rada: Cinderella syndrome: Children who simulate neglect. *Am J Psychiatry* 137(10):1223-1225, 1980.

10. Halmi, Katherine A., Harry Dekirmenjian, John M. Davis, Regina Casper, and Solomon Goldberg: Catecholamine metabolism in anorexia nervosa. *Arch Gen Psychiatry* 35:458-460, 1978.

11. Johnson, Craig, and David J. Berndt: Preliminary investigation of bulimia and life adjustment. *Am J Psychiatry* 140(6):774-777, 1983.

12. Kashani, Javad H., Robert O. McGee, Sarah E. Clarkson, Jessie C. Anderson, Lester A. Walton, Sheila Williams, Phil A. Silva, Arthur J. Robins, Leon Cytryn, and Donald H. McKnew: Depression in a sample of 9-year-old children: Prevalence and associated characteristics. *Arch Gen Psychiatry* 40(11):1217-1223, 1983.

13. Klee, Steven H., and Barry D. Garfinkel: A comparison of residual and non-residual attention deficit disorder in adolescents. *Psychiatr Hosp* 14(3):167-170, 1983.

14. Kovacs, Maria, Terry L. Feinberg, Mary Ann Crouse-Novak, Stana L. Paulauskas, and Richard Finkelstein: Depressive disorders in childhood. I: A longitudinal prospective study of characteristics and recovery. *Arch Gen Psychiatry* 41(3):229-237, 1984.

15. Lowe, Thomas L., Donald J. Cohen, Jill Detlor, Martin W. Kremenitzer, and Bennett A. Shaywitz: Stimulant medications precipitate Tourette's syndrome. *JAMA* 247(12):1729-1731, 1982.

16. Rosenthal, Perihan A., and Stuart Rosenthal: Suicidal behavior by preschool children. *Am J Psychiatry* 141(4):520-525, 1984.

17. Satterfield, James H., Dennis P. Cantwell, Ann Schell, and Thomas Blaschke: Growth of hyperactive children treated with methylphenidate. *Arch Gen Psychiatry* 36:212-217, 1979.

18. Satterfield, James H., Christiane M. Hoppe, and Anne M. Schell: A prospective study of delinquency in 110 adolescent boys with attention deficit disorder and 88 normal adolescent boys. *Am J Psychiatry* 139(6):795-798, 1982.

19. Thomas, Alexander, and Stella Chess: Genesis and evolution of behavioral disorders: From infancy to early adult life. *Am J Psychiatry* 141(1):1-9, 1984.

20. Walsh, B. Timothy, Jonathan W. Stewart, Louise Wright, Wilma Harrison, Steven P. Roose, and Alexander H. Glassman: Treatment of bulimia with monoamine oxidase inhibitors. *Am J Psychiatry* 139(12):1629-1630, 1982.

21. Weiss, Gabrielle, Lily Hechtman, Terrye Perlman, Joyce Hopkins, and Albert Wener: Hyperactives as young adults. *Arch Gen Psychiatry* 36:675-681, 1979.

22. Wold, Patricia Neely: Anorexic syndromes and affective disorder. *Psychiatr J Univ Ottawa* 8(3):116-119, 1983.

Chapter 18

DIFFERENTIAL DIAGNOSIS IN PSYCHIATRY

THE PURPOSES OF DIAGNOSIS

Differential diagnosis in psychiatry is used for:

1. Correct classification (cf. Chapter 4)
2. Ascertaining information necessary for patient management which is not supplied by classification

RELIABILITY OF PSYCHIATRIC DIAGNOSIS

Questions are raised from time to time about the validity and reliability of psychiatric diagnoses. These are based partly on the infinite variety and complexity of human problems. Also, the presence of different personality theories and the variety of ways used in examining and evaluating patients might raise a question as to whether there could be a reasonable consensus in diagnosis. Actually, there is. There is probably as much concurrence in diagnosing psychiatric conditions among different psychiatrists as there is between specialists in any other branch of medicine.

Any study of the reliability of psychiatric diagnosis must take into account the descriptive nature of most categories and, accordingly, the fact that there will be borderline states between diagnostic entities, so that in some instances two different first choice diagnoses may not actually represent much difference of professional opinion. This is analogous to the problem that might be encountered if one were to classify people in terms of physical attributes such as height. One would expect a high level of concurrence in describing a very short person as short or a very tall person as tall, but with some subjects the difference between a very tall short person or a very short tall person is a meaningless distinction.

Since the publication of the third edition of the *Diagnostic and Statistical Manual of Mental Disorders* in 1980 the degree of reliability (concurrence) in psychiatric diagnoses has greatly increased. This is due to the widespread use of uniform diagnostic criteria. Reliability, but not necessary validity, can be further increased by using standardized interviewing and other diagnostic procedures.

THE APPROACH TO DIFFERENTIAL DIAGNOSIS

At the time of one's initial contact with a patient it may be necessary to make a tentative diagnosis. Sometimes this has to be done during a relatively brief interview. Often there are signs or clues that immediately suggest a diagnostic possibility. In that case, one forms a hypothesis about the diagnosis and tests it by looking for the various other features of the disorder and determining whether the established diagnostic criteria are present. Even if all findings support one's hypothesis, one goes on to consider other diagnostic possibilities, not only because one may be mistaken, but also because the patient may have more than one disorder.

When a probable diagnosis is not easily selected, or in the further evaluation of a patient who is tentatively diagnosed, one can quickly review the entire gamut of psychiatric illness. There are several ways of doing this. A problem-oriented method can be used. Another method is to use a flow sheet starting with a symptom or group of symptoms and using questions to rule various diagnoses in or out as is done in the decision trees included in the third edition of the *Diagnostic and Statistical Manual of Mental Disorders*. Still another is to consider the main groups of disorders identifying those in which the patient's condition may fall, and tentatively excluding others so as to limit the scope of investigations to a small group of disorders, the criteria for each of which can be compared to the available information about the patient.

To make a diagnosis one must first think of the possibility. Some of the more serious disorders are so important that they must be thought of in all cases, though often they may be tentatively eliminated from consideration in the first few minutes of an interview.

ORGANIC MENTAL DISORDERS

The possibility of a brain disorder must be considered in nearly all patients. Usually it can be tentatively excluded on the basis of initial interview without performing a detailed sensorium examination. Clinicians are properly concerned about the possibility of missing the diagnosis of a serious brain disorder (e.g., brain tumor) but this concern does not justify extensive studies in cases where there are no clues to give rise to suspicion of such a disorder if another diagnosis can be made on its own merits. However, in the initial interview, one should be alert to the presence of any of the main findings of Organic Mental Disorders, and if any are present, a detailed sensorium examination, neurological and physical examinations, and possibly psychological testing are indicated. The main clues which suggest the possibility of an Organic Mental Disorder are:

1. Any signs of sensorium impairment. This includes subjective complaints of memory loss as well as difficulties in remembering, focusing attention, or maintaining a mental set observed during the interview.
2. Emotional lability. An Organic Mental Disorder must be considered in the presence of emotional lability or instability even though the instability is lifelong, and in that case more likely to represent a Personality Disorder.

3. History or evidence of a sudden change in character or personality other than those changes definitely associated with specific emotional disorders (e.g., if a normally calm and polite person becomes rude and irritable, one must think of the possibility of brain disease; however, if a normally cheerful person becomes depressed, the possibility does not need to receive strong initial consideration unless there is some other clue suggestive of brain disease).
4. Symptoms, whether associated with the psychiatric complaint or not, which are characteristic of neurological disorders (e.g., headache, convulsions) or systemic diseases which are known to produce brain syndromes.

One should be certain that the signs of Organic Mental Disorder are absent even if a patient presents fairly characteristic symptoms of some other psychiatric disorder (e.g., Anxiety Disorder; Schizophrenic Disorder). Patients who have maintained mental health, or at least adequate adjustment in spite of having intrapsychic conflicts or personality characteristics which would make them susceptible to a psychosis or neurosis may have a weakening of ego defenses accompanying brain damage which allows the functional disorder to become clinically overt. Not only neurosyphilis, but any brain syndrome can be "the great imitator." Moreover, the use (and misuse) of potentially toxic substances is so common in contemporary society that this possible cause of an Organic Mental Disorder must be considered in almost every case one sees. On the other hand, the presence of a mild Organic Mental Disorder which can be diagnosed on its own merits (e.g., a senile dementia, some minimal signs of which might be found in many well-adjusted elderly people) does not exclude the possibility of a patient's having an entirely unrelated psychiatric condition which is also to be diagnosed on its merits. Sometimes there is a problem in determining whether the functional disorder is simply secondary to an Organic Mental Disorder or is a separate condition.

MENTAL RETARDATION

The possibility of Mental Retardation as a consideration in differential diagnosis is often suggested by the presenting complaint. In adult patients it is often easy to exclude this diagnosis early in an interview. History of a school record or an occupation incompatible with retardation is often available. The patient's vocabulary and ability at concept formation may also quickly exclude the possibility from consideration.

When there is reason to suspect Mental Retardation, one must distinguish between this as a primary disorder on one hand, or an apparent retardation based on failure to learn, whether this is due to lack of opportunities or to an early onset of an emotional disorder which interferes with learning and acculturation. There are also adult patients of normal intelligence who use "acting stupid" as a coping mechanism (If I appear dull, nothing will be expected of me); these are often persons with severe Personality Disorders.

The presence of symptoms of another mental disease does not exclude Mental Retardation from consideration. Intellectual handicaps limit coping powers and defenses and make the person subject to a variety of secondary disorders.

Diagnosis of Mental Retardation in the adult as well as in the child requires a complete psychiatric examination, social and developmental history, and sensorium examination. It is not accomplished by tests of intelligence alone.

PRELIMINARY GROUPING OF FUNCTIONAL DISORDERS

If the patient's psychiatric symptoms are not the result of Organic Mental Disorder or Mental Retardation, the field of diagnostic enquiry may be narrowed by placing the case tentatively in one of the main groups of functional psychiatric disorders. These main groups are:

1. The Psychoses (Major Affective Disorders; Schizophrenic, Schizophreniform, and Schizoaffective Disorders; Paranoid Disorders)
2. The Neuroses (Anxiety, Somatoform, and Dissociative Disorders) and Adjustment Disorders
3. The Personality Disorders

The Personality Disorders may be first separated from the others. The Psychoses, Neuroses, and Adjustment Disorders are all more or less acute illnesses with an identifiable onset. The Personality Disorders are essentially lifelong processes. Also, they are manifested by recurring patterns of maladaptive behavior and disordered interpersonal relationships more than by subjective symptoms. An adequate history is important in diagnosing the Personality Disorders because during the mental examination the patient may show symptoms more suggestive of some other condition. The patient with a Personality Disorder, whether seen in the hospital or as an outpatient, is most likely to come to medical attention when under external stress and/or during an exacerbation of symptoms. Though patients with Personality Disorders have minimal subjective anxiety most of the time, they show anxiety under stress. Also, having limited ego strength, they are subject to relatively transitory psychotic or neurotic episodes. Recognition that a Personality Disorder is the diagnosis or one of the diagnoses aids in making an accurate prognosis and in planning treatment.

The next step in the clinician's diagnostic thinking is the distinction between the Psychoses and the Neuroses and Adjustment Disorders. The Psychoses are generally more severe, involve the total personality, and interfere with reality testing.

After tentatively assigning a patient to one of the three main diagnostic groups, one may then consider the possibilities within the chosen group.

DIFFERENTIAL DIAGNOSIS OF THE PSYCHOSES

If the patient's main symptom is a disorder of mood, depression or elation, one suspects a Major Affective Disorder. On the other hand, if the main findings suggest a thinking disorder (the term formal thought disorder refers to peculiarities in the *form* of the patient's ideas), one thinks of Schizophrenic or Paranoid Disorders.

If there is both a thinking disorder and a significant affective disorder (elation or depression, not flat or inappropriate affect), the condition may be a Schizoaffective Disorder. However, it should be remembered that signs of thought disorder can be found among patients who are in the Manic phase of Bipolar Disorder.

If one suspects a Schizophrenic Disorder, one looks for the primary symptoms of schizophrenia:

1. Autism
2. Ambivalence
3. Affective disturbance (flat or inappropriate affect)
4. Associative disturbance (looseness of associations)

Hallucinations, delusions, and ideas of reference are characteristic of schizophrenia, but may occur in other conditions.

In Paranoid Disorders the main symptom is a persistent delusion, or delusions of persecution or grandeur. However, if persecutory delusions are prominent in a patient who has the primary symptoms of schizophrenia, the condition is probably Schizophrenic Disorder, Paranoid Type. If grandiose delusions are accompanied by a clearly elevated mood, the patient may have the Manic Type of Bipolar Affective Disorder.

When the most likely diagnostic group is identified one looks for the characteristic findings of the various syndromes and subtypes belonging to that group. In the end there are bound to be a few cases that do not fit any of the classifications, and for them it is better to use the diagnosis of Atypical Psychosis than to try to fit each case into the Procrustean bed of specific nomenclatures.

DIFFERENTIAL DIAGNOSIS OF THE NEUROSES AND THE ADJUSTMENT DISORDERS

Though in the system of classification the various Neuroses and the Adjustment Disorders are separate groups, in the process of thinking about differential diagnosis it is convenient to consider them together, since both groups represent relatively mild psychiatric disorders with identifiable onset, and patients in both groups show some free floating anxiety.

One thinks of an Adjustment Disorder if the symptoms appear to result from environmental stress. If history suggests a normal premorbid personality, a stress or combination of stresses should be sufficient to have a major impact on the average healthy person. However, if the patient also has a Personality Disorder, an Organic Mental Disorder, or any other preexisting psychiatric condition, less serious stresses may result in an Adjustment Disorder. When the stress is a major traumatic event one also thinks of Post-Traumatic Stress Disorders.

Of course, the fact that a person has symptoms at the time of or following a stress can be coincidence. Also, stress can precipitate other disorders. One may also be consulted about a stressful situation that is not producing symptoms. In the latter case, the classification of Conditions Not Attributable to a Mental Disorder can be used.

The neuroses, though they may appear following some stressful precipitating event, and may occur in persons who have not been overtly ill, are usually differentiated from Adjustment Disorders in that the precipitating stress, if any, is usually of less magnitude, and careful history reveals evidence of intrapsychic conflicts of more than a minor nature prior to illness. A careful history will usually reveal some difficulties in the early stages of psychosexual development prior to the latency period and occasional manifestations of conflict subsequently. The neuroses as a group are primarily manifested by anxiety and its derivatives. If the patient is diagnosed as having a neurosis, the selection of the type is made with an awareness that most cases are mixed, and one chooses the appropriate diagnostic category on the basis of the most marked symptom. As in choosing the subclassification of schizophrenia, it must be remembered that the intensity of the different symptoms may vary from time to time.

Among the Anxiety Disorders, Panic Disorder and Generalized Anxiety Disorder are manifested by diffuse overt anxiety with physiological concomitants similar to fear. The Phobic Disorders are manifested primarily by pathological fears. The Obsessive-Compulsive Disorders are manifested by obsessions (persistent recurring thoughts which are unwanted and which cannot be voluntarily excluded from consciousness) and/or compulsions (repetitive and essentially irresistible impulses to perform unwanted acts).

Another group of neuroses, the Somatoform Disorders, may not show a great deal of overt anxiety. They are characterized by physical symptoms. As well as distinguishing the various syndromes in this group through the identification of their characteristic symptoms, one must also bear in mind that some other psychiatric disorders may present with somatic symptoms. Depressed patients may have a variety of symptoms and concerns about health. Patients with Passive-Aggressive Personality Disorder often have multiple somatic complaints. Finally, in evaluating a patient who appears to have any of these disorders, the possibility that some or all of the symptoms are *not* the result of a psychiatric disorder must be considered.

The Dissociative Disorders show a form of personality disorganization in which certain mental functions appear to be split off from the mainstream of consciousness. Symptomatic manifestations include amnesias, fugue states, multiple personalities, and feelings of depersonalization.

The Dysthymic Disorder (depressive neurosis), which is classified among the Affective Disorders, is of course primarily manifested by depression. It is important in diagnosing a Dysthymic Disorder to distinguish it from a mild attack of Bipolar Disorder or a Cyclothymic Disorder.

DIFFERENTIAL DIAGNOSIS
OF THE PERSONALITY DISORDERS

The Personality Disorders are all essentially lifelong processes manifested by persistent or recurrent maladaptive behavior. The subclassification of this group is descriptive, and once one determines that a Personality Disorder is present, one rarely has difficulty in assigning the patient to the appropriate category or categories. One is most likely to have difficulty in making the diagnosis of a Personality Disorder when an adequate past history is not available and/or when the patient is seen at a time when he or she is under stress and shows signs of anxiety or transitory psychotic symptoms. Brief psychotic episodes are frequent in the Borderline Personality, but they may occur in any of the Personality Disorders.

One needs to distinguish the Schizotypal Personality from Schizophrenic and Schizophreniform Disorders. The Compulsive Personality has to be distinguished from the Obsessive-Compulsive Disorder. The Cyclothymic Disorder, classified with the Affective Disorders rather than the Personality Disorders, though it is similar to Personality Disorders in that it is usually lifelong and may have primarily behavioral manifestations, must be distinguished from other Affective Disorders.

Care must be used in making a diagnosis of Antisocial Personality. Though one thinks of this diagnosis upon seeing any patient with a history of recurring antisocial activities or criminal offenses beginning before the age of 15, not all habitual offenders are Antisocial Personalities. One must identify the other characteristic findings of the disorder. For some patients a pattern of frequent offenses is dyssocial rather than antisocial; although such people are in conflict with the rules of the mainstream of society, they do adhere to some sort of moral code or system of values. The dyssocial patient is able to form lasting relationships, tolerate stress, and defer pleasure; these are things that the Antisocial Personality cannot do. If a diagnosis is needed for a dyssocial patient, one uses the classification of Adult Antisocial Behavior which is classified among the Conditions Not Attributable to a Mental Disorder that are a Focus of Attention or Treatment. Antisocial behavior may also result from Mental Retardation or from a psychosis. Some patients with Bipolar Affective Disorder become involved in antisocial behavior while in the Manic phase. If the mood disturbance itself is relatively mild, it may be missed and clinical attention may be incorrectly focused on the antisocial behavior.

Sometimes a patient with an Antisocial Personality, or, less frequently, some other Personality Disorder will be seen because of problems related to sexual behavior, alcoholism, or drug misuse, and the underlying Personality Disorder can be overlooked.

SYMPTOM DIAGNOSIS IN PSYCHIATRY

The problem-oriented method of case study is useful in evaluating a psychiatric patient (it makes one aware of the full spectrum of the patient's problems in living). One can also use it as an aid to diagnosis by considering each major symptom as a problem and thinking of all of the conditions that can cause it. This is of only limited use in psychiatry because:

1. The number of possible psychiatric diagnoses is small enough that all of them can be considered. There are possible exceptions in subclassification of Organic Mental Disorders in which symptom diagnosis can be quite useful (e.g., a delirious patient complains that everything he sees looks yellow. What conditions can cause this? Digitalis intoxication and ??).
2. Most psychiatric symptoms (e.g., anxiety; depression) occur not only in those conditions in which they are the predominant signs of disorder but may also be found to some degree in nearly all other psychiatric conditions and even in the healthy individual. Even symptoms as apparently aberrant as hallucinations are not completely outside the realm of normal experience. Some studies report up to 50 percent of apparently healthy subjects have had at least isolated hallucinations (though one may question some of the experiences classified as hallucinatory. Even if one has an unusual name, hearing it called in a crowd and looking around and failing to detect the source is not sufficient evidence that one is hallucinating. It could be an illusion; there could be another person in the crowd with the same name).

However, it may be worthwhile to list a few symptoms together with the conditions in which they most frequently occur (in approximate order of prevalence), adding parenthetically *some* of the other findings which might help suggest the diagnosis.

1. *Anxiety*
    a. Adjustment Disorder (history of healthy premorbid personality identifiable precipitating stress of sufficient magnitude to disturb the average person)
    b. Generalized Anxiety Disorder (acute onset; history of problems in psychosocial development; signs of intrapsychic conflict)
    c. Other Anxiety Disorders, Somatoform Disorders, and Dissociative Disorders (acute onset; history of problems in psychosocial development; signs of intrapsychic conflict; other characteristic symptoms of the specific subtype)
    d. Personality Disorder in which there is a superimposed stress (lifelong history of maladaptive behavior patterns; anxiety usually absent except at times of stress or crisis)
    e. Some cases of Schizophreniform and Schizophrenic Disorder (primary signs of Schizophrenia present)
2. *Depression*
    a. Dysthymic Disorder (depression is mild and chronic; low self-esteem; condition may follow a loss of some sort)

    b. Major Depression (depression is severe and sustained; psychomotor agitation or retardation; sleep disturbances)

    c. Cyclothymic Disorder with depressive episode (mild depression; history of recurring mood swings of greater than normal intensity; onset of depressed episodes often occurs in the absence of identifiable precipitating stress; possibly some psychomotor retardation)

    d. Bipolar Affective Disorder, Depressed (history of mood swings; history of at least one manic episode; depression at psychotic level; psychomotor retardation usual; first attack in adolescence or early adult life; abrupt onset)

    e. Schizoaffective Disorder (primary symptoms of Schizophrenia present; gradual onset)

    f. Depression associated with Organic Mental Disorder (sensorium impairment; character change; depression frequently labile)

    g. Normal grief of sufficient magnitude to require medical attention

3. *Paranoid ideation*

    a. Paranoid Personality (lifelong pattern of suspiciousness and tendency to blame others; paranoid ideas do not reach the delusional level except briefly at times of stress)

    b. Schizophrenia, paranoid type (primary symptoms of schizophrenia present)

    c. Acute Paranoid Disorder (acute onset; paranoid thinking reaches delusional level; delusions not well systematized; primary symptoms of schizophrenia absent)

    d. Paranoia (gradual onset; well-systematized delusions dissociated from the mainstream of consciousness)

4. *Delusions and/or hallucinations*

    a. Schizophrenia (primary symptoms of schizophrenia present; delusions often bizarre; hallucinations if present usually auditory)

    b. Bipolar Affective Disorder and Major Depression (other symptoms of the specific disorder present; delusions in keeping with the manifest affect)

    c. Paranoia and Acute Paranoid Disorder (delusions of persecution or grandeur; delusions well systematized in Paranoia, less so in Acute Paranoid Disorders; primary symptoms of schizophrenia absent; hallucinations unlikely in Paranoia, but auditory hallucinations, usually accusatory, may occur in Acute Paranoid Disorders)

    d. Organic Mental Disorder (sensorium clouding; affective disturbance; character change; visual, tactile, and olfactory hallucinations are more often seen in association with Brain Syndromes than with the other disorders listed here)

5. *Recurring antisocial behavior*

    a. Antisocial Personality (lifelong antisocial tendencies; lack of guilt feelings; lack of anxiety except when under stress; relative absence of neurotic conflict; lack of lasting interpersonal relationships; inability to tolerate frustration or defer pleasure)

    b. Dyssocial behavior (lifelong process; aberrant moral code or value system; identification with socially deviant groups; lack of guilt feelings based on behavior being ego-syntonic; capable of lasting interpersonal relationships; capable of deferring pleasure and tolerating frustration)

    c. Neurosis with acting-out tendency (identifiable onset; evidences of neurotic conflict; guilt feelings follow antisocial behavior; some free-floating anxiety usually present; mounting tension precedes acting-out)

    d. Organic Mental Disorder with behavioral disorder (identifiable onset of character change; sensorium clouding; affective disturbance)

e. Cyclothymic Disorder and mild Bipolar Affective Disorder (lifelong history of recurring mood swings or cyclic behavior changes suggestive of mood swings; antisocial behavior, possibly accompanied by increased use of alcohol or drugs, in one phase of cycle)

INFORMATION NOT SUPPLIED BY CLASSIFICATION ALONE

Though sometimes additional studies and special tests are necessary, it is usually possible to classify a patient's psychiatric disorder correctly after the initial interview. There are additional questions of differential appraisal that must also be answered. These include:

1. Does the patient need hospitalization?
2. Are additional diagnostic studies urgently needed?
3. How badly does the patient need treatment?
4. What are the assets and liabilities in the patient's personality?
5. How do psychological, biological, and social or environmental factors contribute to the illness?
6. What is the patient's motivation?
7. Which method of treatment will be most helpful?
8. How will the patient relate to the physician?

NEED FOR HOSPITALIZATION

The strongest indications for hospitalization are:

1. An urgent need for additional diagnostic studies, or observation, which cannot be carried out readily on an outpatient basis
2. Danger to self or others
3. Inability to care for self (meet basic biological needs) at home or in the community
4. Certain environmental crises in which prompt removal of the patient from a stress situation may prevent a serious breakdown, a psychophysiologic reaction (e.g., a heart attack), or acting-out behavior that may have lasting consequences (e.g., an adolescent running away from home)

In evaluating the patient's danger to the self, one first thinks of the suicide risk (cf. Chapter 10). However, there are other dangers to the self. A confused or intensely preoccupied patient may be a real danger to self (as well as others) when driving an automobile. A patient who is neglecting diet and general health may require nursing care. Some alcoholics are unable to function as outpatients and may literally drink themselves to death if not hospitalized. Certain mildly hypomanic patients may be taking serious risks because of unrealistic optimism. Patients whose behavior threatens vocational or educational adjustment or who are making grossly unwise business and financial decisions also need protection.

When danger to the patient is extreme, hospitalization is imperative. However, when the danger is at a borderline level, one must take into account:

1. Other indications and contraindications for hospitalization
2. The extent to which the risk can be expected to diminish during a reasonable period of inpatient care

3.   The ability of family members to protect the patient against risks and to notify the physician promptly of changes in the patient's condition

Evaluation of danger to others presents some problems in differential evaluation. Obviously, those few psychotic patients (often those in a state of panic) who
are openly assaultive need hospitalization. The problem of evaluating the patient
who has fears of harming someone is described in Chapter 8 in the discussion of inhibiting obsessions. Certain paranoid patients may be dangerous to others (cf.
Chapter 12), and some patients with Paraphilia (cf. Chapter 13) need hospitalization for this reason. Other indications for hospitalization include:

1.   Need for treatments that can be given more easily or safely in the hospital
2.   Removal of the patient from an unduly stressful environmental situation even
in the absence of a crisis
3.   Possible benefit from the therapeutic milieu of the hospital
4.   The patient's convenience and preference

This latter group of indications usually represents less urgent needs for hospitalization and definite decisions do not always need to be made at the time of
initial interview.
While the therapeutic milieu of the hospital (cf. Chapter 21) offers many advantages to the emotionally disturbed person, there are also some potential disadvantages to hospitalization that must be weighed against the benefits that can be
obtained from nursing care and activity programs. Potential disadvantages of hospitalization include:

1.   Cost to the individual or to the community.
2.   Interference with family life. Being away from home and family is distressing to many patients (though some may find it a blessing). Prolonged hospital care
is especially disruptive to families; the patient who is away for a long time may in
effect lose a place in the home.
3.   Interference with occupation. In addition to loss of income and risk of loss of
job if hospitalization is long-term, the patient who must quit work because of illness experiences a blow to self-esteem. The requirements of one's job offer some
support to maintenance of emotional control, limit the time available for worries,
fantasies, and preoccupations, and as Freud put it, help bind one to reality. Hence,
unless vocational stress is a major factor in the cause of the illness, removal of
the patient from his or her occupation is likely to be harmful. If a patient is not
able to continue at work or in school and would be idle if not hospitalized, there
is no problem of weighing the advantages of the hospital milieu against those of
the working situation.
4.   Emotional impact of hospitalization. Having to go to a hospital forces upon
the patient an admission of illness and dependence upon others which is more likely to be harmful than helpful. The only alternative to the admission of helplessness lies in massive denial and rationalization (I'm not sick, I was railroaded")
which operates against a working therapeutic relationship. Outpatient care is less
damaging to ego and self-esteem; the average person can accept a need for professional advice and treatment. Hospitalization, even on an open ward, interferes
with one's feeling of freedom and independence. There is also likely to be concern
over the attitude of others, a fear of being regarded as "insane."
5.   The stigma of having been hospitalized for mental illness. Studies have shown
that most people regard mental illnesses as sicknesses requiring the care of physicians and believe that mental patients can be cured with proper treatment.

Investigations of social distance show that people usually accept rather than reject the formerly mentally ill. Most employers will not reject an applicant solely because of a history of psychiatric hospitalization. Nevertheless, a person with a history of hospitalization for any mental illness, however complete recovery may have been, sometimes does encounter discrimination when seeking employment, wishing to enter a professional school, wanting to buy insurance, or upon becoming a candidate for public office.

Though there are disadvantages to hospitalization, some patients who may not need hospitalization for strictly clinical reasons elect it. Sometimes this is a matter of convenience. The patient from a community without outpatient psychiatric facilities may find it impractical to commute and may view the prospect of temporarily moving to the city for treatment, and perhaps living alone, as undesirable.

In addition, while most patients prefer to avoid hospitalization, some see the security, freedom from daily responsibilities, special attention, service, and activities of the hospital as pleasant. This creates no problem if one is considering elective hospitalization of the patient at his or her own expense. It does create some problems in evaluating the justification for using public facilities or obtaining insurance benefits for hospitalization. However, while the patient who would *rather* be in the hospital must sometimes be discouraged, most conservative clinicians will, in cases of reasonable doubt, respect a patient's feeling of a *need* for hospital care. After all, even hospitalitis can be cured within inpatient rather than outpatient treatment.

While the advisability of inpatient care may be evaluated clinically, there are certain constraints on the implementation of such a recommendation. First, there is the matter of the patient's willingness to accept the recommendation. If it is refused and involuntary hospitalization is considered, one must conform to the legal criteria for this (cf. Chapter 23). Second, patients admitted to hospitals caring for Medicare and Medicaid beneficiaries must meet established admissions criteria. Under these rules, the justification for admission of a patient with a given disorder usually requires the presence of the major symptom (or one of the major symptoms) usually associated with that disorder plus one or more elements from a list of additional characteristic findings and/or one or more elements from a list of reasons why inpatient care might be necessary (e.g., impaired social, familial, or occupational functioning; need for high-dose medication; inaccessibility of outpatient psychiatric care). These criteria should not be regarded as mere bureaucratic red tape to be implemented solely by marking the right answers on a check list or getting the magic phrases into the admission note (though this is part of it), but they should be used to clarify one's own thinking about why the patient must indeed be in the hospital. On the other hand, taking these criteria seriously does not imply treating them as a textbook on differential diagnosis.

URGENCY OF DIAGNOSTIC STUDIES

If there is doubt about diagnosis, one may sometimes defer further studies pending observation during a trial period of therapy. This is particularly true if the therapy to be used is an expressive or investigative psychotherapy during which one would reasonably expect to learn a great deal more about the patient. A greater concern about differential diagnosis exists when there are alarming symptoms or elements in the history that are not compatible with the most likely tentative diagnosis. Examples: (1) A patient appears to have a mild Anxiety Disorder; no subjective complaints of depression are elicited and there are no outward signs of depression. However, the referring physician reports that the patient has made repeated suicide threats. (2) A patient who has beyond reasonable doubt a Passive-Aggressive Personality also reports symptoms vaguely suggestive of brain tumor. In these cases, the most important factors in deciding whether to proceed at once with further studies or await observations are:

1. Duration of the alarming symptom(s). If the patient has had the same symptoms for months or years and no disasters have occurred, a clinician cannot just dismiss them, but he or she can temporize with greater comfort.
2. Rate of increase in severity of illness. Even with chronic symptoms, the patient who is getting worse rapidly may need prompt studies.

Another factor which may make it necessary to complete any studies quickly so as to select and implement a treatment program is the presence of a crisis in the patient's life situation which involves a decision that cannot easily be deferred.

If the patient tends to be hypochrondriacal and/or presents numerous somatic complaints which are believed to be functional, it is desirable to do all studies promptly and to notify the patient of any plans for routine repetition of follow-up studies. Otherwise, introduction of new tests and procedures at various times may make the patient feel that the physician is uncertain of diagnosis and may reactivate somatic concern.

NEED FOR TREATMENT

Not all patients who consult the psychiatrist need treatment. Some are not ill, but because of some particular experience, need reassurance. Others who are diagnosable may have chronic nonprogressive illnesses that do not cause enough discomfort or disability to warrant treatment (i.e., a patient whose discomfort is minimal may elect treatment; on the other hand, he may want nothing more than reassurance that he is not losing his mind, about to have a nervous breakdown, or something of the sort). In evaluating discomfort, one must be aware of the patient's attitude, culturally and personally determined, toward complaint. Patients may minimize discomfort because of value judgments about being brave, not complaining, or being able to take it.

In evaluating disability, one must remember that illness may interfere in the patient's life in ways of which she or he is not always fully aware. Achievement and adjustment in various phases of living (vocational; domestic; social) must be evaluated in reference to potentialities and goals.

In cases in which there is doubt as to whether disability is great enough to require treatment, the prognosis for effecting changes is taken into account.

ASSETS AND LIABILITIES
IN THE PATIENT'S PERSONALITY

Assessment of the assets as well as the liabilities in the patient's personality is an essential part of diagnostic study. In patients who show features of both a Personality Disorder and a more acute psychiatric disease, this helps one select the more important diagnosis, arrive at a reasonable prognosis, and choose the best methods of treatment and rehabilitation.

History often offers measures of ego strength. It may give a measure of the patient's ability to function in a variety of environmental situations, achievements, and capacity for tolerating stress without using symptomatic defences or maladaptive coping mechanisms. Sometimes the way stress is tolerated is difficult to evaluate (e.g., a patient has experienced a number of tragedies, frustrations, and failures; all apparently unavoidable and irrevocable. His reaction to these events has apparently been unemotional, objective, stoical. Is he facing facts and making the best of bad situations? Or is he utilizing denial, dissociation, isolation, and/or rationalization?).

Though there are few treatment methods that require superior intelligence on the part of the patient, and although a high level of intelligence is not essential for a satisfactory adjustment to life, an accurate clinical estimate of intelligence is essential to full diagnostic evaluation.

If one uses multiaxial diagnoses, one rates the highest level of adaptive functioning of the patient in the year prior to evaluation on Axis V on a seven-point scale.

ASSESSMENT OF PSYCHOLOGICAL, BIOLOGICAL, AND SOCIAL FACTORS

Psychiatric disorders, like most other illnesses, do not usually result from a single cause. They are brought about by a combination of psychological, biological, and social or environmental factors. The relative importance of the various factors differs even within the same diagnostic category. To understand the patient and the patient's illness, the role of each must be recognized. This understanding contributes to the treatment plan, though it does not dictate the treatment. A primarily psychogenic disorder may respond to a biological intervention; a primarily biological disorder may be helped by psychotherapy.

One notes psychological factors, including evidence of intrapsychic conflicts. Prevailing ego defense mechanisms are identified. Personality traits originating in various stages of psychosocial development are recognized. The stage at which the first significant deviation from normal development occurred is obtained from the history.

Biological factors include hereditary predisposition and biochemical, including neurotransmitter, imbalances. Systemic diseases and exogenous toxins may play a part in some psychiatric disorders.

Social and environmental factors include stresses. One looks not only for specific major stresses but also for accumulations of lesser stresses. One is aware of the cultural background of the patient. One looks at the habits and life style of the person and evaluates the influence of his or her social milieu on them.

A psychobiosocial formulation puts together the various contributing factors and indicates their relative importance.

MOTIVATION

Motivation is important to case evaluation. It is difficult to assess. The concept of motivation is often abused. Poor motivation or inappropriate motivation can be a reason for patients failing to keep appointments, dropping out of therapy, or just not getting well. On the other hand, it is all too easy to rationalize clinical failures by placing the blame upon poor motivation and, if motivational problems themselves are a product of the illness, this can be as absurd as blaming the patient for being sick.

A patient who minimizes symptoms and disability may want help badly but be reluctant to admit the need. Comments suggestive of inadequate motivation may be used to save face.

Frightened patients may appear uncooperative or even hostile to therapy. Patients who are crude and sarcastic to the therapist and about therapy may be defending themselves against fears. Others may be revealing habitual maladaptive, symptomatic ways of relating to others (some emotionally disturbed people are expert in the art of losing friends and alienating people).

In evaluating motivation, there are three basic questions one asks one's self (and directly or indirectly asks the patient).

1.   Does the patient really want to change? Is he or she dissatisfied? Uncomfortable? There are patients who come to the psychiatrist without actually wanting treatment. Some come under duress (e.g., the adolescent who has a behavior problem and is *brought* to treatment by her parents; the sex offender who is *ordered* by the court to obtain therapy; the employee who is *told* by his supervisor to attend the clinic). Others come with an ulterior motive (e.g., the student who believes that being in treatment will gain sympathy for him, excuse his failures, and keep him from being kicked out of school; the husband who believes his wife will divorce him unless he appears to be trying to do something about his problem; the wife who has already decided upon a divorce but wants to tell her family, her minister, and even herself that she has tried everything to save the marriage — even psychiatry).

This aspect of motivation is not always easy to evaluate. The patient who comes under duress may arrange for the appointment personally without mentioning being under pressure to do so. The patient who is referred by someone in authority may have initiated or requested referral, or if not, may at least have welcomed it. Patients often make an effort to conceal ulterior motives.

Duress or ulterior motive is not necessarily a bar to successful treatment. Patient and therapist may find mutually acceptable treatment goals and the patient may be helped to see a need for treatment. However, to accomplish this, the nature of the motivation must be recognized, made explicit, and discussed in order to prevent therapy from degenerating into something of a game.

2.   What is the patient's reason for wanting to change? Usually this is related to discomfort; either that directly resulting from symptoms or indirectly from the consequences of maladaptive behavior. However, some patients may wish to change a behavior pattern for other reasons (e.g., to please another person. This differs from the ulterior motives previously discussed, since the patient actually does want to change. The hope of some benefit expected, realistically or otherwise, from changing, such as that of the obese girl who believes that if she gets help losing weight she will be popular, can be a factor).

3.   How badly does the patient want to change? This cannot always be estimated from the apparent degree of discomfort and disability. There are patients who may wish to be rid of a symptom only if the change can be made easily. In some elective cases this is a perfectly legitimate and healthy approach to treatment. There are many analogous situations in daily life; many of us would like to acquire new skills if they could be learned without too much expenditure of energy, time, and money.

When treatment is elective, that is when disability is not, and is not likely to become great, and the patient's life is not endangered, inadequate motivation may be a reason for discouraging (but not prohibiting) entrance into treatment. Sometimes treatment is deferred pending reevaluation. However, when disability is marked, poor motivation, while it must be recognized and dealt with, does not prevent treatment. Initial goals must then be related to motivation, not to change itself.

DIFFERENTIAL DIAGNOSIS
AND THE CHOICE OF TREATMENT METHODS

Correct classification alone is not generally a sufficient guide in the selection of the most appropriate treatment method. In some cases of Organic Mental Disorder, a knowledge of the correct diagnosis permits the use of a specific treatment directed against the etiological agent. Some other conditions frequently respond to a particular treatment (e.g., most patients with involutional melancholia benefit from electroconvulsive therapy; Bipolar Affective Disorder, Manic Type usually responds to lithium).

For patients in most diagnostic groups, a variety of treatments are possible (cf. Chapters 19 and 20). To select the best treatment, a knowledge of the other factors which have been discussed is essential. If symptomatic relief is urgently needed, one cannot rely exclusively on a treatment that will offer benefit only after weeks or months of therapy. Some techniques of psychotherapy and the appropriate use of some medications (e.g., disulfiram for the alcoholic) require that the patient have at least moderate ego strength. Other methods require a certain level of intelligence for patient participation. The nature of a patient's motivation may have a great deal to do with whether psychotherapy and/or medication should be aimed primarily at symptomatic relief or at an extensive revision of the personality structure.

PREDICTION OF NATURE OF THE
DOCTOR–PATIENT RELATIONSHIP

With any form of treatment, results usually depend in part upon patient cooperation. Long-term psychotherapy involves a close working relationship, a cooperative endeavor between patient and therapist. Likewise the use of medication requires patient collaboration. The patient needs to take the medicine as directed and report results, including side effects, accurately. In general medical practice it has been estimated that half or more of the patients fail to receive full benefit from prescribed medication because of failures in adhering to the treatment plan. One would expect a similar problem in working with psychiatric patients.

The therapist should be able to predict how well the patient will cooperate. If advice is given, will it be followed? Will medication be taken according to directions? Will appointments be kept? The therapist should also be able to predict the sort of working relationship that will develop in therapy, the nature of problems that may arise, and the steps necessary to achieve adequate doctor-patient collaboration.

Transference, countertransference, and resistance will be discussed in Chapter 19. The initial assessment of probable cooperation and of the sort of treatment relationship likely to develop is part of diagnostic study. Classification helps to predict these factors, as does interview behavior and motivation. In addition, much can be learned from history.

1.   What has been the patient's attitude toward significant people in the past? How did he or she relate to father and mother, to teachers, to employers? To what extent have feelings toward such people (with or without obvious good reason) included respect, affection, dependence, competitiveness, fear, and hostility?
2.   What has happened to potentially close, cooperative relationships in adult life? Has he or she avoided them? Have they worked out well? Is there any common denominator, recurring pattern in the way they terminate (e.g., do close

relationships usually end in a violent quarrel?)? Is there any recurring unpleasant complication to close relationships (e.g., an employed woman reports that several employers have made sexual advances toward her. At this point, though it may be chance, the clinician suspects a recurring pattern. It is unlikely that one can have more than tentative hypotheses as to whether the patient for some unconscious (?) reason elects to go to work for predatory males, flirts with men in positions of authority, provokes seductive behavior, or has a vivid imagination. Nevertheless, one is alerted to a *possible* pattern which may complicate treatment).

3. How has the patient worked with physicians in the past? Has there been a tendency to change doctors or for doctor shopping? Has the patient rejected previous medical advice? Is there a tendency not to take prescribed medication, or not to take it as prescribed? If any of these questions are answered in the affirmative, what seem to be the reasons involved in the failure of patient-doctor collaboration?

Predictions about the treatment relationship may influence the choice of treatment method. However, the clinician in some cases may feel that the patient's expectations and patterns of relationship can be modified, and one may choose a treatment knowing that there will be problems. One is alert to those potential problems and is ready to take steps to prevent them from interfering with treatment.

REVIEW QUESTIONS

1. Make a schematic diagram of the steps in preliminary differential diagnosis outlined in the first part of this chapter.
2. If multiaxial diagnosis (cf. Chapter 4) is used, what contributions do Axes IV and V make to differential diagnosis? Prognosis? Treatment planning?
3. If you were the chief medical officer for an insurance company and knew that an applicant for a large policy had had a psychiatric illness, what would you like to know about it besides the classification, dates of illness, and condition at the time of discharge?
4. Construct a table showing the different disorders in which depression is a major symptom. In the table compare age ranges, premorbid personality, rate of onset, and the presence or absence of the symptoms and findings that you consider most important in differential diagnosis.
5. Construct a table comparing the different disorders in which suspiciousness and jealousy may be among the presenting symptoms.
6. Compare the types of affective disturbance associated with Organic Mental Disorders with those of the Dysthymic Disorders. What are the major points in the differential diagnosis between Organic Brain Syndromes (with depression) and Dysthymic Disorder?
7. In addition to the presence or absence of the primary symptoms of Schizophrenia, what findings would be helpful in differentiating between Schizoaffective Disorder and Bipolar Affective Disorder?
8. A patient has tremor, restlessness, and tachycardia. What nonpsychiatric conditions could produce this?
9. Why does a thorough diagnostic study include an estimate of intelligence? Ego strength? Motivation?
10. Why must psychological, biological, and social factors all be identified and evaluated even if one factor appears primarily responsible for a disorder?

SELECTED REFERENCES

1. Akiskal, Hagop S., Robert M. A. Hirschfeld, and Boghos I. Yerevanian: The relationship of personality to affective disorders. *Arch Gen Psychiatry* 40(7): 801-810, 1983.

2. Baldessarini, Ross J., Seth Finklestein, and George W. Arana: The predictive power of diagnostic tests and the effect of prevalence of illness. *Arch Gen Psychiatry* 40(5):569-573, 1983.

3. Beck, Aaron T., C. H. Ward, M. Mendelson, J. E. Mock, and J. K. Erbaugh: Reliability of psychiatric diagnoses: A study of consistency of clinical judgments and ratings. *Am J Psychiatry* 119(4):351-357, 1962.

4. Caveny, E. L., C. L. Wittson, W. A. Hunt, and R. S. Herrman: Psychiatric diagnosis, its nature and function. *J Nerv Ment Dis* 121(1):367-373, 1955.

5. Crocetti, Guido, Herzl R. Spiro, and Iradj Siassi: Are the ranks closed? Attitudinal social distance and mental illness. *Am J Psychiatry* 127(9):1121-1127, 1971.

6. *Diagnostic and Statistical Manual of Mental Disorders.* 3rd ed. Prepared by the Committee on Nomenclature and Statistics of the American Psychiatric Association, Washington, D.C., American Psychiatric Association, 1980.

7. Eraker, Stephen A., John P. Kirscht, and Marshall H. Becker: Understanding and improving patient compliance. *Ann Intern Med* 100(2):258-268, 1984.

8. Grove, William M., Nancy C. Andreasen, Patricia McDonald-Scott, Martin B. Keller, and Robert W. Shapiro: Reliability studies of psychiatric diagnosis. *Arch Gen Psychiatry* 38(4):408-413, 1981.

9. Harrow, Martin, Linda S. Grossman, Marshall L. Silverstein, and Herbert Y. Meltzer: Thought pathology in manic and schizophrenic patients. *Arch Gen Psychiatry* 39(6):665-671, 1982.

10. Mackenzie, Thomas B., and Michael K. Popkin: Organic anxiety syndrome. *Am J Psychiatry* 140(3):342-344, 1983.

11. Olin, Harry S., and Avery D. Weisman: Psychiatric misdiagnosis in early neurological disease. *JAMA* 189(7):533-538, 1964.

12. Prusoff, Brigitt, and Gerald L. Klerman: Differentiating depressed from anxious neurotic outpatients. *Arch Gen Psychiatry* 30(3):302-309, 1974.

Part III

TREATMENT

Chapter 19

A METHOD OF TREATMENT

Sullivan defined the psychiatric interview as:

> a situation of primarily *vocal* communication in a *two-group,* more or less voluntarily integrated, on a progressively unfolding *expert-client* basis for the purpose of elucidating *characteristic patterns of living* of the subject person, patient or client, which patterns he experiences as particularly troublesome or especially valuable, and in the revealing of which he expects to derive *benefit.*

Not every psychiatrist would accept this as a working definition of psychotherapy, but then it would be hard to find any definition that would encompass all of the methods of psychotherapy now in use.

Whatever the definition, psychotherapy plays a central role in psychiatric practice. Psychotherapy, including therapeutic listening, occurs in 95 percent of office visits to psychiatrists by persons having a primary diagnosis of a mental disorder. Drug therapy is involved in only about a third of such visits. Patients seeing primary practitioners for mental disorders are less likely to receive psychotherapy, but its use is increasing. In 1975 22 percent of visits to primary practitioners by such patients included psychotherapy; in 1980 29 percent did.

If a psychiatric symptom or problem is the result of an individual's difficulty in achieving certain basic biological goals within the environment, there are three possible ways of helping him or her:

1. Producing a basic change in the individual
2. Changing the environment
3. Helping the person find a more effective way of dealing with the environment

The first might be done with medication or other somatic therapy (cf. Chapter 21); the second is largely in the purview of social and community psychiatry (cf. Chapter 22), though environmental manipulation may be undertaken to a limited extent in industrial psychiatry and to a greater extent in child psychiatry, and the third is in the main objective of most of the treatment methods we call psychotherapy.

Psychotherapy is a form of treatment; as such, it is purposeful and, to some degree at least, systematic. Its goal is benefit, as Sullivan said, but not all things that benefit the person or the mind are properly described as therapy. If an attractive person of the opposite sex smiles at you, you feel better; this may be in a sense therapeutic, but it is not therapy (unless the person is your nurse and the smile has been prescribed). It is a treat, not a treatment, if we may borrow the phrase.

TECHNIQUES OF PSYCHOTHERAPY

Many different ways of helping emotionally disturbed people feel better and live more effectively have been described, and a number are in widespread use. Some are highly complex; others are relatively simple. Some are recommended for a wide range of disorders, others for specific problems or syndromes.

Comments on the relative merits of methods of psychotherapy should be (but are not always) made with some reservation and a great deal of humility. Most such statements, here and elsewhere, are based upon opinion and experience, not scientific proof. There are very few well-constructed scientific studies comparing results of different methods in specific conditions or in general use. Research in this field poses major problems in design. These include:

1. Time required for completion of treatment and adequate follow-up
2. Difficulty in selecting truly comparable series of cases
3. Problems in choosing measurements of improvement (especially in evaluating techniques not directly aimed at relief of one specific symptom)
4. Individual variations in the skill of clinicians
5. Difficulty in eliminating bias, especially unconscious bias, in evaluating results

Therapeutic techniques are sometimes named and classified on the basis of the theories of personality development, psychosexual or psychosocial development, implicit in their use. However, differences in these theoretical bases are often relatively superficial and are more a matter of terminology and emphasis than anything else. Even granting theoretical differences, the actual interview methods of experienced clinicians from different schools do not vary as much as one might expect.

Another classification of methods is based upon goals; on this basis one may speak of therapy as being one of the following.

Symptomatic

The goal of therapy is the relief of specific symptoms or the solution of a particular problem. Symptomatic therapy is most indicated for the patient who has a clearly definable symptom and in the absence of it would, presumably, feel well and function effectively (e.g., a patient has a phobic dread of cats and young women. In their absence he feels fine. His achievements in various spheres of activity are adequate. Perhaps if he can learn to tolerate these creatures, all will be well).

An objection to most symptomatic techniques, certainly valid in some cases, is that they do not resolve underlying conflicts, if present, and there is a likelihood either of relapse or of the emergence of new symptoms. On the other hand, aspirin does not do anything about the basic problems that cause a tension headache, but if tension headaches are not too frequent, many of us would prefer it to a more definitive therapy. A second objection is that often the presenting symptom is only one of many problems the patient has, and removing it alone could not be expected to leave the patient feeling well and functioning effectively. However, even granting this, symptomatic treatment may still be worth considering. Not only is there some value in eliminating an unpleasant symptom, but once the ego is free of the added stress the symptom causes, the patient may be able to resolve some of the other difficulties unassisted (or with less assistance).

Supportive

The goal of supportive therapy may be to help a patient tolerate a period of stress, to help a patient with chronic emotional problems continue to function in the community, in spite of them, or to help the patient function better by strengthening some ego defenses and encouraging healthful activities.

Hence, the "support" in supportive therapy may be a rather general moral support or it may be a highly specific support of an adaptive pattern of behavior. Supportive therapy may also be aimed at increasing self-esteem and self-confidence so that the patient may cope with problems, environmental and intrapsychic, more effectively and with greater *ego strength.*

Those supportive therapies which strengthen defenses in order to keep conflictual material repressed or which aim at helping the patient suppress disturbing material are sometimes spoken of as *repressive* therapies.

Reconstructive or Investigative

The goals of these therapies include helping the patient achieve self-understanding, analyze emotional conflicts, and acquire *insight.* With insight, one is able to achieve a reorganization, revision, or reconstruction of the personality.

Another way of classifying therapies is on the basis of technique. However, in some therapies, technique as such is deemphasized. The rationale for this is that if the therapist understands basic principles of psychopathology, the precise way that material is elicited, attitudes and feelings are communicated, and suggestions or interpretations are made is irrelevant. However, most therapies can be classified as *directive* or *expressive* (the term nondirective is the antonym of directive, but there is also a specific technique so named).

In a directive therapy, the patient is in one way or another told what to do about a problem. The telling may be in the form of advice and prescriptions for action. It may involve persuasion, exhortation, or suggestion. A directive therapy may include interpretations or explanations of the patient's behavior, including symptoms; if it does, these are usually furnished as statements.

Expressive therapies are those in which the patient does most of the talking. The therapist may furnish information, but he or she rarely advises. In expressive, less directive therapies, the patient is helped to arrive at his or her own interpretations, though the therapist may introduce possibilities, usually in the form of questions. Some expressive therapies deemphasize interpretation altogether with the assumption that freedom from repression, abreactive reexperiencing of past traumas, or simply the ability to express the true emotion freely is in itself curative. In speaking of therapist behavior, the terms authoritarian, directive, and active are sometimes interchanged as are permissive, nondirective, and passive. Though authoritarian therapists are usually directive and active, and permissive therapists tend to be nondirective and passive, the terms are not always truly interchangeable. One can offer a great deal of direction without being authoritarian. The therapist can be highly active, say a great deal, without being very directive or authoritarian; or can say very little but be quite authoritarian.

THE COMPONENTS OF PSYCHOTHERAPY

Various techniques of therapy have, to a greater or lesser degree, certain beneficial components in common. These may be divided into three main groups:

1. Benefits derived from talking freely to a noncritical listener
2. The effects of adding the therapist to the patient's environment
3. The products of the therapist's activity

Talking to a noncritical listener is a feature of many therapies. There are several ways in which this is helpful to patients:

1. Confession. Most of us have had the experience of feeling better after confessing something. This stems from childhood experience, is related to guilt feelings and superego values, and is entered into with some expectation of punishment (at least a scolding). After it is all over and the punishment either does not materialize or does and is survived, there is a feeling of relief, an absence of fear. (Religious confession differs from confession as a component of psychotherapy in its goals and areas of interest. Much of what is confessed in therapy is not "sinful" in any sense of the word. Also, psychiatrists are usually not regarded as qualified to grant absolution.)
2. Catharsis and ventilation. The expression of thoughts and feelings that are generally suppressed helps one feel better much as does confession. Anyone can think of times when he or she has felt better getting something "off his chest" or "out of her system."
3. Desensitization. As a disturbing topic is talked about, it often becomes more familiar and less frightening. When it can be thought of without anxiety, it can be dealt with more objectively.
4. Clarification and reformulation. Telling someone about a problem helps one understand it better oneself. The therapist's noncritical attitude helps make reformulation possible, since the patient is better able to inspect his or her ideas when there is no reason to feel a need to defend them.
5. Uncovering and abreaction. As a patient talks about past experiences, incidents may be recalled that have been forgotten (or repressed?). If an incident is recalled, and in a sense reexperienced with feeling, the emotional discharge is called abreaction. Desensitization then becomes possible. Uncovered material often contributes to clarification and reformulation.

It might be asked whether the benefits of talking to a noncritical listener could not equally well be obtained if the patient would talk about the problems to family members, friends, or other nonprofessional people. It does sometimes help to talk with friends about certain problems. However, few people are good listeners; most have suggestions to make, opinions to offer, and problems of their own to describe. The patient may be reluctant, often with good reason, to tell people about feelings lest they react negatively to them. One may fear exploitation if one's emotional needs and "weaknesses" are known. There may be concern about confidentiality.

One might also question the appropriateness of being noncritical when the patient discusses behavior that is socially undesirable and detrimental to his or her well-being. The therapist does, and should, have value judgments, but reserves judgment until a situation is completely understood. One does not attempt to bring about changes until one is sure that they are desirable and that there are effective means for helping the patient change. Telling a person who has a recurring symptomatic behavior pattern that it is bad, and he or she should stop, is about as likely to be effective as telling the same thing to someone with a headache.

Adding the therapist to the environment is in itself a potent ingredient of therapy. To the patient it means:

1.   Relief of loneliness. Many patients, because of symptoms and difficulties in interpersonal relationships, feel acutely lonely.
2.   Someone to turn to at a time of crisis. The feeling that there is someone available if things go wrong, a strong person who can and will do something, is often reassuring.
3.   A feeling of being understood. Sometimes it is only a feeling that someone is trying to understand. This furnishes hope and may add something to self-esteem.
4.   An implied suggestion that the illness is not hopeless. If the therapist recommends treatment, the implication is that change is possible. Closely related is the fact that in accepting therapy, the patient, unless there are ulterior motives, is acknowledging a need for change and committing himself or herself to make an effort.
5.   Sometimes an effect upon other people in the environment. If the patient elects, or for some reason finds it necessary to tell others that she or he is in therapy, the results are not always favorable. The patient may be rejected as unstable or neurotic, may encounter curiosity rather than interest, or may be overprotected. In some instances, however, the reaction is more constructive. Examples: (1) A husband who has previously ignored or denied the fact that his wife is ill recognizes when she goes into therapy that she has problems and begins making an effort to be more helpful to her. (2) The father of an adolescent patient starts to spend more time with the boy after the latter begins treatment.

Sometimes family members modify aggressive or deviant behavior simply because they know it will be talked about in therapy. This is usually not because they believe the therapist would do anything about the behavior, or because they care what the therapist as a person thinks of them, but for much the same reasons that they might stop certain activities if a stranger should look in the window.

Just as the advantages of talking freely to a noncritical listener are lost if the therapist talks too much (asks too many questions, offers frequent comments, or makes premature value judgments) some of the benefits from the therapeutic relationship are lost if the therapist demonstrates a lack of availability or understanding. Ideally, the therapeutic relationship offers a corrective emotional experience in interpersonal relationships. The patient who has encountered a lack of understanding and has experienced rejection, exploitation, or domination by others learns that another human being can be accepting and treat one with understanding and respect.

These first two basic components of therapy are common to nearly all techniques. Even techniques which are ultimately directive rather than expressive (e.g., deconditioning or desensitization in the treatment of a phobia) offer an initial opportunity to discuss the problem freely and even if somewhat mechanical procedures are introduced, the doctor is present and personally involved.

The therapist's activity varies more with the specific method employed but may include some of the following:

1.   Interpretation. This term is roughly synonymous with explanation. The therapist explains to the patient or helps the patient discover explanations for recurring patterns of behavior, including that which is symptomatic or maladaptive. *Dynamic* explanations attempt to account for behavior in terms of its basic goals and the ego defense mechanisms involved. *Psychogenetic* interpretations trace the origin of conflicts and patterns of behavior. Sometimes things other than intrapsychic phenomena are interpreted. Sometimes a patient may need an explanation of physiology, an understanding of the emotional reactions of others, or some interpretation of the social milieu.

   Interpretation can be helpful in several ways. Sometimes simply knowing the reason for a symptom robs it of a frightening or uncanny quality. Understanding the nature of a conflict helps one resolve it. Recognizing a goal clearly helps one find an easier method of attaining it. A patient may recognize that the factors that originally accounted for a behavior pattern are no longer operative and accordingly be able to modify it.

2.   Furnishing information. The therapist may recognize that the patient's effort to find a workable solution to a problem in living is hampered by a lack of some type of information. Sometimes all that is necessary is to make the patient aware of a need for information. At other times, the therapist may be in a position to furnish the information or to direct the patient to an appropriate source.

3.   Advice. This may take the form of a direct prescription for action or simply the suggestion of possible courses of action for the patient's consideration. As in the case of interpretation, more often the therapist helps the patient arrive at his or her own advice. This is done by making sure, usually through questioning, that the patient has actually thought of all of the possible things that one might do about the difficulty. The therapist then helps the patient weigh the advantages and disadvantages of each.

4.   Influencing behavior by attitude. Most therapists prefer to help the patient produce changes in behavior through insight. Sometimes, when this is impossible, behavior may be modified by showing approval or disapproval. To do this, the therapist has to modify the original noncritical and nonjudgmental attitude. For example, if one thinks that a patient will be benefited by more social activities, one may simply show increased interest whenever the patient does mention going out socially. The influence of the therapist's attitude is greatest when there is a strong positive relationship. However, sometimes a patient's negativism can be utilized. If the negativistic patient is told in effect that he or she should not or cannot do something, the patient may do it to "show" the therapist.

5.   Other activities of the therapist. These include the introduction of a number of specific treatment techniques.

   It should be emphasized that in most therapies which are classifiable as investigative, reconstructive, or expressive the main activity of the therapist consists of asking those questions which help the patient arrive at a better understanding of self, problems, and society so that she or he can make useful interpretations and achieve insight. Some of the other activities mentioned may play an ancillary role in these therapies, but together with reassurance, encouragement, and sometimes persuasion or suggestion they play a greater part in symptomatic, supportive, or directive therapies.

A BASIC METHOD OF INVESTIGATIVE PSYCHOTHERAPY

There is no one therapeutic method suitable for all patients and all disorders. However, a general technique of brief investigative psychotherapy based upon psychogenetic and dynamic principles can be offered.

The patients are seen for regularly scheduled appointments of fixed duration. Most patients can be seen once weekly. Some patients who feel quite uncomfortable may need to be seen more often initially. There are times when a need for observation requires more frequent appointments. More frequent appointments are necessary when a patient needs to cope promptly with a stress situation or crisis. Less frequent than weekly appointments are usually inadequate, since they do not allow for sufficient continuity for an investigative therapy.

The usual duration of appointments is 45 or 50 minutes. Some patients cannot comfortably tolerate appointments of this length, and others have so much difficulty in expressing themselves that they require longer appointments. Some modifications of scheduling are discussed in Chapter 23.

Therapy can be conducted in any office in which both patient and therapist can be seated comfortably and have reasonable privacy. Chairs are usually placed somewhat at an angle so that the patient does not have to look directly at the therapist except by choice. The therapist should have a clock placed so that she or he can note the time without the patient being aware of it. If the therapist looks at a watch, the patient may feel that he or she is bored or that the interview is nearly over, though the therapist may actually only want to know how long a particular topic has been discussed or whether there is sufficient time to undertake a new line of questioning.

The therapeutic process may be divided, somewhat arbitrarily, into four stages:

1.   Initial interview
2.   General exploration
3.   Investigation of specific problems
4.   Interpretation and formulation

Initial Interview

The initial interview usually takes the form of the evaluation described in Chapter 3. While there would be some advantage in letting a patient tell his or her story spontaneously and beginning at once with work on the patient's problem, this is offset by the advantages of some questioning of the patient in order to obtain a history and mental examination. In some settings, this is essential for purposes of differential diagnosis. However, even if the patient is referred for therapy and has already had adequate diagnostic study, or for some other reason diagnosis is not necessary, a brief history of present illness and past life is a good beginning. It helps the therapist understand and organize subsequent data provided by the patient.

If there is no reason to suspect a need for prompt differential diagnosis (including evaluation of possible need for hospitalization) history-taking may sometimes be deferred. This is done if the patient

1.   Is too upset to answer questions
2.   Has a great deal that he or she is very eager to tell the therapist
3.   Needs immediate help in arriving at a decision or coping with a crisis

The initial interview begins with identification of the patient's purpose in coming and the way(s) he or she hopes to benefit. It ends, if psychotherapy is indicated, with a clearly understandable recommendation which is acceptable to the patient, and a consensus as to the purpose of interviews. The basic implied questions of the first interview are:

1. What can I do for you?
2. Tell me about your illness (or problem), including the things you think caused it and the ways you have tried to overcome it.
3. Give me a brief biographical sketch so that I may begin to know and understand you as well as your problems.
4. Are you prepared to come for a series of interviews to attempt to understand yourself better and to try to attain the objectives which were your purpose in coming?

General Exploration

General exploration follows the initial interview. At the end of the evaluation, the therapist has at least a general idea of the patient's problem, has identified some of the difficulties in living, past and present, together with some of the dynamic and psychogenetic factors associated with them, but he or she has not explored these in depth. The therapist needs to know more about the patient in order to decide what things need detailed discussion and in what order they should be undertaken.

Further information may be obtained by systematic questioning or by permitting (or encouraging) the patient to tell more things about life experiences and problems spontaneously. At this stage there are advantages to letting the patient do most of the talking, to listening, and to assuming a passive role:

1. It permits the patient to have the fullest possible benefit from catharsis, ventilation, desensitization, etc.
2. Relevant material may be elicited about which one might not think of asking.
3. The patient may approach painful or embarrassing subjects at his or her own rate.
4. The patient establishes a "set" or expectation of doing most of the talking. This may be useful later in therapy if something comes up about which the therapist prefers to defer comment (one of the best rules of therapy is if you do not know what to say, keep your mouth shut. This is easier to follow if the patient goes on talking rather than pausing to await the next question or comment).

The patient is asked to talk about herself or himself. An introductory comment can be made to the effect that in the first appointment a number of questions had been asked, but that for the *next few* appointments there will be very few questions or comments. One may add the instruction to think aloud or to say whatever comes to mind. Sometimes this is qualified by a phrase appropriate to the particular patient such as:

1. "Even if you think of something impolite or not socially acceptable" (for a shy, inhibited person)
2. "Without editing your thoughts" (for the patient who appears to pause and choose words carefully)

3.   "Even if things occur to you that do not *seem* important" (for the patient who appears to be trying too hard to focus on significant things)
4.   "If you think something that is not true, go ahead and say it; another thought will come along later to correct it" (for the patient who appears to be less than candid about some aspects of the history. The permission to lie makes it easier to tell the truth later)

Some patients are able to talk rather easily. Others have trouble getting started. If there are difficulties at first, the therapist must try to determine the reason for them. Does the patient understand what he or she has been asked to do? Is the patient trying but finding it difficult? If so, why? Or is he or she uncooperative? Again, why?

If there is difficulty or resistance, this can be discussed with the patient. One words questions about it cautiously. To say something like, "You seem to be having trouble talking about yourself" misses the point if the patient, rather than having trouble is not trying because the whole idea is regarded as ridiculous. Sometimes it is necessary to change modes of therapy and/or reevaluate goals and motivation. However, if the patient truly finds it difficult to talk, patience and encouragement are indicated.

Some patients are uncomfortable if the therapist is silent too long. Most patients are more productive if they are sure that the therapist is listening and if they occasionally get some response. Hence, the therapist is not altogether silent, but murmurs from time to time. Now and then one asks a minor question that neither focuses the patient's attention on the subject nor directs the subsequent course of the interview.

If there are silences, one may ask, "What are you thinking?", or say, "Go on." This is to be avoided if the patient seems to be trying to put a thought into words or is catching a moment's rest. It is not done often enough to be nagging. If the patient expresses concern about silence, he or she may be asked the reasons for the silences, or may be assured that silence is all right and that one will think of things to talk about in time.

The patient's production may at first seem repetitive or uninformative. If so, one proceeds to the next stage after three or four appointments. On the other hand, this stage may be continued for many appointments if the patient continues to show subjective and objective improvement, or even in the absence of improvement if appointments continue to provide new and therapeutically relevant information.

Beginning therapists often defeat the purpose of this stage of therapy by becoming too eager to discuss some of the things the patient brings up early in treatment.

Though during this stage the therapist is primarily a good listener, there are times when intervention is necessary:

1.   If the patient needs help in making a decision that cannot be deferred or in coping with a crisis.
2.   When it is necessary to avoid giving tacit consent to a truly dangerous idea that is likely to be carried into action. An idea that is dangerous for one person may not be for another (e.g., if a man is thinking of doing something that may cost him his job, the "danger" depends upon what the emotional impact of loss of job may be, his need for the income, and his probable difficulties in finding an equally good position). Patients may express dangerous ideas they do not intend to act upon. They may do this to test the therapist's reaction. It may simply be the result of following instructions to think aloud by reporting a fantasy.

In dealing with a dangerous idea, one asks questions about possible consequences, advantages and disadvantages, and alternate courses of action. The patient may change his or her mind after looking over the situation. If necessary the
therapist may state the consequences that will probably occur. It is rarely practical or desirable to forbid an unwise act, and patients, like anyone else, have a right
to expose themselves to some danger if they know what they are doing. However,
there are times (e.g., serious suicide threats) when one prevents the dangerous act
or at least forces its postponement by insisting on hospitalization. A patient who
is about to act on an unwise but less dangerous decision, and who underrates or denies the consequences, can be asked to postpone action for at least a stated period
of time for further therapy.

3.   To keep anxiety within tolerable limits. Emotion expressed during abreaction
is helpful. However, if a patient is discussing highly disturbing material, he or she
may become more anxious than is desirable. Also, if the patient reveals too much
of an embarrassing nature too soon, he or she may be overconcerned about having
done so. At worst, overwhelming anxiety can lead to panic, psychotic decompensation, or development of new symptoms. It may also cause a patient to discontinue
therapy. Mounting anxiety is best handled by changing the subject. This should
not be done abruptly, but by gradual transition to a related, less disturbing topic.
One can stop the patient to ask for a factual detail (e.g., where were you living at
the time?) and then follow up the question with others based on the answer.

4.   To avoid misunderstandings. For example, if the patient says, "Since your religion is the same as mine" in introducing a topic, and it is not, the therapist should
say so. Otherwise, the patient will make some assumptions about the therapist's
knowledge of the subject that may be contrary to fact. Also, if the patient later
discovers the truth, she or he is likely to feel that the therapist has been disingenu-
ous, if not dishonest.

Conducting this stage of therapy passively is impractical in patients who are
not capable of at least moderate verbal fluency (e.g., many depressives; some normally taciturn people). It is contraindicated in Schizophrenics and borderline
Schizophrenics with loose associations, as it tends to make that symptom worse.
Though it may be tried, its usefulness is likely to be limited in obsessional and hypochondriacal patients who are often highly repetitive or circumstantial.

An alternate to passivity is systematic questioning, either based on the life
history (Sullivan's detailed inquiry) or based on the problem areas identified in the
initial interview.

In some cases, remission occurs during this stage, and if the patient is asymptomatic, the basic problems and treatment goals must be reevaluated to see whether
further therapy is indicated. The basic implied question or instruction in this stage
of therapy is: Tell me more about yourself.

Investigation of Specific Problems

An investigation of specific problems follows general exploration. In certain cases, first there is a transitional period of increased activity that is still a part of
general exploration. Some patients speak almost exclusively about current hap-
penings, while others talk only of the past. The patients who dwell on the past are
encouraged to talk about the present with such questions as, "How does this affect
you now?", "What is the most recent experience like that which you have had?",
"What is the nearest thing to that which you experience nowadays?" phrased so as
to avoid an abrupt change of subject. Similarly, the patient who talks only of today
is led to discuss yesterdays as well.

Patients who speak in generalities (My sister was always mean to me) are asked for examples, and those who present only concrete data are asked for generalization, abstractions, and concepts.

Those whose spontaneous production is usually limited to one problem, a preoccupation, or specific symptoms are systematically drawn away from the subject (except in cases in which it is believed that proceeding directly to work on that problem would be fruitful). One does not do this by abrupt changes of the subject which, in most cases, would only antagonize the patient, but by a series of smooth transitions whose goal is to reach *any* subject other than the stereotyped one (e.g., a patient talks only of a disturbed relationship with a woman friend; it is obvious that there are other significant problems that are not being mentioned; efforts to discuss the relationship realistically have led to a series of repetitive moves and countermoves. The patient tells of being at a party with the friend; the therapist asks who else was there, then asks about one of the people mentioned, uses several open-ended questions, and falls into attentive silence as soon as the patient begins talking at any length about a new subject.

A selection of specific problems to investigate is made from the content of the initial interview and the subsequent general exploration. Subjects include:

1. Topics introduced by the patient
    a. Things the patient feels to be important, including the problem or complaint that initiated therapy, current stresses, and past experiences that are regarded as having influenced personality development
    b. Situations past and present that would be important in the life of the average person even though the patient deemphasizes them
    c. Things that are mentioned with strong feeling
    d. Things that are repeated, recurring themes and evidences of repetitive patterns of behavior
    e. Subjects that apparently undergo distortions as the patient tells about them as suggested by contradictions, anachronisms, improbabilities, etc.
2. Subjects the patient does not mention spontaneously. These may be excluded because they are unimportant to the purpose of therapy or because they evoke anxiety-provoking associations
    a. Gaps in the life history
    b. Significant people in the environment, current and past, who are rarely mentioned
    c. Parts of daily living that are not discussed (e.g., an employed patient has discussed a variety of problems but has never talked about work)
3. Topics selected because they are often important in the psychopathology of persons in the patient's diagnostic category

The therapist should be able to list mentally or on paper, in order of probable importance, several topics that require additional investigation. Next, in planning strategy, one should choose the order in which they are to be investigated. Possibilities include:

1. The order in which they emerge. This is workable if the topics to be investigated are mainly those which the patient mentioned spontaneously, with fair frequency. It has the advantage of being the least directive method.
2. Beginning with the most central or important topics. This is preferable when one has reason to anticipate a brief therapy, when the patient has good ego strength, and when resistance and defensiveness are minimal. It makes sense to the patient to begin with the main problems. However, these may be the

most anxiety-provoking and the most hedged around by defenses. Also, they may be difficult to understand before a broader knowledge of the total personality is obtained.

3. Beginning with peripheral or less important topics. This is indicated if a long-term therapy is anticipated, if the patient has poor ego strength or is highly defensive. These topics add to one's knowledge of the patient and are less anxiety-provoking. Also, the familiarity with working through relatively minor problems prepares the patient for the type of exploration that will be used in the more central ones.

While the strategy of this phase of therapy involves a systematic exploration of chosen topics in detail, the tactical handling of a particular appointment may depart from this. One may begin the appointment intending to draw the patient out on a particular topic (or whichever of several topics comes up first); however, if the patient is obviously eager to talk about something else or brings up something of apparently greater importance, the plan for the appointment is quickly revised. Also, it is necessary to be constantly aware of the patient's mood. If the patient is unusually anxious, irritable, angry, or even tired, it may be a poor time to try to investigate a touchy subject.

Most investigation, especially of difficult subjects, takes place in the middle half of the appointment. The first few minutes are used listening to the patient to see what is on his or her mind and to evaluate mood; then one looks for a good opening to begin exploration. During the last few minutes, if the patient has been at all anxious, it is desirable to discuss less troublesome material so that she or he will leave the appointment reasonably comfortable. Once exploration of a subject is started it should be continued until:

1. The therapist feels that enough has been learned to dismiss the subject tentatively as irrelevant.
2. All available information concerning it has been elicited (or at least all that is necessary to understand and interpret it).
3. It is felt that further exploration would provoke excessive anxiety or resistance.
4. A topic of greater importance or more immediate relevance is introduced by the patient.

Failure to complete a topic leads to repetition. Often the beginning therapist will go over the same sort of material repeatedly; different examples of a repetitive pattern will be discussed, each superficially, with the result that therapy is unnecessarily prolonged.

With repetitive patterns one does need several examples, usually from the previous stage of therapy, to begin to recognize the common denominator. Recent examples are easier to recall completely, but the patient may find it easier to be objective about something that is all over. An example involving an important relationship may seem more relevant to the patient, and he or she may work harder to understand and explain it, but one concerning a less important relationship causes less anxiety.

The technique of exploration should be as unobtrusive as possible. If the patient is unaware or only minimally aware that the therapist is drawing him or her out:

1. It is easier for the therapist to drop a topic after deciding it is irrelevant. If the questioning labels it as important, the patient is more likely to keep thinking and talking about it.

2. The patient is less likely to feel anxious, defensive, or resistive, and does not have a feeling of being cross-examined.

3. The patient is less dependent on the therapist. If one ends therapy feeling that one worked out most of one's own problems, one will feel more confident in using the methods of therapy in solving future problems unassisted. It might appeal to the therapist's narcissism to have patients leave each hour thinking, "I would never have thought of those things had that brilliant, intuitive doctor not asked about them"; but the therapist's mission is to help the patient, not to be impressive.

If the topics for exploration are those the patient mentions from time to time, it is relatively easy to investigate them unobtrusively. Often, just showing increased interest and attention nonverbally or with a murmur is sufficient to cause the patient to elaborate. Repeating a key word or phrase in a questioning tone usually draws the patient out on a subject.

If displaying special interest and repeating phrases is not enough, general questions (of the sort that might begin, "Tell me more about _____") can be used, and if necessary, more specific questions are added.

Questions beginning with Why are generally avoided. If pursued, they are unanswerable. They are more likely to elicit a rationalization than a reason. The implication of "Why did you do that" is often critical and puts people on the defensive. In addition to getting information about *what* happened and *how,* one can ask what led up to the happening, what the patient was thinking and feeling, what was expected to occur. Questions using the words *always* and *never* may be useful and often elicit significant exceptions. An admission that the therapist does not fully understand something that has been said often leads to clarification.

Material that does not come up frequently in the patient's spontaneous production can be reached most easily through a related subject by a series of smooth transitions similar to those described for use in the transitional period at the beginning of this stage of therapy.

Sometimes, knowing the facts (including consciously recalled thoughts and feelings) is not enough. To understand some defense mechanisms (e.g., symbolization; complex formation) it is necessary to know the special meanings words and situations have for the patient. This requires the use of associative techniques. Associations are the ideas suggested by or connected with a subject. One way to obtain associations is to keep the patient talking about a specific subject or event. In time the patient will run out of facts and begin to furnish related ideas. This is time consuming, but it is effective with relatively verbal patients who tend to continue talking about a subject as long as interest is shown in it. Other less verbal patients need considerable encouragement, and there is the risk that efforts to keep to the subject will interfere with the basically collaborative therapeutic relationship. The patient feels pushed and, naturally, resists.

One alternative is to ask the patient, "What does it remind you of?" Another is to ask her or him to keep a particular thought in mind and express whatever other thoughts come to mind while doing this (whether they seem really connected or not).

Still another way of getting associations and, perhaps the most useful if one expects to need them often, is simply to ask, "What are your associations to _____?" and explain what is wanted if the patient appears to hesitate or not to understand.

If in response to any type of request for associations the patient gives a sequence of thoughts or recollections, it is sometimes helpful to return to the original stimulus one or more times and compare the sequences obtained. One looks not only for individually significant associations, but also for themes and trends (e.g., a patient is asked to associate to an activity he has described as being important and particularly pleasant. All of his associations are to generally unpleasant things. This suggests that his presumably sincere statement that he enjoys the activity requires further study and is likely to represent rationalization, reaction formation, compensation, or perhaps some other counterphobic mechanisms).

Other methods of obtaining associations, though more obtrusive and less often used, are sometimes indicated. A modification of the Word Association test (cf. Chapter 3), introducing some words related to the topic under investigation, may be used. The patient may be asked to answer the next question with the very first thought that comes to mind, whether it actually represents a considered judgment or not.

A patient may be asked to complete a sentence in a stated number of ways (or as many ways as you can think of). Usually, the first few thoughts are commonplace; significant associations may follow. During therapy, a patient may talk about a book, a movie, or a television program. Sometimes there is a connection between some aspect of the personality and one of the characters in the story, or between the patient's problem and the theme. It may be worthwhile to draw him or her out about the story and perhaps obtain some associations to things in it. If the therapist is familiar with the story, she or he must be careful not to assume that the patient's ideas about it are the same as one's own.

Dreams and fantasies are mentioned sooner or later by most patients. Though dreams provide important clues to unconscious processes, the use of dream material is too time-consuming to be warranted in brief therapy unless there is a definite need for associative material to help with an understanding of the patient's problems. Often, when dreams are first mentioned, the therapist may be uncertain as to whether he or she will need to use them. In any case, it may be desirable to show an interest in the first dream reported, since it is often closely related to the patient's main problem. Also, the interest in the first dream will encourage the patient to keep reporting dreams which later may be used or not as the therapist sees fit.

Dream material is most useful in the therapy of patients with Neuroses. It is probably of little value in the treatment of schizophrenic patients and may be contraindicated in any patient who has difficulty in reality testing. Dreams are unreal; dwelling upon them may be harmful to anyone who has trouble recognizing their unreality. This includes the patient who wonders if the dream is an omen of some sort. The very unreality of the dream makes possible one of its uses. If a patient has difficulty in talking about a subject because it is not acceptable (e.g., a minister with hostile impulses), one can talk about a dream in which the subject is represented (directly or symbolically) with much greater comfort. After all, it *is* only a dream. The dream can be used as a starting point for discussion of a relevant subject.

In other cases, one may want to have the patient associate to various elements of the dream. One should not attempt to interpret dreams (even to oneself, let alone to the patient) without knowing the associations to them. Because something in a dream is a common symbol, it cannot be assumed that it has that meaning in a particular dream or for a particular patient (Santa Claus is not always a father figure, nor is George Washington, "father of his country" notwithstanding; and church steeples are not always phallic).

During the investigation of specific problems, they may be clarified enough that the patient obtains insight and/or finds solutions to them without specific interpretive activity by the therapist. This stage of therapy is continued until the patient has an adequate remission, or failing that, until the therapist has a clear enough understanding of the patient's difficulties to begin the next stage of work. The basic implied question or instruction in this stage of therapy is: Tell me all about these specific aspects of your life.

Interpretation and Formulation

Interpretation, formulation, and advice can rarely be given early in therapy. Human life is too complicated. One needs to know a great deal about the patient before one can be helpful. Sometimes an explanation of the patient's difficulty and an apparently workable solution is seen early in therapy, perhaps even in the first interview. Occasionally, most often in Adjustment Disorders, this is valid. However, the therapist should view these preliminary interpretations with caution. If the therapist can see explanations so readily, why has not the patient grasped them? Have they been suggested by members of the patient's family or friends? If so, why has this not helped?

Early interpretations are likely to be incorrect or at least incomplete. If they are correct, there is often a reason, which must be discovered, for the patient not being able to accept them. If the patient accepts the explanation, there may be reasons for its failure to be useful. When there seems to be an obvious explanation, or an apparent solution, it is appropriate to ask the patient if she or he has thought of it or if anyone has suggested it. This should, in wording and tone, be clearly a question and not an indirect way of advising. If the idea is new to the patient, it can be discussed. If it has been rejected or has failed to help, the reasons can be ascertained.

There are times when one must seek an interpretation in the absence of adequate background information. This is indicated when the patient has to make prompt decisions, when a crisis must be resolved, or when immediate relief is needed for a highly destructive symptom.

Usually, during the first three stages of therapy a number of hypotheses can be formed about the psychogenesis and dynamics of the illness. As the time for interpretation nears, the therapist begins to seek additional examples to verify impressions about repetitive patterns. The therapist seeks data to confirm or refute hypotheses. During this period the patient may reach conclusions before the therapist does. If not, before one makes an effort to help the patient see an explanation and solution, one must validate it. In addition to being right, an interpretation should be useful. If one sees an explanation, one asks oneself, "What good will it do the patient to know this?"

The therapist may then be ready to ask for connections between past experiences and present ones (e.g., similarities between feelings about mother and about wife; connection between childhood experiences of rejection and recent anxiety attacks). The therapist asks about purposes and goals of behavior as well as the meaning of symptoms and behavior patterns.

To a large extent, the process is one of helping the patient think psychologically, in terms of meaning and of cause and effect, rather than descriptively. The patient is helped not only to see *the* explanation, but to think of and weigh all possible explanations. Human behavior is overdetermined; several factors may be involved in producing a symptom. There are enough possible explanations for even the simplest act that if neither patient nor therapist can think of more than one, two people are blocking.

Interpretation is principally achieved by raising relevant questions. However, if the patient omits possible explanations, one may ask about them specifically. Sometimes, early in the interpretive phase, it may be useful in dealing with a particular incident to suggest several alternate hypotheses and ask the patient to discuss each possibility with an open mind. This is not so much intended to help achieve the correct explanation of that incident as it is to teach a problem-solving approach.

In short-term therapy, in explaining behavior, one goes no further than necessary in the chain of causality. For example, a woman patient has anxiety attacks which are caused (in part) by disturbed relationships with women friends (her need to please these women has been explored but not interpreted). Disturbance in the relationships usually stems, directly or indirectly, from her tendency to flirt with her friends' husbands (the friends' resentment of this is compounded by the patient's guilt feelings and projections). It is established that a main reason for the seductive behavior is that she is seeking proof of attractiveness and femininity (not trying to make her own husband jealous, not leading men on so as to reject and punish them, not attempting in an aim-inhibited way to satisfy a frustrated sex drive, etc.).

Concern over being attractive is traced to childhood competition with an unusually pretty younger sister (as a result of reaction formation this is her favorite sister and she has no idea she was ever a rival). Perhaps it is enough for her to recognize that her flirting is a factor in interpersonal difficulties. If she can stop it, or do it more discreetly with relative comfort, her problem may be solved for all practical purposes. On the other hand, she may need to go a step further and see that she is trying to prove something that does not need proof. It may be necessary for her to understand her sibling rivalry and its implications. However, the therapist takes one step at a time in helping the patient understand herself and her problem.

Sometimes a patient will arrive at a useful interpretation and then repress it. It may have to be elicited again in another context. An initial enthusiasm for an apparent insight is of limited significance. The patient may later reject it for valid reasons or because of defenses. Conversely, the patient sometimes rejects an apparently correct explanation only to reconsider it between appointments. Some people have a life style of initially rejecting new ideas, even their own.

When a number of interpretations have been made, the therapist may combine them into a formulation. If this is done, the therapist should be careful not to introduce new interpretations, but to use only those already developed jointly with the patient.

Not all interpretations need implementation. If symptoms stem from an unrealistic fear (a basic one, not the displaced fear of a phobia) and this is recognized, the symptoms stop. The same is true of unwarranted guilt feelings. Once a goal is clarified, self-defeating behavior when recognized is almost automatically eliminated.

Some authors feel that this is true of all symptoms and problems; once they are understood, they go away. This may be true if there is enough insight. In brief therapy, however, there are times when even after a problem is understood, the question what can be done about it remains.

This is the place for advice. The technique of advising is, like that of interpretation, one of helping the patient see all the possible solutions and their consequences so that he or she may make a rational, not a rationalized, choice. The basic implied questions in this stage of therapy are:

1. What causes the symptom or problem?
2. What is the goal of symptomatic behavior?
3. What does it mean?
4. What is the best solution for the identified problems in living?

The doctor-patient relationship, including manifestations of transference and resistance, is important throughout therapy. The therapist is constantly alert to the patient's mood, attitude toward therapy, and attitude toward the doctor.

The patient does not need to *like* the doctor. However, to work effectively, one needs to respect the doctor's ability and integrity. A patient may have confidence and trust in the doctor from the beginning. Often the patient does not, and the therapist can only earn it by being worthy of it. Likewise, the patient does not need to believe in therapy. If the patient is willing to give it a try, he or she may be doubtful or skeptical. The therapist welcomes open expressions of hostility. If they are expressed, they can be studied and handled. The patient's ability to put anger into words indicates a degree of confidence in the therapist; one feels free to say what one thinks and does not fear reprisal or rejection. There are ambivalent feelings in most relationships; the sooner the negative ones come into the open and are dealt with, the less they will interfere with the subsequent course of treatment and the firmer the ultimate working relationship will be.

The therapist need not *like* the patient. In fact, if one likes the patient too well, one may be overprotective. One must recognize the patient's needs and respect his or her rights as a person. If there are things about the patient's behavior that anger or annoy the therapist, one must be objective about them. If they are symptomatic, one must view them as problems to be solved. If they are essentially irrelevant, one must keep one's reaction to them from interfering with the care of the patient.

A patient may show a prevailing attitude toward the therapist. In addition, there may be attitudes which appear in a particular appointment. Both prevailing attitudes, and transient ones are recognized and studied. Patients may show a positive, friendly, trusting, or affectionate attitude. They may be dependent and compliant or competitive and negativistic. There may be fear, hostility, or anger. There are several possible explanations for any emotional reaction the patient may display. Among the possibilities are:

1. The patient is reacting more or less appropriately to something the therapist has done (e.g., an angry patient may be reacting to a tactless remark).
2. The manifest feeling is a reaction formation or a conscious method of coping with another feeling (e.g., a patient is behaving hostilely because he cannot tolerate his positive feeling; a patient is acting friendly to placate a therapist he fears).
3. The interview behavior represents a displacement (e.g., a patient expresses anger at the therapist; he is actually angry at his employer).
4. The interview behavior stems from anxiety aroused by something the patient is talking about in therapy (e.g., many patients are irritable when anxious; the patient may be moving too rapidly in a discussion of disturbing material).
5. The patient is displaying an habitual way of relating to others (e.g., a man who is highly critical of everyone will be critical of his therapist; a woman who behaves seductively toward all men behaves that way in therapy).
6. The behavior is a manifestation of transference and is specific to the doctor-patient relationship.

Transference

Transference is the mechanism by which a person reacts to someone as if he or she were a significant figure in the individual's past, usually a parent. Transference is spoken of as *positive* if the feelings transferred are warm and affectionate, *negative* if they are hostile. Ambivalence and indifference are also attitudes that can be transferred.

The sex and age of the therapist have little to do with whether the feelings and attitudes transferred are ones originally directed toward mother, father, or sibling. The relative significance of the original person in the patient's emotional growth and development is usually the determining factor. If feelings about both parents were about equally important in personality development, the sex of the therapist may still not be as much a deciding factor as mannerisms and other superficial similarities to one parent or the other. In such cases, a fairly active therapist is more likely to be seen as "father" and a passive one as "mother" since in our culture, activity, including verbal productivity, is regarded as a masculine characteristic!

The diagnostic evaluation (cf. Chapters 3 and 19) usually enables the therapist to predict both the general nature of the transference (e.g., "This patient may never say, 'you are exactly like my mother,' may never even consciously think it, but she will behave as if it were so") and specific transference problems that are likely to arise (e.g., "If this young woman talks about a boyfriend and I show a lot of interest, she will think I'm trying to marry her off"; or, conversely, depending on how mother's behavior was perceived, "She will think I'm trying to break up the relationship").

Prepared in this way, the therapist modifies the handling of certain situations which might otherwise lead to misunderstandings or to an impasse in therapy. The therapist is also in a position to lessen the intensity of transference if he or she chooses. To lessen the intensity of the transference, the therapist may elect to behave differently from a parent. Also, one may show more of one's own personality than is otherwise indicated. Transference occurs in many relationships other than the therapeutic; its effects are less profound (usually) because differences are constantly perceived between the present and past relationship (e.g., an employer who is dealt with mainly through intermediaries may be treated, felt about, reacted to, as if he were father; an employer with whom one has daily contact says and does enough things different from father's behavior to keep the reality of the current relationship in the foreground. This would be less true if the employer greatly resembled father. Sometimes defense mechanisms keep a person from seeing obvious differences; perception of them is repressed, dissociated, or rationalized away).

In brief therapy, transference is not interpreted systematically. However, when transference problems interfere with therapy, the distortions of the reality of the relationship must be explored, brought into the open, and explained.

Countertransference is the term applied to the mechanism by which the therapist reacts to the patient as if he or she were some other person from the therapist's own life. Not all positive or negative feelings a patient has toward the therapist are manifestations of transference; likewise, not all feelings the physician has about the patient result from countertransference. Many patients are at times, intentionally or otherwise, downright annoying; many are at times appealing and likable. The therapist, though attempting to control words and nonverbal communication, should seek to understand rather than suppress positive or negative feelings. If one finds oneself looking forward to or dreading certain appointments, if one thinks of the patient very often between appointments when there seems to be no need to review or study the case, one must look for the explanation. Are the feelings disproportionate? Do they interfere with therapy? Is one reacting to symptomatic behavior as if it were something personal? Is one blaming the patient for being sick or for not getting well? Is one displacing? Is the feeling a result of countertransference? Does the patient remind one of anyone else he or she has known? Is there anything about the patient that is reminiscent of a significant person from one's own past? What are one's associations to the patient; to those things the patient does which evoke the most feeling?

Resistance

Resistance is a concept that is often misunderstood. If represents an effort of the ego and superego to maintain repression. The patient is not struggling with the therapist and resisting *him* or *her*. The patient is not resisting getting well; it is not that he (or she) wants to stay sick. He *is* resisting change. He *does* resist giving up behavior patterns that have, albeit infrequently and uneconomically, led to some satisfaction or helped prevent some discomfort. He *does* resist giving up a defense that has protected him, even at great cost to his personality, from intolerable thoughts and impulses, from anxiety.

Overcoming resistance is a collaborative effort of patient and therapist. Resistance is suspected when the patient's behavior seems to impede the progress of therapy. However, alternate explanations must be considered (e.g., the patient who is habitually late for appointments may have very real difficulties in adjusting activities to the schedule, or may be symptomatically late to everything). Sometimes resistance is readily suspected; the patient who appears to avoid answering certain questions, who cannot see a fairly obvious interpretation even when all the data are organized, and who finds a dozen specious reasons for not even considering it, alerts the therapist to the possibility of resistance among other potential causes for the negativism. However, other manifestations are more subtle. If may take a while to recognize that a patient suddenly presents an interesting dream, a startling childhood recollection, or an urgent new problem whenever a certain, perhaps apparently innocuous topic is approached.

The possibility of resistance is thought of readily when a patient seems angry or hostile; one may be less quick to think of it when the patient behaves flirtatiously or seductively, though such behavior can be used to avoid working on problems or even to embarrass the therapist, or make one uncomfortable.

Silences are quickly interpreted (sometimes incorrectly) as resistance; but an intense, animated discussion of a clinically interesting subject may not be recognized as a filibuster.

Sometimes, after therapy has progressed well for a time, a plateau seems to be reached. While this may mean that goals have been reached and that it is time to summarize what has gone on and, if necessary, select new goals, it can also mean resistance. Sometimes this is a strong resistance that needs special attention. It may be rather mild resistance complicated by poor technique. The therapist may have been drawn into a repetitive interaction, a stalemate, a merry-go-round, in which the patient repeatedly offers the same or similar data (recollections, problems, questions) and therapist makes more or less identical responses.

When resistance is suspected, one must determine the extent, if any, to which the patient is conscious of it. Then the subjects that evoke the resistance are identified. What changes are feared? Is the source of the resistance in the superego, the ego, or the id?

In brief therapy, a general tendency toward resistance is handled by efforts to clarify goals and motivation and to improve the doctor-patient relationship. It is also often a signal to proceed more slowly. Resistance to specific areas of investigation or interpretation generally indicates that the patient is not ready for them and that other subjects need handling first. Sometimes the disturbing material can be approached in a different context. Resistances may also be investigated and interpreted; however, when possible, in brief therapy it is usually better to work around a resistance than to attack it directly. Resistance, like other defense mechanisms, serves a purpose and should be treated with respect.

Termination

Termination of therapy is usually by mutual consent. If the patient introduces the subject directly, one wonders, regardless of apparent progress, if this could result from resistance (including resistance manifested by a flight into health), negative transference, or a wish to test the therapist's interest and attitude. Sometimes one also wonders about pressure from family members, concern over cost of therapy, or other reality-based problems. It is wise to explore the reasons for and feelings about termination. Usually, it is better not to terminate at the appointment in which termination is first discussed, but to recommend at least two additional appointments. The first of these can be used for summarization and consideration of remaining problems. Some remaining problems may prove to be indications for further therapy; others may lend themselves to advice. In bringing out remaining problems, the therapist's goal is to have the patient see the problems clearly; it is up to the patient to decide whether to work on them. If there are dangerous or highly destructive symptoms remaining, of course, much more effort is made to help the patient see a need for change.

The patient may bring up termination indirectly through a discussion of progress or through complaints about the inconvenience of keeping appointments. A question can then be raised about thoughts of discontinuing therapy, and the subsequent investigation follows the same pattern as if termination had been mentioned directly. If the therapist feels that the patient does not need further therapy, but the patient makes no reference to quitting, it is appropriate for the therapist to summarize what has happened in therapy, inquire about progress, and discuss further goals. This usually leads to the patient's expressing feelings about termination.

Some patients are reluctant to terminate. Insecurity, fears of relapse, enjoyment of the interviews, dependent needs, and/or transference difficulties may be involved. One may investigate and interpret these problems. Alternatively, they may be handled by gradually decreasing the frequency of interviews. One must be careful not to press for termination in a way that the patient feels (consciously or unconsciously) a need to develop new symptoms to stay in treatment. Many therapists, after relatively long contact with a patient, prefer to arrange periodic follow-up appointments, or at least correspondence. An objection to this is sometimes made on the basis that transference is not resolved and the patient is not allowed to function independently. This may not be altogether valid. A young adult who has resolved dependence on a parent and formed a life of his or her own, or a student who no longer needs to turn to a teacher for instruction and advice, does not necessarily break off the relationship completely.

The successfully treated patient ought to be able to solve new problems independently, but he or she should feel free to return for more therapy without a feeling of failure or of letting the therapist down. Likewise, the patient who drops out of therapy more or less against advice should feel comfortable about returning. The latter is more likely if the patient's feelings have been recognized and discussed than if he or she just quits coming.

Modifications in technique for different syndromes are indicated. In treating Adjustment Disorders, one may move directly from the first stage, initial interview, to activities of the third or fourth stage, focusing on exploration of the presenting problem, and discussing alternate possibilities for coping with it.

In treating Personality Disorders, the emphasis in the third stage, specific investigation, is on identification of recurring behavior patterns, finding out the ways that they are maladaptive, and determining their goals. In the fourth stage, the patient is helped to see what he or she is doing and why, and is assisted in finding more effective ways of attaining his or her objectives.

With the Neuroses, there is much more emphasis in the third stage on the search for psychogenetic factors, significant developmental experiences, and intra-psychic conflicts. Investigation of defense mechanisms is important. Associative techniques are often needed. In Conversion Disorders, dream material may be especially useful. One looks for dissociated behavior and for symbolism. In Obsessive-Compulsive Disorders, technique is often more active, since the spontaneous production tends to be repetitive, circumstantial, or unrelated to basic problems. Both psychogenetic and dynamic interpretations are usually necessary for neurotic patients.

In treating schizophrenic and borderline schizophrenic patients, a passive second stage may be contraindicated either because of a tendency toward increasing looseness of association or to mounting anxiety. Investigation is extremely cautious because of the patient's low ego strength. Usually, work with dreams and fantasies is avoided because of problems in reality testing.

When Alcoholics or patients with other Substance Use Disorders are treated, exploration is also done with extreme caution and anxiety is kept minimal, since any increase in anxiety is likely to lead to increased use of alcohol or drugs (or to symptomatic relapse if the patient is not drinking or using drugs at the time).

In treating persons with Organic Mental Disorders, and in working with elderly patients who have some organic impairment in addition to whatever other conditions are present, one must keep in mind the degree to which memory is impaired. One may need to review material that has been covered more frequently and may need to repeat interpretations and advice. When indicated, psychotherapy should be accompanied by programs of reeducation and resocialization.

When psychoactive medication is used along with psychotherapy, the patient needs to know the purpose of each treatment modality, how the purposes differ, and how they complement one another. The patient's attitude toward taking medication must be explored lest it complicate the transference.

OTHER TECHNIQUES OF PSYCHOTHERAPY

Psychoanalysis

Psychoanalysis is a method of treatment based on the work of Sigmund Freud. Its basic assumptions include the theory of the unconscious, the Libido Theory, and the concept of psychosexual development (cf. Chapters 1 and 2). It employs *free association* as a basic therapeutic tool. Transference and resistance are *systematically* analyzed. Psychoanalysis is a long-term therapy. It requires interviews daily (or at least four or five times a week) for from 1 to several years.

Largely because of the problems of systematically interpreting transference and resistance, the technique is quite complex. The American Psychoanalytic Association essentially requires that the analyst be a physician trained in psychiatry, who has also graduated from a Psychoanalytic Institute, and who has had a personal psychoanalysis. It is not a technique that can be learned or should be attempted without special training. It is very possibly the treatment of choice for certain chronic Neuroses. However, it has some limitations. It is highly time consuming and accordingly is impractical for many patients. Results are slow. Patient participation usually requires average or better intelligence and ego strength. In many instances, one would not recommend it without a prior trial of brief psychotherapy.

Modifications of Psychoanalysis

Modifications of psychoanalysis, including those described by Adler, Jung, Horney, Rank, Sullivan, and others, differ from psychoanalysis largely in their underlying theories of personality development and their emphasis on different human problems. Some reject a portion of psychoanalytic theory, such as the concept of the libido. Others deemphasize the sexual elements in early personality development. These differences in theoretical bases do not lead to as much difference in technique (and perhaps results) as one might first think when reading about them. Naturally, a therapist who feels that inferiority feelings, efforts at compensation, and a struggle for power are especially important in the lives of most people (as would the student of Adler), or one who feels that a need for religious belief is particularly important (Jung), or one who feels that most difficulties are related to problems in interpersonal relations (Sullivan), or one who feels that practically all of us have a central concern over the problem of being or not being (the existential analyst), would be alert to different facets of a patient's problems, would explore these more deeply, and would be more likely to interpret them. However, since all of these therapies are largely expressive, investigative, and ultimately reconstructive, the therapist, regardless of theoretical bias, seeks data and interprets data.

In actual practice, Sullivan's methods probably differ more from orthodox psychoanalysis than any of the others. Sullivan made limited use of free association, preferring to elicit information by detailed inquiry. He did not systematically interpret transference as such, but he did interpret the patient's distortions of the doctor–patient relationship along with other distortions of realistic, consensually validated thinking.

Analytically Oriented Therapy

Analytically Oriented Therapy is a phrase that can be used to describe any psychotherapy based primarily on psychoanalytic theory. The general technique of therapy described in this chapter could be termed psychoanalytically oriented if the therapist uses analytic concepts in selecting material for investigation and interpretation. However, techniques could be quite different and still be described as psychoanalytically oriented. For example, an analytically oriented method could begin by eliciting the patient's associations to the presenting problem and various things related to it. Psychoanalytically oriented therapies can be brief or long term. They are investigative and usually expressive.

Psychobiological Therapies

Psychobiological Therapies are based on the theories and methods of Adolf Meyer. Psychobiology is a psychogenetic and dynamic approach to the understanding of the total personality, including a study of all aspects of the patient's physical health, psychological functioning, and social adaptation. Especial attention is paid to progressive adaptations and maladaptations.

Hypnosis, Hypnotherapy, and Hypnoanalysis

Hypnosis, Hypnotherapy, and Hypnoanalysis are not in wide use in modern psychiatry. Probably less than 15 percent of psychiatrists utilize hypnosis, and most of these use it only in a few selected cases. In hypnosis, the patient is put into a trancelike state by narrowing the field of consciousness. This is usually accomplished by having the patient look at an object (a coin, a beam of light, a revolving ball, or a card with two contrasting colors), relax, and pay attention only to what the hypnotist is saying, while the hypnotist repeatedly suggests relaxation and sleepiness. During hypnotic trances, suggestions can be given that symptoms will become less severe or will go away, or suggestions may be made concerning changes in attitude. The main objections to this symptomatic use of hypnotherapy is that it fails to solve underlying problems and that there may be a considerable risk of relapse or of development of new symptoms. Using hypnosis to modify a symptom, even though further therapy may be necessary, should have special consideration when symptoms must be relieved promptly for the patient's safety and general health (e.g., hysterical vomiting) or when they prevent communication (e.g., aphonia).

In hypnoanalysis, hypnosis is not used to suggest the remission of symptoms but to gain a better understanding of them more quickly. The technique is used to uncover repressed memories and to minimize certain resistances.

The use of hypnosis may create problems in the doctor-patient relationship. Some of these relate to dependence and others to the patient's feelings about authority. Erotic fantasies may occur during hypnosis. Information obtained under hypnosis is not necessarily accurate. Some patients, particularly passive dependent and prepsychotic individuals, may be harmed by hypnosis. Psychotic episodes are sometimes precipitated.

Research is still going on in hypnotherapy and it may in the future prove a more useful tool, but at present, hypnotherapies are recommended only for those persons especially trained not only in the techniques but in recognition of contraindications and management of complications associated with this method. This, of course, does not necessarily apply to the use of hypnosis for symptomatic purposes in nonpsychiatric cases (e.g., for the relief of pain in patients who have had extensive burns) or for the use of hypnosis as a method of anesthesia in patients with good ego strength.

A stage of restricted consciousness and heightened suggestibility similar to hypnosis can be obtained with amobarbital or thiopental sodium interviews. These can be used in much the same way as hypnosis. Interviews of this sort may be of value not only in confirming diagnosis, but also in beginning treatment of some hospitalized patients who are mute (including catatonics), some who have an apparent amnesia, and others with dissociative disorders.

Conditioning, Operant Conditioning, and Learning Theory

Conditioning, Operant Conditioning, and Learning Theory as bases for psychotherapeutic technique are receiving increasing attention. These techniques essentially enable the person to choose healthy responses to environmental stimuli and reject unhealthy ones. An early use of conditioning in psychiatric treatment was the conditioned reflex treatment of Alcoholism. Hospitalized patients were given alcohol along with an emetic. In time they became nauseated upon tasting or even smelling alcohol. After the conditioned reflex was established, the patient could be brought back from time to time to have it reinforced by repetition of the initial conditioning procedure, though many patients found it so unpleasant that they refused to do this. The full procedure was bound to fail unless the patient was strongly motivated and fully cooperative. Example: A patient who had not really wanted the treatment but yielded to persuasion described spending several days after discharge from a hospital deconditioning himself. At first he was nauseated even standing outside a tavern; gradually he became able to enter, then to have a drink placed in front of him while he had a glass of water, then to take a few sips, and finally to drink again with unnauseated bliss. Development of other treatment methods for Alcoholism led to this method's virtually dropping out of use. However, there have been recent experiments with other conditioning techniques in the treatment of Alcoholism, and it is possible that a modified conditioned reflex treatment will come back into general use.

Similar techniques have been used in treating some cases of Paraphilia. The patient is conditioned to respond negatively to stimuli which would previously have been erotic and to respond positively to stimuli evoking thoughts of the desired form of heterosexual activity.

A gradual desensitization of phobic patients so that things once feared can be tolerated with comfort has produced some favorable results. Wolpe's technique of *reciprocal inhibition* combines a stimulus that evokes anxiety with a response opposite to anxiety (relaxation). Systematic desensitization for Phobias begins with inducing relaxation by direct instruction, hypnosis, medication, or other methods. Then a hierarchy of anxiety-provoking stimuli is constructed, ranging from the sort of stimulus that causes the patient the least anxiety up to those which cause the most. This is followed by a step-wise pairing of relaxation with imagined anxiety-provoking scenes.

In addition to the above, there are a number of other techniques based on learning theory. These behavior therapies attempt to modify observable and quantifiable performance. Responses are strengthened by *reinforcement*. A positive reinforcement is one that rewards a response by adding something to the environment (i.e., a pleasant stimulus); a negative reinforcement removes something (i.e., an undesirable stimulus) from the environment. Behavior that is not reinforced in some way ceases (becomes extinguished). Operant conditioning consists of *shaping* behavior through differential reinforcement. Aversive control, using unpleasant stimuli (including punishment) to modify undesirable behavior, is also used but raises medicolegal issues and requires informed consent.

In an inpatient or day patient setting, various behavioral techniques may be combined into a behavior modification program. Such programs may include token economies in which desirable behavior is rewarded by tokens which can be exchanged for privileges or things that the patient wants. Another device, contingency contracting, has the patient work on behaviors that can be counted or measured, select and agree to goals, and receive rewards for fulfilling the "contracts."

Other behavior therapies, or components of behavior modification programs include assertiveness training (teaching patients appropriate responses to use in various interpersonal situations), implosion (a method in which the patient is exposed to repeated horrifying accounts of a phobic object until desensitization takes place), and flooding (another way of desensitizing phobic patients using aversive stimuli).

Response prevention and thought stopping are behavioral interventions that have been used with obsessive compulsive patients. Response prevention exposes the patient to a situation that would usually evoke ritualistic behavior and actively prevents the behavior from taking place. This is done repeatedly. Thought stopping has the patient, relaxed and with eyes closed, verbalize an obsession and interrupts this with commands to stop. At first the commands are shouted. Ultimately the patient gives his or her own commands silently.

Behavioral therapies are symptomatic. Underlying problems, if any, are not resolved. Needs for therapy in addition to the relief of presenting symptoms must be evaluated.

Client-Centered Therapy

Client-Centered Therapy (nondirective counseling) is a treatment technique developed by Carl Rogers. It emphasizes the importance of the therapist's personality characteristics (which, to some extent, may be acquired). The important characteristics are: (1) genuineness, (2) a capacity for unconditional positive regard and total acceptance of the patient, and (3) a capacity for empathy. The therapist asks no questions and makes no interpretations, but accepts what the patient says. He or she gives verbal recognition to the fact that a message has been received and the feelings associated with it are understood. The message is reflected by repeating it to the patient without essential alteration. The recognition and reflection of what the patient says and feels is relatively systematic. The rights of the patient are respected and this includes the right to have incorrect ideas, the right to be sick, the right to be peculiar, and even the right to commit suicide (though one can use the technique without going quite that far).

This form of treatment is particularly useful in the treatment of hypochondriacal and complaining patients. It may also be useful in other patients who resist efforts at investigation and persist in talking about presenting problems. Often, when it is used, one sees rapid improvement for a few interviews and then a relapse. The therapist may become alarmed by the relapse and violate the principles of treatment. Though this is sometimes necessary, usually it is better to continue despite the relapse, and after this, improvement again takes place, usually more gradually but more permanently.

Cognitive Therapy

Cognitive Therapy is used primarily in the treatment of depressions, especially Dysthymic Disorders. It is problem oriented, structured, and directive. It is short term (12 to 20 weeks). It attempts to help the patient identify and correct unrealistic negative views of the self and the life situation. Correcting self-defeating thoughts and assumptions is used to bring undesired emotions under control. Outcome studies have shown cognitive therapy to be among the effective treatments for depression. Its use requires special training in the technique and in patient selection.

Interpersonal Psychotherapy

Interpersonal Psychotherapy (IPT) is also used in treating depressions. Though based in part on Sullivan's theories, it is a relatively new treatment method that focuses on grief, interpersonal conflicts, role transitions, and interpersonal deficits.

Logotherapy, Primal Therapy, Rational-Emotive Therapy, and Reality Therapy are among other therapeutic methods which have been developed in recent years and are more frequently used by nonmedical therapists than by physicians. However, the physician may wish to become familiar with them in order to be able to make appropriate referrals (and avoid inappropriate ones) or to advise patients considering entering a treatment program. One may also wish to master some of the techniques so as to utilize them in selected cases or to adapt certain features of them to an eclectic therapy.

Logotherapy

Developed by Victor Frankl, Logotherapy is based on existentialism. Patients are thought to have symptoms because they have lost meaning in their lives. The therapist exposes the patient's existential frustration and assists in finding meaning for the patient's life. Paradoxical intention, one of the techniques used in Logotherapy, can be adapted to other treatment methods. In effect, a patient is asked to *wish* for the very thing that is feared most. Example: A patient troubled by stage fright who has to make a speech fears that he will shake, stammer, forget his speech, and generally make a fool of himself. Just before speaking, he is asked to wish earnestly to have all of these things happen and to think, "I will show them what real stage fright is like." This particular device may be suggested to some patients as something that people sometimes find helpful. Another major technique in Logotherapy is dereflection, in which the patient removes the center of attention from the self to the external.

Primal Therapy

Primal Therapy was introduced by Arthur Janov. Its underlying theory is in effect that Neurosis results from failure in meeting infantile needs. In order to control these infantile needs, the patient uses repression. Primal Therapy helps the patient regress to a very early stage in psychosexual development so as to reexperience the feelings caused by having the unmet infantile needs and to scream with anger about them. Its main elements are abreaction and catharsis.

Rational-Emotive Therapy

Rational-Emotive Therapy is described by Albert Ellis. He believes that people become neurotic because they indoctrinate themselves with irrational ideas. Therapy is directed toward logic and rational thinking. Emphasis is placed on what the patient *tells himself (or herself)* in various situations, and the patient is taught more logical and effective substitutes.

Reality Therapy

William Glasser's Reality Therapy rejects the concepts of mental illness, the unconscious and transference, and the usefulness of past history. It stresses "the morality of behavior," attempting to teach patients (who are not sick?) better ways to meet their needs.

Group Therapy

Group Psychotherapy

Group Psychotherapy, in which the therapist meets for regularly scheduled appointments with several patients in a group rather than with a single patient has several potential advantages, including:

1.   Expediency. It conserves the therapist's time and permits one to serve more patients. This in itself is not generally sufficient indication for its use. A patient should have the best treatment regardless of convenience to the doctor. However, in any case in which group therapy is equally suitable convenience can be a deciding factor. Also, extensive use of group therapy may be the only way to meet treatment needs in some institutional settings.

2.   Opportunity for the patient to develop skills in interacting with others. Some patients have more problems in their lives in dealing with groups of people than in one-to-one relationships. Such a patient can benefit from the experience in the group and from the opportunity to study his or her own behavior in the context of the group.

3.   Help in overcoming feelings of isolation, alienation, and uniqueness. It is comforting to some patients to learn that others have similar feelings and problems. Likewise, such a patient may be less shy in discussing some feelings if other group members acknowledge them. One can profit by solutions that others have found for difficulties similar to some of one's own.

4.   For a few patients the group gives a feeling of safety, perhaps from vague fears of the therapist, perhaps from fears of their own hostile or erotic impulses.

5.   Many patients learn problem solving, including investigative techniques that may help them work with their own difficulties as they participate in studying problems of other group members.

6.   The group may point out the patient's maladaptive behavior more readily than this can be done in individual therapy. In individual therapy, if the therapist confronts the patient with something unpleasant too bluntly or abruptly, there are often undesirable consequences. The patient feels hurt or angry; may discontinue therapy; may become less cooperative; or may simply feel very unhappy until some new defenses can be established. The therapist cannot very well say, for instance, "Lady, you are a dominating, interfering mother-in-law, and it's a wonder your daughter-in-law hasn't kicked you in the slats long ago." Instead, one must take weeks or months of painstaking work to arrive at the point where the patient says it about herself. On the other hand, a fellow patient in a group *can* say something of the sort. Naturally the patient rejects it, and is either angry or hurt, or both; but she is not angry at her therapist, who can then ask her or some other group member, "What do you suppose may have given him that impression?," and a discussion of the topic is underway. Likewise, another group member can suggest a course of action at times when the therapist might hesitate even to ask about the possibility, lest the patient take it as definite advice. Again, the patient reacts less because of the source, and a discussion of the topic can be opened. It is probably of less clinical importance, too, but a comfort to the therapist at times, that one cannot be quoted as having said or asked something relevant and needing to be said, but offensive to some significant third party, if it is uttered by a group member.

These and other advantages of group therapy vary in importance with the patient's needs and with the technique being used. In addition to advantages, there are some disadvantages and limitations:

1.   The patient gets less individual attention. The problems of some patients are so complex as to need undivided attention.   Undivided attention may be needed for ongoing evaluation of differential diagnosis or of suicide risk.

2.   There may be more embarrassment in discussing some problems before a group, especially a group of one's peers, than in privacy with one person.

3.   Confidentiality cannot be assured. Group members may agree not to discuss each other outside the group, but the patient cannot have as much confidence in this as one would in the physician's own promise reinforced by the ethics of the profession and the law. Obviously, the presenting problem may very well exclude a patient from group therapy (e.g., a homosexual employed by the state department; a minister upset by an affair with a girl in the choir). However, a patient whose *main* problems could be aired freely in public may omit some important bits of data because of possible gossip.

4.   Some patients who function very well in group settings need help in a one-to-one relationship that only an individual therapeutic experience can provide.

The size and composition of groups depend on the technique employed. The most usual number of members is six or eight. Members may all have similar problems (e.g., all Alcoholic; all with marital difficulties), or they may have different problems. Most methods require that the group be fairly well matched for degree of illness, intellectual capacity, and education. Matching for age range and socio-economic class is also sometimes done. Groups may run for a set period (with the option of prolonging the series of meetings or reconstituting the group before beginning a new series) or indefinitely. Groups may add new members from time to time or remain closed until the series terminates.

In psychiatric practice, most group therapy is either analytically oriented or essentially nondirective. In the former, an investigative, expressive problem-solving approach is used to explore the problems of individual members, and especial attention is paid to the significance of interactions between members. In the latter, emphases are placed on the acceptance of each member by the therapist and the group and each patient's capacity to solve her or his own problems. The group's ability to work out its own procedure is assumed, and the therapist's activity is largely limited to recognizing and reflecting back to patients the essence of their communications.

There are several forms of group therapy that are centered around activities (e.g., Slavson's activity group therapy; Remotivation groups). In these, the promotion of group activity and interaction is emphasized, with discussion of personal problems being largely incidental. The purpose may be socialization or resocialization (e.g., a substitute for gang activity and a step toward mature socialization in delinquent adolescents; a treatment for the shy, the withdrawn, or the social isolate) or it may be the development of new interests, hobbies, and recreations helpful to patients with Compulsive Personalities, among others. The goal can be reawakening an interest in living in chronically ill, hospitalized patients.

Closely related to activity group therapies and remotivation programs are a variety of programs for training persons in social skills. Mentally retarded persons and chronic schizophrenics who are being rehabilitated need instruction and experience in a variety of skills needed for independent living. Among these, they need experience in dealing and communicating with people in a variety of situations. Modeling, role playing, and active practice, with feedback concerning performance and with positive reenforcement of effective performance, are features of social skills training. Less seriously ill patients may sometimes benefit from similar training programs for enhancing specific social skills such as assertiveness.

Transactional Analysis

Transactional Analysis, in group therapy, focuses upon certain aspects of group interaction. To indicate what is studied and interpreted in this method, it is necessary to summarize some of Eric Berne's concepts. One of the goals of human interaction is seen as obtaining "stroking"; this in effect symbolizes attention, recognition, intimacy, and/or affection. An act that acknowledges another's presence is a stroke. Hence, strokes are the units of interaction. An exchange of them is a *transaction.* All people communicate and react on three different levels (at different times) or assume three different roles: parent, adult, child. These roles are referred to as Ego States. Regardless of age, if people communicate on a parent-to-parent, adult-to-adult, child-to-child, or parent-to-child level a *complementary transaction* exists. A *crossed transaction* occurs when one person communicates or reacts on a level inappropriate to the other's communication (e.g., an adult, operating on the adult level, asks a simple favor of a friend. Instead of responding adult-to-adult by agreeing to fulfill the request, setting conditions, or refusing politely, the other person reacts on the level of child-to-parent, behaving as a petulant child reacting to one too many parental demands). A group of goal-directed complementary transactions constitutes a *procedure* (e.g., asking for directions; planning a party). Some series of transactions are not directed to their apparent goal but have ulterior, in a sense dishonest, aims. Recurring series (repetitive patterns) of ulterior transactions are called *games*. The concealed purpose of the game may be learned from its recurring result or "pay-off". Example: A person who frequently asks for advice, and considers it seriously, whether planning on following it or not, is engaging in a procedure. A person who repeatedly asks for advice and then offers reasons why it will not work is probably playing a game. Berne called this game Why Don't You? Yes, But, and interprets its usual purpose as seeking reassurance.

Reinforcers which perpetuate behavior are referred to as *stamps,* using an analogy to trading stamps which can then be exchanged for something. Positive reinforcers are called gold stamps (or sometimes, warm fuzzies) and negative ones are called brown stamps (or cold pricklies). These imaginary stamps can be "cashed in" periodically (e.g., one collects and treasures a series of real or imagined slights — brown stamps — and cashes them in for a free drunk, a free divorce, or even a free suicide attempt).

The pattern of a patient's games, and of the reinforcers which help perpetuate them, reveals a lifelong pattern referred to as the *life script.* Life scripts may identify a role similar to that of characters in legends or fairy tales.

In Transactional Analysis, the patient examines his or her games and the life script so as to make changes which fit more closely with conscious goals and desires. This method, while applicable to a number of problems, offers special potential value in the treatment of Personality Disorders. One must be cautious, however, that the patient does not use the therapy as a sanction for socially unacceptable behavior through deciding in inappropriate circumstances to let the natural child out.

Gestalt Therapy

Gestalt Therapy was developed by Fritz Perls and is based (partially) on the gestalt school of psychology, which evolved from Wertheimer's studies on perception in the early part of the century. Gestalt Therapy was described by Perls as an experiential rather than a verbal or interpretive therapy. Patients are asked to reexperience problems and to bring them to a satisfactory conclusion (complete the gestalt) by acting them out in fantasy. In the group setting, role playing is used to facilitate this.

Other techniques of group therapy include Psychodrama (Jacob Moreno) and Adlerian family counseling, both rather complex methods. There are also a variety of didactic (educational) groups, inspirational groups, and self-help groups.

Conjoint Family Therapy

Conjoint Family Therapy treats the family as a functioning natural group. This differs from most marriage counseling and some other family therapies in which members of a family may work together to solve a mutually recognized problem. Conjoint Family Therapy was first applied to the treatment of schizophrenic patients and their families. The two basic concepts from which interpretive activity derive are:

1.   The double bind hypothesis (cf. Chapter 11)
2.   A concept of family homeostasis

This mode of therapy has been used with other conditions. However, in many conditions, possible advantages over individual therapy are less apparent. For example, the neurotic adolescent or young adult can learn to cope with parents or be emancipated during individual therapy. The married person does not have to continue in an unhealthy symbiotic relationship; as an individual he or she can modify it or even dissolve it. The individual often has major problems which antedate marriage and has difficulties in living outside as well as within the family circle. The schizophrenic and certain others may be caught in the double bind; all coping methods are wrong and the injunction not to leave the field is reinforced by the disability.

Among the many methods of psychotherapy only a few have been reviewed. There are others equally useful (and still others which appear to have no discernible merit). Some clinicians master one technique (e.g., psychoanalysis) and refer to someone else patients for whom it is not suitable. The general psychiatrist should develop skill in several methods of treatment so that he or she can choose the one best suited to the patient's personality, needs, and illness.

REVIEW QUESTIONS

1.   What is your concept of psychotherapy? Definition? Purpose?
2.   What are the indications for supportive therapy? What is supported?
3.   How does desensitization take place in a series of psychotherapeutic interviews in which the therapist is relatively passive? How does this differ from desensitization as a technique of treating phobic patients?
4.   What are some of the advantages of group psychotherapy?
5.   Describe a hypothetical case in which you might offer interpretation and advice in the first interview.
6.   What are associations? How are they obtained in brief psychotherapy? What is meant by free association? In what method of therapy is free association a principal tool?
7.   Define psychoanalysis. What are the indications for it?
8.   Give a short description of two techniques of brief psychotherapy.
9.   Why is Conjoint Family Therapy called conjoint? Who introduced this term?
10.   Look up Eric Berne's description of games. Describe three different games in transactional terms. Describe these same games and explain them without using transactional terminology.

SELECTED REFERENCES

1.   Ackerman, Nathan W.: *The Psychodynamics of Family Life.* New York, Basic Books, 1958.

2.   American Psychiatric Association: *Economic Fact Book for Psychiatry.* Washington, D.C., American Psychiatric Press, 1983, p. 48, chart 22.

3.   Berne, Eric: *Games People Play.* New York, Grove Press, 1964.

4.   Bordin, Edward S.: *Research Strategies in Psychotherapy.* New York, Wiley, 1974.

5. Brady, John Paul: Social skills training for psychiatric patients. II: Clinical outcome studies. *Am J Psychiatry* 141(4):491–498, 1984.

6. Fromm-Reichmann, Frieda: *Principles of Intensive Psychotherapy.* Chicago, University of Chicago Press, 1950.

7. Hsu, L.K. George, and Stuart Lieberman: Paradoxical intention in the treatment of chronic anorexia nervosa. *Am J Psychiatry* 139(5):650–654, 1982.

8. Jackson, Don D., and John H. Weakland: Conjoint family therapy. *Psychiatry* 24(2):30–45, 1961.

9. Kaplan, Harold I., and Benjamin J. Sadock (Eds.): *Comprehensive Group Psychotherapy.* 2nd ed. Baltimore, Williams & Wilkins, 1983.

10. Karasu, Toksoz B.: Psychotherapies: An overview. *Am J Psychiatry* 134(8): 851–863, 1977.

11. Karasu, Toksoz B.: Recent developments in individual psychotherapy. *Hosp Community Psychiatry* 35(1):29–39, 1984.

12. Klerman, Gerald, Myrna M. Weissman, Bruce Rounsaville, and Eve Chevron: *Interpersonal Psychotherapy of Depression.* New York, Basic Books, 1984.

13. Kovacs, Maria: The efficacy of cognitive and behavior therapies for depression. *Am J Psychiatry* 137(12):1495–1501, 1980.

14. O'Neill, George W., and Russell Gardner, Jr.: Behavior therapy: An overview. *Hosp Community Psychiatry* 34(8):709–715, 1983.

15. Perls, Frederick S.: *The Gestalt Approach: An Eye Witness to Therapy.* Ben Lomond, California, Science and Behavior Books, 1973.

16. Rogers, Carl R.: *Client-Centered Therapy, Its Current Practice, Implications and Theory.* Boston, Houghton Mifflin, 1951.

17. Rush, A. John (Ed.): *Short Term Psychotherapies for Depression.* New York, Guilford Press, 1982.

18. Steketee, Gail, Edna B. Foa, and Jonathan B. Grayson: Recent advances in the behavioral treatment of obsessive-compulsives. *Arch Gen Psychiatry* 39(12):1365–1371, 1982.

19. Sullivan, Harry Stack: *The Psychiatric Interview.* New York, Norton, 1954.

20. Wolpe, Joseph: *Psychotherapy by Reciprocal Inhibition.* Stanford, California, Stanford University Press, 1958.

21. Wright, Jesse H., and Aaron T. Beck: Cognitive therapy of depression: Theory and practice. *Hosp Community Psychiatry* 34(12):1119–1127, 1983.

Chapter 20

SOMATIC THERAPIES

THE NATURE OF SOMATIC TREATMENT

Psychiatrists often protest the dichotomy of psyche and soma, insisting that structure, chemistry, and function are inseparably interrelated. However, these same psychiatrists, being no more consistent nor rational than other humans, habitually refer to certain therapies as somatic. These are treatments designed to produce structural or biochemical change in the hope of modifying symptoms and symptomatic behavior.

Somatic therapies include various medications and certain other treatments including electroconvulsive therapy and psychosurgery. Though one might make a case for calling them somatic, behavioral therapies employing relaxation techniques and biofeedback are generally included among the psychotherapies.

In ordinary clinical use, no treatments are exclusively somatic. The attitudes and expectations of patient and therapist, the relationship during treatment, and communication at the time of appointments introduce elements of psychotherapy even if specific psychotherapeutic techniques are not being used.

There is no theoretical objection to using psychotherapy and somatic treatment concurrently. A decision to use either one, or both, may be independent of theories concerning etiology. Undoubtedly, biochemical alterations accompany symptoms; modifying these may be helpful whether the biochemical abnormality is a primary factor in causing the disease or is secondary to experiential factors. Likewise, psychotherapy can be helpful in disorders that are not, or not exclusively, psychogenic.

There may be occasional practical incompatibilities between somatic treatment and psychotherapy if:

1. The patient's attitude toward the treatment imperils the collaborative psychotherapeutic relationship.

2. The treatment interferes with participation in the form of psychotherapy chosen (e.g., treatments producing clouding of sensorium or memory impairment interfere with investigative psychotherapy).
3. Symptomatic relief reduces motivation (a problem only if something more than symptomatic relief is needed).

MEDICATION

A number of medications are used in the treatment of specific psychiatric symptoms and for the relief of certain target symptoms. However, the four most important groups of psychotropic drugs are:

1. Antianxiety agents (anxiolytics; minor tranquilizers)
2. Antipsychotics (major tranquilizers; neuroleptics)
3. Antidepressants
4. Lithium carbonate

Antianxiety Agents

The benzodiazepines are the most widely used and generally the most effective antianxiety agents. Their mode of action is unknown. Benzodiazepine receptors are closely related to gamma-aminobutyric acid (GABA) receptors. Benzodiazepines are used for moderate or severe anxiety and are useful in the treatment of Generalized Anxiety Disorders, Adjustment Disorders with anxious mood, and sometimes for generalized anxiety accompanying other disorders. They can be used for Panic Disorders and Agoraphobia with panic attacks but with the exception of alprazolam are somewhat less effective.

Available benzodiazepines include: alprazolam (Xanax), chlorazepate (Tranxene; Azene), chlordiazepoxide (Librium), clonazepan (Clonapin), diazepam (Valium), flurazepam (Dalmane), lorazepam (Ativan), oxazepam (Serax), prazepam (Centrax), and temazapam (Restoril). Among these there are minor chemical differences together with differences in potency and, accordingly, dose. Practically, the main difference is in plasma half-life, so that they may be classified as short acting (e.g., alprazolam; lorazepam; oxazepam) or long acting (e.g., chlorazepate; chlordiazepoxide; diazepam). Longer-acting ones are usually preferred as they give a smoother control of anxiety, have less withdrawal effects, and are less likely to produce habituation. Shorter-acting ones, however, are used for elderly patients in whom the half-life of drugs is prolonged and for patients with liver disease. Another difference among the benzodiazepines is the speed of onset of effects of a single dose. Though diazepam is long acting, it has a rapid onset of action, and might be chosen if one were using a benzodiazepine for episodic anxiety or for anxiety accompanying a Social Phobia.

In using any benzodiazepine one should be familiar with the contraindications, possible drug interactions, and side effects of the group and of the specific drug chosen. Benzodiazepines are contraindicated in acute narrow-angle glaucoma, and because of an increased risk of congenital malformations are nearly always to be avoided during the first trimester of pregnancy. Common side effects include drowsiness, fatigue, and ataxia. Less common side effects include constipation, headache, skin rashes, jaundice, and neutropenia. Central Nervous System depressants, including alcohol, have an additive effect to that of benzodiazepines and this may represent a danger to some patients. On the other hand, stimulants, including caffeine, reduce the effect of benzodiazepines. Cimetidine, a drug used in the treatment of peptic ulcer and one of the most commonly prescribed drugs currently, increases blood levels of long-acting benzodiazepines; therefore, one would use caution, and lower doses, in prescribing benzodiazepine for persons taking cimetidine.

The main disadvantage of the benzodiazepines lies in the development of tolerance and the risk of drug dependence. Though it may take 5 to 6 months for tolerance to the anxiolytic effects of diazepam, for example, to develop, these drugs are best used in acute situations in which treatment can be completed in a few days or at most a few weeks. If used in chronic cases, the benzodiazepines can be used intermittently with drug-free periods or periods in which another type of drug is used. Whenever benzodiazepines are withdrawn, it should be done gradually.

Mild withdrawal symptoms include nervousness and insomnia. More serious withdrawal symptoms include hypotension and hyperthermia. Convulsions and psychotic episodes may occur.

Though one may use benzodiazepines briefly during alcohol withdrawal to lessen discomfort and prevent Withdrawal Delirium, one would not otherwise use these drugs for persons with a history of alcoholism or with other signs of a potential for drug dependence. The risks of habituation should be discussed with patients before benzodiazepines are started. Prescriptions should be limited to the actual amounts needed between visits. With generalized anxiety one may wish to maintain a steady state, but if a patient has attacks of anxiety or fluctuations of anxiety and needs medication only at certain times, a modified dose schedule that encourages use only when needed may be preferable to a fixed schedule. In such cases one chooses a drug with prompt initial action from the long-acting group.

Benzodiazepines, when used, should be part of an overall treatment plan. Unless anxiety resolves promptly and does not recur when the benzodiazepines are gradually withdrawn, psychotherapy must also be used. While short-term or intermittent use is preferred, in selected cases long-term use of benzodiazepines may be justified. These are cases in which anxiety regularly recurs when the drugs are withdrawn (this is to be distinguished from withdrawal symptoms) and for which other interventions have proven ineffective.

One should be alert for behavioral side effects when using any benzodiazepine. These include irritability, aggressiveness, and displays of hostility. If these effects occur with a long-acting benzodiazepine and are not eliminated by a reduction in dose, a short-acting one may be tried, or some other drug may be substituted.

The fact that a few clinicians have overused benzodiazepines, or used them carelessly, has given the drugs a bad name. Casual use and overuse are to be avoided. However, underutilization is also to be avoided. One need not deny severely anxious patients the relief that short-term use of these drugs will give because long-term use and poor case selection can result in addiction.

Other antianxiety agents are considered when the benzodiazepines are contraindicated or have been tried and have proven ineffective. They are also used when benzodiazepines are used intermittently and another agent is needed during the periods when the benzodiazepines are withdrawn. Other anxiolytics include barbiturates, propanediols, antipsychotics, antihistamines, antidepressants, and beta-adrenergic blockers.

Though the use of barbiturates for anxiety is often regarded as obsolete, small doses of a long-acting barbiturate such as phenobarbital can sometimes be effective in controlling anxiety. Disadvantages include the sedative effects of the barbiturates. Drug dependence is also a problem with barbiturates, though it is more common with the short-acting ones. Behavioral side effects such as displays of hostility may be less frequent with barbiturates than with benzodiazepines.

The effects of meprobamate, a propanediol, are similar to those of the barbiturates. Withdrawal symptoms and risks of habituation are among the disadvantages of meprobamate.

The antipsychotics, especially those with some sedative effect, are effective antianxiety agents. Patient acceptance of these drugs is limited because of annoying side effects. The risk of serious side effects such as tardive dyskinesia also limits their usefulness. However, a short period of use of chlorpromazine, for example, to control severe anxiety may be warranted. Since the withdrawal of benzodiazepines or barbiturates, drugs which raise the convulsive threshold, carries some risk of seizures, and since phenothiazines lower the convulsive threshold, one must avoid a sudden change from benzodiazepines or barbiturates to these drugs.

Antihistamines have mild sedative and anxiolytic effects. They are not used in the elderly because of possible anticholinergic toxicity. Like the antipsychotics they lower the convulsive threshold.

Tricyclic antidepressants, especially those with sedative effects such as amitriptyline, have some anxiolytic effects. Certainly they are to be considered when patients have both anxiety and depression. Antidepressants are also sometimes effective for panic attacks.

Propranolol, a beta-noradrenergic blocker, though not approved by the FDA for use in psychiatric conditions, is widely used in the treatment of panic attacks. Informed consent should be obtained and one should be familiar with risks and side effects. Propranolol cannot be used in patients with asthma and is usually to be avoided in patients with diabetes. In addition to its use for panic attacks it may be helpful in cases of generalized anxiety in which tachycardia or palpitation is a prominent symptom.

Antipsychotics

Though antipsychotic is the most widely used term for this group of agents, it is a trifle overoptimistic. These drugs are primarily used in the treatment of Schizophrenia. They frequently ameliorate the secondary and/or positive symptoms, including hallucinations and delusions, and they reduce agitation. They do not cure Schizophrenia, but as a part of an overall treatment program are of considerable value. They are also effective in some Schizoaffective and Paranoid Disorders and in the early phases of the management of Manic episodes in which they reduce hyperactivity. This is necessary in some cases as lithium is slow acting. The antipsychotics can be used to treat Manic patients for whom lithium is contraindicated or has proven ineffective. They may also be useful when Schizophrenia-like symptoms accompany Organic Brain Syndromes or Mental Retardation. They may control disturbed behavior in such patients, but the use for that purpose alone raises some ethical questions in view of possible side effects, though there are cases in which it is clearly warranted. If a patient's behavior is truly harmful to himself or herself, achieving some degree of tranquility and greater comfort may be worth some risk. Antipsychotics have been used in the treatment of Borderline Personality and in Tourette's Disorder. Many of the antipsychotic agents are effective anxiolytics, but because of their side effects they have limited use in the treatment of anxiety.

Antipsychotic agents include:

1. Phenothiazines
   a. Aliphatics (dimethylamines)
      (1) Chlorpromazine (Thorazine)

      (2) Promazine (Sparine)
      (3) Triflupromazine (Vesprin)
    b. Piperidines
      (1) Mesoridazine (Serentil)
      (2) Piperacetazine (Quide)
      (3) Thioridazine (Mellaril)
    c. Piperazines
      (1) Acetophenazine (Tindal)
      (2) Butaperazine (Repoise)
      (3) Carphenazine (Proketazine)
      (4) Fluphenazine (Prolixin, Permitil)
      (5) Perphenazine (Trilafon)
      (6) Prochlorperazine (Compazine)
      (7) Thiopropazate (Dartal)
      (8) Trifluoperazine (Stelazine)
2. Butyrophenones
    a. Haloperidol (Haldol)
3. Thioxanthines
    a. Chlorprothixene (Taractan)
    b. Thiothixene (Navane)
4. Rauwolfia alkaloids
    a. Alseroxylon (Rauwiloid)
    b. Deserpidine (Harmonyl)
    c. Rescinnamine (Moderil)
    d. Reserpine (Serpasil)
5. Dihydroindolones
    a. Molindone (Moban)
6. Dibenzoxazepines
    a. Loxapine (Loxitane)

In comparing the effects of different antipsychotics, one must take into account possible differences in potency and be sure that comparable doses are being studied. There are differences in the effects and side effects of these drugs, but the similarities are more striking than the differences.

The phenothiazines, butyrophenones, and thioxanthenes stimulate the amygdaloid nucleus in the limbic system and depress both the hypothalamus and the reticular activating system. All of these medications block central adrenergic and dopaminergic synapses in the brain. The specific receptors blocked are those which are sensitive to norepinephrine and dopamine in the postsynaptic cleft. The beneficial effect in Schizophrenic Disorder is probably related to the ability to block the dopamine receptors. These drugs also accelerate the transformation of tyrosine into dopamine. It is hypothesized that this occurs because the dopamine receptors are blocked so the brain tries to make more to replace the deficit. In acute Schizophrenic Disorders, serotonin levels are elevated in the brain. When patients respond to treatment with antipsychotics, the serotonin levels return to normal, suggesting that the medications may also facilitate the metabolism of serotonin (LSD, which has an antiserotonin effect, produces an Organic Brain Syndrome which is similar to Schizophrenia in some of its symptoms).

Phenothiazines produce numerous other effects including: (1) psychic dampening of the midbrain (decreased affective response due to reduced activity of the limbic system); (2) inhibition of both the cholinergic and adrenergic systems; (3) inhibition of the vomiting center; (4) inhibition of blood pressure regulation; (5) inhibition of temperature regulation; (6) potentiation of analgesic and narcotic effects; (7) an antihistaminic effect; and (8) lowering of the seizure threshold.

Phenothiazines, butyrophenones, and thioxanthenes have all been shown to be more effective than placebos in well-controlled, double-blind studies. There are probably more studies demonstrating the effectiveness of chlorpromazine, trifluo-perazine, and thioridazine than any of the other phenothiazines.

Rauwolfia derivatives were among the first antipsychotics to be used. They were generally less effective than the phenothiazines and have largely been re-placed by them and by newer drugs. Their mode of action is somewhat different in that they reduce the amount of norepinephrine and serotonin at the synapses. One of their side effects, a tendency to precipitate depressive episodes, is a fac-tor in their not being widely used in contemporary psychiatric practice. Also, there have been reports that reserpine is an animal tumorigen, though the risk to humans is uncertain. One may still consider this group of drugs for patients who do not respond to the more usually used ones.

In choosing an antipsychotic for the treatment of a Schizophrenic Disorder, one should carefully study the side effects most common for each drug and select one medication which is most appropriate for the individual patient. Though the antipsychotics are similar in action, some patients who fail to respond to one do respond to another. Hence, if one antipsychotic has had an adequate trial, suf-ficient doses over a sufficient length of time and enough benefit has not resulted from its use, one may try others, preferably from different groups.

Obviously if a patient has a past history of responding or not responding to certain antipsychotics, this will influence drug choice. There is no evidence that combinations of antipsychotics are more effective than the use of a single agent. Though many clinicians routinely use larger doses, most patients do not show short-term or long-term benefits from doses over the equivalent of 300 mg of chlorpro-mazine daily. However, individual patients may respond to higher doses, and since the antipsychotic drugs have a high therapeutic index (ratio of toxic to therapeu-tic dose), higher than usual doses may be tried. If one does increase the dose and further benefit fails to occur, one should reduce it. Likewise, a patient on main-tenance medication who needs increased medication during an exacerbation of symptoms or a period of stress should have a subsequent reduction in dosage. Schizophrenic patients are often overmedicated.

The phenothiazines produce undesirable effects as well as desirable ones. Some of the side effects are sufficiently frequent and potentially serious that they should be discussed carefully with patients before treatment is started so that informed consent can be obtained. For involuntary patients who are unable or unwilling to give informed consent the physician must conform to legal requirements for using medication without consent (cf. Chapter 23). Side effects are discussed in the fol-lowing paragraphs.

Subjective discomfort

Patients often complain of drowsiness, dry mouth, stuffy nose, weight gain, blurred vision (associated with mydriasis), and dizziness when changing body posi-tions rapidly (orthostatic hypotension).

Dermatological complications

Photosensitivity is most common. Though sometimes severe, it is usually relative-ly mild (discoloration of the skin with itching and burning). Patients should be warned of this possibility and cautioned about exposure to sunlight. In addition to photosensitivity, allergic skin rashes sometimes occur. In a few instances of long-term treatment (over 3 years) with high doses of chlorpromazine (over 500 mg/day) patients have developed a slate-gray color induced by the chronic stimulation of tyrosinase. The skin discoloration can be treated with oral penicillamine.

Blood dyscrasias

Over 200 cases of agranulocytosis, including some that were fatal, have been reported in association with the use of chlorpromazine. This complication has been reported with other phenothiazines. Since it is not a common complication, and since chlorpromazine has been used longer than the other phenothiazines, reports indicating fewer cases of agranulocytosis with another preparation may be inconclusive. While agranulocytosis is uncommon, leukopenia is not. This may contribute to a lowered resistance to infections. Hemolytic anemia, thrombocytopenic purpura, and pancytopenia also occur in rare circumstances. Mild eosinophilia (4 to 6 percent) is almost universal.

Blood dyscrasias usually occur within the first few weeks (4 to 10) a phenothiazine is used but may appear after more than a year. Some clinicians obtain frequent blood counts while patients are taking phenothiazines; others do not. The onset of agranulocytosis is usually rapid and even weekly blood counts may not warn that it is impending. Patients should be cautioned to report fevers and infections (e.g., sore throat) promptly. Blood counts are then obtained and if a dyscrasia is present, the phenothiazine is stopped and treatment for the infection is initiated.

Jaundice

Jaundice is a relatively infrequent complication. Some authors report that it occurs in less than 1 percent of cases, but other authors estimate it as occurring in up to 4 percent of patients receiving phenothiazines. Most cases of jaundice occurring in the first few weeks of chlorpromazine administration are obstructive and cholestatic in character. It is possible that other types of liver damage may occur with long-term use of phenothiazines. Phenothiazines should be discontinued if jaundice appears. Very few clinicians use frequent routine liver function tests on patients receiving these medications.

Extrapyramidal syndromes

There are five different neurological sequelae which can develop in patients on Antipsychotics. They are:

1. Akinesia (weakness and muscle fatigue)
2. Akathisia (motor restlessness with inability to sit or lie still)
3. Acute Dystonia (a disordered tonicity of muscle, one feature of which may be an oculogyric crisis)
4. Parkinsonism
5. Tardive Dyskinesia (a late-occurring impairment of the power of voluntary movement often manifested by the buccal-oral masticatory syndrome)

Akinesia

Akinesia is the most common of the syndromes. The patient complains of muscle weakness, lethargy, and easy fatigability. Decreasing the dose of the medication is sometimes of benefit.

Akathisia

Akathisia occurs in about one of five patients and is twice as common in women. It usually begins relatively early in treatment, e.g., in the first 2 months. Patients sometimes notice it more when in bed and complain of difficulty sleeping because they are unable to keep their legs still (restless legs syndrome). Treatment with anticholinergics, e.g., benztropine mesylate (Cogentin) or trihexyphenidyl (Artane) or antihistaminic agents, e.g., diphenylhydramine (Benadryl) usually helps in the acute phase.

Acute Dystonia

Acute Dystonia affects men twice as often as women, occurs very early in treatment (usually less than 1 week), and is more common in younger patients, especially children and adolescents. It is very dramatic in appearance. Various involuntary movements may occur, but the patient often appears frozen in position with torticollis and the eyes open and rolled upward. Occasionally, opisthotonos occurs and the patient can be misdiagnosed as having tetanus or strychnine poisoning. Another error in diagnosis is in suspecting catatonic type of Schizophrenic Disorder. In dystonia the body is very stiff, while in catatonia there is waxy flexibility and posturing. The differential is important for two reasons: (1) the patient can swallow his or her tongue in Acute Dystonia and choke to death; and (2) increased tranquilizer dosage which might be used for catatonia would make Dystonia worse. The treatment of Acute Dystonia is an anticholinergic or antihistaminic agent either intramuscularly (takes 2 to 5 minutes) or intravenously (takes about 30 seconds). The patient is usually very frightened by this experience and may refuse future medications despite encouragement from the physician.

Parkinsonism

Parkinsonism occurs in about one in six patients, is twice as common in women, and usually occurs within the first 3 months of therapy. The Parkinson Syndrome responds to anticholinergic or antihistaminic medications as well as reduction in dosage of the Antipsychotics.

Tardive Dyskinesia

Tardive Dyskinesia (buccal-oral-masticatory syndrome) is one of the serious problems which can be associated with the use of antipsychotics. The patient develops rhythmical involuntary movements of the face, mouth, jaw, and tongue (vermiform in type). This complication is related to dose and duration of administration. Using the lowest effective dose for the shortest possible time reduces the risk. Up to 20 percent of patients who take an antipsychotic for over a year will develop Tardive Dyskinesia. The syndrome is sometimes relieved by stopping the antipsychotic, but may get even worse. It is not improved by anticholinergic or antihistaminic agents. The following medications have been tried in the treatment of Tardive Dyskinesia with varying results: (1) tetrabenazine and reserpine (to deplete norepinephrine), (2) haloperidol (a potent dopamine blocker which can mask the movement disorder), (3) lithium (increases tryptophan metabolism and decreases serotonin production), (4) alpha-methyldopa, (5) amitriptyline (blocks serotonin reuptake), (6) imipramine (blocks both serotonin and norepinephrine reuptake), (7) deanol (a presumed stimulant), (8) lecithin and choline, (9) valproate and baclofen (gamma-aminobutyric acid agonists), (10) apomorphine (a dopamine agonist), (11) tryptophan, (12) benzodiazepines, and (13) tacrine (an orally active anticholinesterase). Although each of these treatments, including combinations of them, has good theoretical rationale, results have been disappointing and leave the treatment of Tardive Dyskinesia primarily empirical.

Neuroleptic Malignant Syndrome

A rare but serious effect of antipsychotics is the Neuroleptic Malignant Syndrome. It is most likely to occur with highly potent dopamine blockers such as halperidol. It is manifested by fever, autonomic instability, and general muscular rigidity or severe extrapyramidal dysfunction. The condition is fatal in 20 percent or more of cases. It is usually treated supportively, but it is said to respond to bromocriptine, a dopamine agonist, and to dantrolene sodium, a drug used for other types of malignant hyperthermia.

Convulsions

Phenothiazines reduce the convulsive threshold and in susceptible patients spontaneous convulsions may occur. Convulsions are particularly likely to occur if there is a withdrawal of an anticonvulsant medication or an antianxiety agent with anticonvulsant properties followed by the administration of a phenothiazine. The combination of the withdrawal symptoms and the effect of the phenothiazine on the convulsive threshold may be dangerous.

Failure of autonomic reflexes

Phenothiazines interfere with the autonomic responses to stress necessary to raise blood pressure and increase cardiac output. This may endanger the patient who is exposed to an unexpected stress. Incidentally, it provides a contraindication for the combining of large doses of phenothiazines with the use of electric shock therapy.

Accident risks

In some cases antipsychotics interfere with visual, auditory, and kinesthetic perceptions. There may be also some interference with motor skills and coordination. These drugs have been implicated in some motor vehicle and other accidents. In view of the large number of people taking them on an outpatient basis, it would appear unrealistic and futile to recommend that all people using them should not drive cars or work around machinery. After all, people who drink alcoholic beverages have thus far not been completely discouraged from driving. However, patients should be warned to use extra caution and to use their own judgment as to whether or not they are safe drivers when using these medications. In selected cases, of course, it may be obvious that a patient should be advised not to drive.

Adverse psychological effects

While antipsychotics make many patients feel better, some experience no subjective reaction to medication, and others experience dysphoria. If dysphoria occurs, it is likely to be noted shortly after medication is started. If the medicine makes the patient feel worse from the beginning, he or she is likely to be reluctant to take it. Initial dysphoria is also reported to be associated with poor outcome. If it occurs (and one should ask about the perceived effects of medication), one should consider a change of drugs. Other behavioral and psychological side effects include those related to sedation such as drowsiness and apathy or occasional irritability. Depression and toxic-confusional states sometimes occur.

A number of other side effects have been reported at least occasionally with antipsychotics. Interference with the menstrual cycle is relatively common and the pregnancy test can be falsely positive (this can create real problems; is she or is she not pregnant?). Women in child-bearing age may lactate while on phenothiazines, especially thioridazine, while men may get gynecomastia. Thioridazine often delays orgasm in men and sometimes causes retrograde ejaculation into the bladder. It is to the advantage of both the physician and the patient to discuss the side effects which affect sexual function in order to prevent the patient from stopping the medications and getting an exacerbation of symptoms. Pigmentary retinopathy has been reported after prolonged (over 2 years) high doses (more than 800 mg/day) of thioridazine. Phenothiazines can also cause corneal and lens opacities. Sudden death has been reported with chlorpromazine, but a review of the cases suggests another etiology besides the medication. Some patients report that they get cold more easily or become hot when they usually would not. This is presumably the result of inhibition of the temperature regulatory mechanism in the hypothalamus. Q and T wave distortion on the electrocardiogram has also been reported.

It is difficult to generalize on the differential incidence of side effects with the various antipsychotics. As a rule, as the milligram potency of the drug increases, the risk of movement disorders increases and the risk of orthostatic hypotension decreases. For example, haloperidol (1 mg is equivalent to 50 mg of chlorpromazine) is likely to produce a movement disorder (extrapyramidal syndrome) and unlikely to cause orthostatic hypotension. The reverse is true of chlorpromazine. The choice of the antipsychotic should be individualized to achieve the maximum balance between therapeutic effectiveness and the fewest side effects.

Fluphenazine (enanthate or decanoate), which is the only phenothiazine currently available in the United States that has long-acting injectable forms (depot), has the advantage of only being necessary once every 2 weeks or so. It is recommended for patients who are unreliable at taking oral medications. The decanoate form of fluphenazine has a slightly longer duration of action and slightly fewer side effects than the enanthate form.

Abrupt cessation of treatment with most antipsychotics is associated with gastritis, nausea, vomiting, dizziness, and tremulousness, in varying degrees, in some patients. A more serious withdrawal effect is the supersensitivity, rebound, or withdrawal psychosis. There is some question as to how often this occurs, but it has been estimated that it happens in as many as a third of patients whose medication is stopped abruptly after a prolonged period on full therapeutic doses. The withdrawal psychosis may be confused with a recurrence of the illness for which the antipsychotic was originally given. However, withdrawal psychoses begin within a few days after medication is stopped and recurrences usually do not take place for a month or more. Unless the patient is experiencing serious side effects, antipsychotics should be withdrawn gradually rather than stopped abruptly.

Some clinicians suggest drug holidays — times when the medications are omitted for brief periods of time, e.g., 1 or 2 days. This does not usually lead to patients having withdrawal symptoms.

All patients deserve periodic review of their medications and appropriate adjustment of dosage. Even patients who have long required medication for maintenance may be able to do without it.

If it is necessary to use anticholinergic or antihistaminic drugs to treat extrapyramidal symptoms produced by the antipsychotics, these medications do not have to be continued indefinitely. Once the extrapyramidal symptoms are under control, the drugs can be stopped and in a majority of cases (possibly 9 out of 10) the symptoms will not recur.

Though the antipsychotics are valuable drugs, the incidence of side effects is high enough that this should always be considered before prescription, and they should not be used casually in the treatment of minor symptoms.

Precautions and warnings

In prescribing antipsychotics, caution should be taken if there is preexisting cardiovascular, respiratory, or liver disease. Antipsychotics potentiate anesthetics, antianxiety agents, narcotics, and alcohol. Thus, if a patient is on an antipsychotic, less anesthetic or narcotic will be necessary for induction of sleep or relief of pain and alcohol tolerance will be decreased. The seizure threshold is lowered, so dosage adjustment of Anticonvulsant Medication is likely to be necessary in epileptics who need antipsychotics. Hyperpyrexia (fever) can occur in patients who are exposed to high environmental temperatures. Exposure to organophosophorus insecticides should be avoided, as should the use of atropine (patients can develop atropine poisoning from the cumulative anticholinergic effects). The antiemetic effects can mask symptoms of various diseases. Patients who have a history of jaundice or blood dyscrasia should be carefully evaluated to weigh benefits against hazards. Phenothiazines counteract the antihypertensive effect of guanethidine.

Contraindications

Antipsychotics are contraindicated in comatose states, in the presence of large amounts of central nervous system depressants, and in the presence of bone marrow depression.

Antidepressants

Available antidepressants include: (1) the tricyclic antidepressants, (2) a group of second generation antidepressants, including some heterocyclics (tricyclics and tetracyclics) and some other compounds with more diverse chemical structures but similar effects, (3) the monoamine oxidase (MAO) inhibitors, and (4) various stimulants.

Tricyclic antidepressants

The first generation of tricyclics includes the most widely used antidepressants, and the ones that one would usually consider first in choosing a medication for a depressed patient. Available first generation tricyclics include:

1.   Amitryptyline (Elavil; Endep)
2.   Desipramine (Pertofrane; Norpramin)
3.   Doxepin (Adapin; Sinequan)
4.   Nortriptyline (Aventyl)
5.   Protriptyline (Vivactil)

The tricyclics are useful in the treatment of Major Depression and for the depressed phase of Bipolar Disorder. They are sometimes useful in treating Dysthymic Disorder and in treating depression as a symptom of other psychiatric illnesses. They also have some uses in the management of conditions other than depressions, including Attention Deficit Disorder, Panic Disorder, Enuresis, Anorexia Nervosa, and Bulimia.

For depression, they are good drugs but not great drugs. In unselected groups of depressives they can be said to be effective in 60 to 80 percent of cases, but effectiveness often means improvement, not complete recovery. Only about a third of patients get enduring, completely satisfactory results. Better results can be obtained by careful patient selection and by not using drug treatment, or at least not drug treatment alone, when other interventions are indicated.

Response to most of the tricyclics tends to be slow. At best, it takes 1 to 4 weeks. Some investigators suggest that for adult patients at least the equivalent of 150 mg/day of imipramine for 60 to 90 days is necessary before the patient can be considered a treatment failure.

Mechanism of action

Tricyclic antidepressants block the reuptake of norepinephrine and/or serotonin at the synapses and, hence, raise the levels of these neurotransmitters. It is widely believed that this accounts for their effectiveness in relieving depressions. However, this is by no means proven. One argument against it is that the neurotransmitter-blocking effect of the drugs is prompt and the clinical response to them is slow.

At any rate, the various tricyclics are not identical in their effects on the reuptake of the two neurotransmitters. Amitryptyline, for example, is effective in blocking the reuptake of serotonin but is a weak norepinephrine blocker. Desipramine, on the other hand, is highly efficient at blocking the reuptake of norepinephrine, but it has little or no effect on serotonin. Imipramine is moderately effective for both.

The differential effect on norepinephrine and serotonin is significant, if the depression heterogeneity hypothesis (cf. Chapter 10) is valid, and if increasing neurotransmitter levels is really the way these drugs work. On that basis, desipramine might be the tricyclic antidepressant of choice for Bipolar Disorder, depressed type, or for that matter any retarded depression, since it increases norepinephrine levels; and amitriptyline would be preferred for agitated depressions because it has the greatest ability to raise serotonin levels. Even if one does not accept the depression heterogeneity hypothesis, one might make the same choices because of relative sedative effects.

In order of decreasing sedative effect the tricyclic antidepressants are: doxepin, amitriptyline, imipramine, and desipramine. A sedative effect may be desirable for a depressed patient who is agitated, irritable, or nervous or who has difficulty in sleeping. In other cases, a sedative effect may be undesirable. Of course, if one chooses a tricyclic with sedative effects, but regards daytime sedative as undesirable for the patient, one can give the total dose at bedtime. Doing this will also to some extent reduce the discomfort from anticholinergic side effects.

Precautions, side effects, and contraindications

In an occasional patient, one finds a "manic shift" after therapy with the tricyclic antidepressants. Some investigators believe this occurs because of a missed diagnosis (Schizophrenic Disorders are sometimes made worse by tricyclics, perhaps especially those that elevate norepinephrine) and others believe the drug causes the patient with Bipolar Disorder, mixed type, to shift from the depressed to the manic state.

Caution must be exercised in estimation of suicide risk in any patient considered to be a candidate for tricyclic antidepressants. The physician should continue to evaluate the patient for suicide risk while tricyclic antidepressants are being given, even though the patient begins to show improvement. Between the second and fourth week of treatment, the patient just might get well enough to commit suicide.

Do not combine tricyclic antidepressants and MAO Inhibitors. While this is sometimes done in Europe, it is rarely done in the United States, and is to be avoided unless one has special experience in managing this combination of drugs (and recognizes the medicolegal risks involved), as there is a serious danger of hypertensive crises accompanied by restlessness, hyperpyrexia, and convulsions. A 2-week drug-free period is required before switching from tricyclic antidepressants to MAO Inhibitors or vice versa.

Akathisia, tremor, muscle twitches, ataxia, increased muscle tone, hyperreflexia, and convulsions can all occur secondary to tricyclics.

Autonomic nervous system effects are numerous, including: orthostatic hypotension, blurred vision (especially close vision), dry mouth, constipation, urinary retention (prostatic hypertrophy is a relative contraindication), increased tension of the anterior chamber angle in the eye (contraindicated in glaucoma). Allergic or toxic reactions include cholestatic jaundice (like chlorpromazine) and rarely agranulocytosis. Cardiac effects include flattening of T waves, prolongation of the Q-T interval, and depression of the S-T segment in the electrocardiogram (tricyclics, especially imipramine, are contraindicated within 6 weeks of an acute myocardial infarction).

Among the first generation tricyclics, desipramine probably has the least anticholinergic effect; doxepin the fewest cardiovascular side effects.

In using tricyclics it is desirable to begin with small doses and increase to therapeutic levels over the course of a few days. In that way, sensitivities and side effects may be recognized early. Though withdrawal symptoms are usually mild, tricyclics should also be withdrawn gradually.

The effect of tricyclics may be increased by thyroid preparations and by stimulants. It is diminished by sedatives and antianxiety agents.

Overdose syndrome

Tricyclic Antidepressants have become popular agents for suicide attempts. These drugs are lethal in 20 to 50 times the daily therapeutic dose. Avoid prescribing large amounts for potentially suicidal patients. Overdose symptoms include: delirium or deep coma with clonic movements or seizures, hyperpyrexia, depressed respiration, and cardiac conduction and rhythm defects as described above. The syndrome is clinically very similar to atropine poisoning (anticholinergic crisis). The treatment of choice is gastric lavage and physostigmine (Antilirium) in the dose of 1 mg intramuscularly. The patient should then be admitted for observation. The physostigmine may have to be repeated one or two times. Alternatively, slow intravenous administration of physostigmine salicylate, 1 to 3 mg for adults, can be used. If sedation is desired, use antianxiety agents, e.g., diazepam, and avoid antipsychotics, e.g., chlorpromazine, since the latter aggravate the anticholinergic symptoms.

Second Generation Antidepressants

Overall, the newer antidepressants have not been shown to be any more effective than the original tricyclics. Nevertheless they may be considered for some patients on the basis of side effects one wishes to avoid or because of previous treatment failures with established drugs. Amoxipine (Asendin), a second generation tricyclic, is said to be faster acting than other tricyclics. It has little sedative effect. A high mortality rate from overdose has been reported with this drug.

Trimipramine (Surmontil), another tricyclic, has a relatively high sedative effect. It is said to be well tolerated by elderly patients. Maprotiline (Ludiomil), a tetracyclic, probably has fewer anticholinergic side effects and less cardiotoxic effect than most tricyclics. It reduces aggressivity in animals and one might wonder if it would be helpful for depressed patients who are also hostile or aggressive. Seizures have been reported with large doses and/or rapidly increased dosage.

Tradozone (Desyrel), chemically unrelated to the heterocyclics but similar in effect, has no major anticholinergic side effects. It has been reported to cause arrhythmias; it should be avoided or used with extreme caution in patients with preexisting cardiac disease. It has a moderate sedative effect. Alprazolam (Xanax), a benzodiazepine, may have some antidepressant effects. It has the side effects and disadvantages of the other benzodiazepines, but one might consider it for certain anxious, moderately depressed, neurotic patients. There are several other second generation antidepressants that may or may not be shown to have special advantages.

The Monoamine Oxidase Inhibitors

The Monoamine Oxidase Inhibitors include hydrazine compounds such as phenelzine (Nardil) and nonhydrazine compounds such as tranylcypromine (Parnate). The Monoamine Oxidase Inhibitors work by increasing the brain concentrations of norepinephrine through blocking of mitochondrial monoamine oxidase. The MAO Inhibitors are potent drugs. There are a number of studies that show that they are more effective than placebos in treating severe depressions. They are probably less effective than imipramine or amitriptyline. However, some atypical depressions may respond to MAO Inhibitors that do not respond to the other medications. Phenelzine is also used in the treatment of panic disorders. It is not as quick to produce results as alprazolam nor is it demonstrably better in controlling panic as such, but patients who do respond to phenelzine are sometimes more satisfied with overall results. The hydrazine MAO Inhibitors are slower-acting than the iminodibenzyl derivatives and may take several weeks to produce a clinical effect. Tranylcypromine is relatively fast acting; results are usually apparent within a week or two.

The MAO Inhibitors have frequent and rather serious side effects. Quite a number have been introduced and then subsequently withdrawn from the market. In fact, tranylcypromine, among the most effective of the group, was withdrawn temporarily because of side effects.

Jaundice is among the side effects associated with the MAO Inhibitors. This is sometimes associated with hepatitis and sometimes with severe hepatic necrosis which may be fatal. It may be desirable to order liver enzyme studies (SGOT, etc.) before MAO Inhibitors are prescribed. If they are abnormal, a different treatment should be chosen. Agranulocytosis has been reported. Hypertensive crises, sometimes with brain hemorrhages, have occurred with MAO Inhibitors. The concomitant administration of iminodibenzyl derivatives or sympathomimetics may produce such crises and may be fatal. If one is going to shift from the use of a member of one of these groups of drugs to a member of the other in the treatment of depression, at least 2 weeks' medication-free interval must be allowed between medications for safety. Even then caution must be used. The MAO Inhibitors as well as being incompatible with some medications are incompatible with some foods which are high in tyramine content. Hypertensive crises have occurred as a result of ingesting cheese, wine, sardines, beer, and other substances with high tyramine content while on these medications. The physician should consult a dietician or the *Physicians' Desk Reference* (PDR) for a complete list of foods and beverages to be avoided. The MAO Inhibitors potentiate the effects of a number of drugs and toxins. Periods of excitement and Brain Syndromes have also been observed in patients taking MAO Inhibitors.

Sympathomimetics and Stimulants

Rapidly acting stimulants, including the amphetamines (Benzedrine; Dexedrine) and other compounds such as methylphenidate (Ritalin), phenmetrazine (Preludin), and pemoline (Cylert), have a limited usefulness in the treatment of depression. Their stimulating effect increases alertness and tends to elevate mood. Their antidepressant effect is rarely marked enough to be helpful in severe depressions at or near the psychotic level. However, the response to a stimulant may be helpful in the choice of antidepressant medication, since a favorable response suggests that norepinephrine rather than serotonin concentrations need to be elevated. They are helpful in the mild depressions characteristic of the Cyclothymic Disorder. In some cases they are helpful in Dysthymic Disorder. In the latter condition not only do they relieve the depression but sometimes reduce the feelings of fatigue experienced by these patients. They tend to increase tension and cause hyperalertness; however, because of the feeling of well-being associated with their use, some nervous patients do not complain of this. Other side effects include increase in blood pressure and pulse rate, sweating, difficulty in concentration, and insomnia. The latter side effect is minimized if patients are warned that the medication will lead to a lowered sleep requirement and are advised to go to bed later than usual. Keeping doses small and adjusting the time of the last dose of the day also helps with this. Amphetamine increases blood pressure and should be used with caution, if at all, for hypertensive patients.

Because of the pleasant effects of stimulants, voluntary overdosage occasionally occurs, and a tendency to misuse the medication may lead to impaired judgment and hypomanic behavior. Schizoid individuals show an increased looseness of associations when they take these medications.

Amphetamine decreases appetite. This may be an undesirable effect in some cases and a desirable one in others. These drugs sometimes decrease sexual desire of women and increase sexual desire but decrease potency of men. Prolonged use of high doses of amphetamines produces an Amphetamine Psychosis (cf. Chapter 14).

Another complication of amphetamine usage in the treatment of Dysthymic Disorders is its short span of action. As the drug wears off, there may be a letdown with sometimes a marked increase in depressive symptoms and an occasional increase in suicide risk. In cases for whom the suicidal potentiality is high, considerable caution must be used in employing these drugs.

The stimulant medications are also used to treat the Attention Deficit Disorder. Methylphenidate is usually regarded as the drug of choice for children 6 years of age or older with Attention Deficit Disorder. If it is ineffective, dextroamphetamine or pemoline can be used. The drug is usually stopped at puberty, since hyperactivity decreases then though other symptoms may persist. These drugs suppress growth in height and weight, but this is usually reversed after the drugs are stopped.

Recent reports suggest that methylphenidate may be useful in testing whether antipsychotics can be discontinued for certain schizophrenics. If amphetamine precipitates a recurrence of positive symptoms, it is suggested that relapse may be likely if antipsychotics are discontinued. On the other hand, if there is no recurrence of those symptoms, and if the patient appears to respond favorably to the stimulant, gradual withdrawal of antipsychotics may be more safely undertaken.

Lithium Carbonate (Eskalith, Lithane, Lithonate)

Lithium was introduced as a treatment of mania by Cade in Australia in 1949. It was used only briefly in the United States because of toxic effects. By the early 1970s it was reintroduced, and it is currently the treatment of choice for Bipolar Affective Disorder, Manic Type.

Therapeutic Considerations

Lithium is a basic element and balances rapidly between intracellular and extracellular fluids by simple exchange with the sodium ion. The mechanism of action for reversal of mania is thought to relate somehow to this exchange. In the acute manic attack, the patient receives a thorough physical and evaluation of cardiac, hepatic, renal, and thyroid function. If all are normal, lithium is given in a dose of 300 mg three times per day. Serum lithium levels are measured 8 hours after the last dose to achieve the most accurate reading (it is absorbed very rapidly and will give a false high reading if one does not wait 8 hours). The dosage is adjusted upward to achieve a serum lithium level between 0.7 and 1.5 mEq/L (milliequivalents per liter). The antimanic effect takes about 7 days. After the symptoms have decreased, the dosage of lithium is usually decreased also, since the maintenance dose is usually one-half or less of the antimanic dose. The patient then has monthly serum lithium levels drawn and is maintained between 0.7 and 1.2 mEq/L. Lithium has a prophylactic effect against recurrent manic attacks and against depressive attacks in bipolar illness. Although all investigators do not agree, some preliminary studies have shown lithium to be equally as effective as Tricyclic Antidepressants in the treatment of retarded depressions. Some clinicians combine lithium with an antipsychotic during the initial stages of therapy. Chlorpromazine was used mostly, but by the mid 1970s, haloperidol became popular. There have been reports of the development of a severe Organic Brain Syndrome with the use of haloperidol and lithium together. Thus, even though it is unlikely that there is a real incompatibility, one might prefer to use another antipsychotic rather than haloperidol.

Side Effects and Intoxication

Toxic effects occur if the serum lithium level exceeds 1.5 mEq/L. They include nausea, vomiting, diarrhea, lethargy, mental confusion, thirst, polyuria, and fine tremor which is worst in the hands. The intoxication syndrome occurs between 1.5 and 2.0 mEq/L. Along with the toxic effects mentioned above, one sees muscle twitches, coarse tremors, slurred speech, and ataxia. The syndrome progresses to coma, convulsions, and death. Since serum lithium levels decrease by 50 percent each 24 hours, presuming adequate sodium intake and normal renal clearance, the treatment for the intoxication syndrome is basically supportive.

The tremor, which is among the more annoying side effects, may respond to propranolol, or if that is contraindicated, possibly metoprolol. Other minor side effects such as thirst, mild gastrointestinal distress, and fatigue or weakness are often related to peak blood levels and can be controlled by using more frequent, smaller doses or controlled-release tablets.

Warnings and Contraindications

Lithium causes a nontoxic goiter in about 10 percent of patients; the hypothyroidism can be treated with thyroid extract. Diuretics are to be utilized with caution and the thiazide type are the agents of choice, since they do not deplete potassium as severely as some agents, e.g., furosemide (Lasix). One dosage of a thiazide in a 24-hour period will raise the serum lithium concentration by about 40 percent, and two doses in the same period will increase it about 70 percent, assuming all else is constant. Thus, one can adjust the dosage of lithium downward by about 300 mg for each dosage of the diuretic and achieve approximately the same blood levels of lithium. There have been reports of lithium causing the syndrome of inappropriate antidiuretic hormone (SIADH) as well as altered kidney function secondary to glomerular precipitates. Serious renal damage as a result of lithium use is not common, but the possibility must be kept in mind.

Renal clearance must be normal. The patient needs to drink adequate water and eat adequate salt (NaCl) to prevent an inadvertant increase in serum lithium. Cardiac status and electrolyte balance should be normal or near normal. The ability to excrete lithium decreases with age and appropriate dosage adjustments should be made in the elderly.

SUGGESTIONS ABOUT THE USE OF PSYCHOTROPIC DRUGS

Before considering the use of drugs, the clinician should review the patient's experience with medication in the current illness and previously. In outpatient practice, psychotropic drugs may be less useful to the psychiatrist than the primary physician; many patients have had adequate trials of medication before referral to a specialist. The patient's attitude toward taking medicine should be assessed. Some patients do not take medication that is prescribed for them; others do not take it as directed. Some are likely to become habituated; others have an excessive fear of depending on medication. Some have a negative view of "having to take your medicine"; for others a prescription is tangibly giving something. Histories of allergies and drug reactions add to the risk of complications.

In each group of drugs there are several relatively similar, though not identical, preparations. The literature on psychotropic drugs is so voluminous that no clinician can keep up with all of it. The practitioner should become familiar with one drug in each major group and make a point of studying all articles concerning it. One should know its indications and contraindications, know the effects, side effects, and subjective symptoms accompanying its use, and become expert in adjusting dosage. At times one will want to use other similar drugs in preference to one's usual choice because of particular benefits, absence of certain side effects, or inadequate response to the drug first chosen. In considering a choice between major groups of drugs that may be effective for a particular condition, we do not as yet have precise ways of determining which drug will be best for a particular patient. In time there may be biochemical, psychophysiological, or psychological tests that will aid in making the choices. Now there is an element of trial and accidental success. If a schizophrenic patient, for example, has had an adequate trial (sufficient time; upward *and* downward adjustments of dose of a phenothiazine without adequate response), rather than next trying another phenothiazine, one may wish to use a drug from a different group (e.g., a butyrophenone). If, later, one elects to try another phenothiazine, one would choose one from a different subgroup than had been used previously (e.g., if the patient had had chlorpromazine, an aliphatic phenothiazine, rather than using another aliphatic, one would use one of the piperidine or piperazine phenothiazines). Sometimes patients who combine symptoms which might respond to an antidepressant with others usually treated by antipsychotics may require trials of both types of drugs before the most satisfactory treatment is found. However, there is little point to prescribing a whole series of similar drugs in hopes of finally finding one that will work in the case.

Combinations of drugs are to be avoided when possible. Often patients are given two or more psychotropic drugs at the same time. There are sometimes good reasons for this. However, there is little research evidence to show the advantage of combinations of drugs over one well-chosen one. Combinations add to the risk of side effects (also undesired potentiation) and make it harder to determine the cause when these effects do occur. Combinations may be antagonistic to one another. While some clinicians prescribe combinations of tricyclics and phenothiazines or butyrophenones, others believe this is irrational because they compete metabolically in the liver, the anticholinergic side effects are additive, and they compete with each other in the synaptic clefts in the brain.

When possible, it is desirable to defer drug therapy for a few appointments. Medication makes evaluation more difficult. Also, many outpatients with anxiety and some psychotic inpatients respond quite rapidly to the beginning of psychotherapy (or to the hospital milieu) and medication may be unnecessary. Of course, if patients are suffering greatly, one must try to relieve this as promptly as possible. The desirability of limiting the length of hospital stay may also be a factor in deciding to start medication promptly.

All other things being equal, a drug that has been in use for some years is preferable initially to a new one, except for research purposes. Side effects may be slow to be reported; this is especially true of some rather rare but serious complications (e.g., tranylcypromine was in use 3 years before the first major hypertensive crises were reported). When a drug is used therapist and patient should understand the goals (expected result; target symptoms), know what constitutes an adequate trial period, and measure results carefully, so that useless medication will not be continued indefinitely. Progress graphs charting a target symptom, or symptoms, can be helpful in adjusting dosage and evaluating drug response. Once a baseline is established, one can measure the response to a new medication or a change of dose. One can have patients rate their own symptoms daily (e.g., rating a continuum between severe depression and euphoria on a 10-point scale) as well as having ratings by the therapist (and by other personnel for hospitalized patients).

Medication may be more freely used when it is expected to be needed for a short time only. Symptomatic medication for Adjustment Disorders and crises, and for other disorders in which there is reason to expect spontaneous remission, remission as a result of drug therapy, or remission from other therapy presents fewer potential hazards than does medication for chronic illness which may have to be given for years or for a lifetime. If one wishes to remove medication, it is often best to do this in a stage of treatment in which close observation is possible (e.g., in inpatients before discharge from the hospital) and can be continued (on inpatient or outpatient basis) until the danger of relapse is minimized. We simply do not know all the risks associated with long-term use of these medications. Most of them have been available generally for a relatively short time. After years of treatment, new complications may arise. There are cases in which that risk is justified; it should be avoided when possible. Certainly, limits should be placed on refilling of prescriptions for psychotropic drugs so that their use remains always under medical supervision.

One tries to use the lowest effective dose and continue medication for the shortest time possible. With most medications, when possible, one wants to start with a small dose and increase gradually. Likewise, one withdraws medications gradually.

Caution must be used in prescribing drugs for women of childbearing age. The fact that a psychotropic drug has been used by a number of pregnant women without complication does not mean total safety. Danger to the fetus may occur in only a brief critical period. Unfortunate experiences abroad with one tranquilizing drug, together with results of some animal experiments with drugs which have been believed to be safe, underline this warning. Again, calculated risks are sometimes justified but should never be undertaken casually.

EVALUATING DRUG STUDIES AND NEW DRUGS

Each year new psychotropic drugs are introduced. One can expect that some of these will prove of special value; that they will have specific indications; that they will do things existing preparations will not; that they will be better; that they will have fewer side effects. It behooves the clinician to select from reports in the literature those drugs that may be valuable. Unfortunately, this is not easy. All too often a new drug is reported with great enthusiasm only to prove worthless or to be withdrawn because of dangerous side effects. One does not need to suspect pharmaceutical houses of avarice or clinicians of an unwholesome eagerness to publish to be skeptical. The people involved are human; wish-fulfilling fantasies produce distortions; idealization and denial play their roles. Some published drug studies are scientifically naive. They are little better than the testimonials for patent medicines. The discriminating reader must reject most drug studies that fail to meet certain essential criteria which are discussed below.

1.   The purpose for which the drug is used, and the way subjects are selected must be clear. Is it for a symptom (e.g., anxiety)? If so, how is the symptom defined and measured for purposes of the research (e.g., subjective complaints by patients? ratings by one examiner? multiple ratings? an objective test?). Is it for patients with a particular syndrome? If so, what diagnostic criteria are used?
2.   The dosage used and the duration of administration must represent a fair test. This is particularly important in evaluating studies with negative results. Earlier in this chapter we cited the fact that well-constructed studies proved certain drugs more effective than placebo; we did not add that other studies (usually fewer) failed to show this. Sometimes the reason lies in case selection; other times in dosage.
3.   There must be an adequate measure of results. How is improvement defined? If the main measure of results is a test, is improvement in test findings a valid measure of improvement of patients?
4.   The effect of suggestion on patients and unconscious bias in interpreting results must be controlled. *The double-blind* technique is the *most widely accepted* way of doing this. Controls are used. These patients receive a placebo (or another drug). Neither the clinician nor the patients know which ones are receiving the preparation under study (unless complications make it necessary to break the code). Of course, if the preparation has some characteristic objective or subjective effects aside from any benefit it may produce, no one is blind (except the editorial board that accepts the study). Sometimes the double-blind design includes cross over; the group that originally has one preparation subsequently takes the other.

The double-blind study is not the only way to eliminate bias. Objective tests of improvement, or the use of independent raters, may control the possible bias of the clinician. The effect of suggestion on the patient can probably be controlled, or at least minimized by a single blind technique. Actually, studies have shown that bias is fairly well-controlled when rating scales, rather than simple, overall subjective judgments of improvement, are used.

Some studies that are not blind more closely approximate the conditions of administration of medication in actual practice than do the double-blind. The interaction between the doctor-patient relationship in prescribing medication and the medication itself is not fully understood. Suggestion, for example, may act synergistically with or potentiate some drugs more than others. It is important that a research design takes into account suggestion and bias and deals with them effectively; the methods of dealing with them may vary.

Even well-constructed studies which have clear results do not fully answer questions of clinical usefulness. Statistical significance, important though it is in research, tells us only the probability that results are not chance. A finding significant to the 0.001 level means that there is only one chance in a thousand the results are accidental. A clinical drug study may have highly significant results (statistically) and, likewise, be significant in opening the way for further research though only a very few patients improve. One must ask not only whether the study is well constructed and the result significant, but also, how many patients appear to benefit how much.

Though in selecting medications one relies on scientific data and recognizes the possible biases of uncontrolled studies, and in the impressions one gets from one's own experience and that of colleagues; individual case studies, anecdotal material, and uncontrolled series of clinical observations are not to be disregarded. They may sometimes provide clues to case selection, to unexpected results, or to precautions needed that have not yet been subject to scientific investigation. The important thing is to keep an open mind, to attempt to validate one's impressions, and to attempt to give one's patients the best treatment available.

OTHER SOMATIC THERAPIES

Aside from drug therapies, electroconvulsive therapy, electric shock therapy, is the most widely used of the somatic therapies. Its mode of action is unknown. However, it is known that the seizure activity is necessary for the treatment to be effective. The neurochemical consequences of electroconvulsive treatment are: (1) an increase in the turnover rate of norepinephrine (which may be why it helps retarded depressions), (2) an increase in serotonin levels (which may be why it improves agitated depressions), (3) an improvement in the sodium transport system in the red blood cells (which is the proposed mechanism of action of lithium and may be why it helps mania), and (4) a decrease in serum calcium concentration at the same time that the antidepressant effect becomes manifest.

The traditional shock machine uses 110-volt alternating current and is equipped with a rheostat which permits delivery of a current anywhere from 70 to 130 volts. There is also an electrical timer which can be set to deliver the current for periods ranging from 0.1 second to 1.0 second. Current is passed through electrodes applied bitemporally (electrode jelly is used to prevent burns). Usually, the lowest amount of current for the shortest time that will produce a generalized tonic and clonic (grand mal) convulsion is selected. Treatment is usually given three times weekly until improvement is noted and then once weekly until the maximum benefit of treatment has been obtained. More frequent treatments can be used initially for highly disturbed patients.

Most modifications of electroshock treatment are aimed at reducing memory loss which is one of the side effects of treatment. Variables include electric waveform (brief pulse or sinusoidal) and electrode placement (bilateral or unilateral using the nondominant hemisphere; a variety of different placements have been used for unilateral treatment). In general, brief pulse current and unilateral placement each cause less memory impairment. On the other hand, some studies suggest that there are more treatment failures when *both* brief pulse current and unilateral placement are used. Also, there are some studies that suggest slightly longer series may be required with unilateral placement. There may be a subgroup of patients who fail to respond to unilateral placement but do respond to bilateral; it has been recommended that if a patient fails to show response by the sixth unilateral treatment, bilateral treatment be substituted. An early change from treatment three times weekly to twice weekly may also lessen memory impairment.

Depressed patients usually begin to show improvement by the fourth treatment. A total of six to 12 treatments is usually required for remission. The clinician should judge the improvement objectively; most patients express the belief that they are well and want to discontinue treatment before reaching maximum benefit. Usually, they will agree to the additional treatments on the physician's recommendation, just to be sure. Patients with Schizoaffective Disorder require more treatments. However, it is rarely worthwhile to give more than 15 to 20 treatments unless definite improvement is taking place.

There are studies that show statistically higher remission rates with longer series, up to 40 treatments. However, it is better to individualize therapy than to give a course of a predetermined number of treatments.

A variety of premedications and treatment routines are employed to reduce the incidence of complications. Many of these are difficult to evaluate, since the complications they are intended to prevent are rare. Usually, atropine is given as one of the premedications. A short-acting barbiturate such as sodium methohexital (Brevital) is injected intravenously to induce sleep. Then the patient is given succinylcholine chloride (Anectine) also intravenously. The succinylcholine functions as a depolarizing muscle relaxant and causes respiratory arrest, so manual respiratory assistance is mandatory. A small percentage of Caucasians, approximately one in 2500, have abnormal pseudocholinesterase and are unable to metabolize succinylcholine in the rapid manner which most people do. A simple screening test for pseudocholinesterase deficiency is available.

Electroconvulsive therapy is a relatively safe procedure. Deaths are rare, but do sometimes occur, usually from cardiac or respiratory complications. It is difficult to estimate the death rate, since it is not high enough for any one hospital's experiences to provide meaningful figures. Probably no more than one patient in 25,000 receiving a series of treatments died, and most deaths were of elderly persons or in cases in which a known risk of complication was recognized. Shock therapy is probably safer than most psychotropic medication; nevertheless, a signed informed consent (cf. Chapter 23) of the patient and usually of the family as well is necessary.

Serious skeletal complications, fractures, resulting from treatment are rare except in cases of osteoporosis. Special care should be taken in treating elderly patients, patients with osteogenesis imperfecta, and those who have been on prolonged corticosteroid treatment. Muscle relaxants, at least as ordinarily used, will not prevent all fractures in such cases.

While serious skeletal complications are rare, vertebral compressions are frequent. They probably occur in about 20 percent of cases treated. Since many are asymptomatic, studies reporting a lower incidence of this complication are meaningless unless routine pretreatment and post-treatment x-rays are compared. If a compression results in back pain, analgesics and a few days rest are usually all that is needed for relief. Treatment can usually be continued, preferably with the use of increased muscle relaxant, even after a symptomatic compression has occurred. Persistent pain and/or disability is extremely rare.

Jaw dislocations occasionally occur. If they are recognized and reduced before the patient begins to awaken from treatment, they are rarely a problem. However, the physician unfamiliar with this procedure is reminded to wrap the thumbs well in a clean towel before placing them on the back teeth, not only for esthetic reasons, but to prevent getting bitten as the jaw snaps shut.

Postshock confusion is rarely sufficiently severe and prolonged to be a complication. On awakening from a treatment, the patient is usually disoriented and has marked memory impairment. In an hour or so memory is largely restored, though some things may still be forgotten. After several treatments, there may be some cumulative memory loss. The patient is most likely to complain of forgetting events immediately prior to the series of treatments and may also complain of difficulty in remembering names, addresses of friends, and telephone numbers. Usually this improves in a few weeks after treatments are stopped. Though residual memory impairment is usually not marked, and often cannot be detected without careful pre- and post-treatment testing, some long-term impairment frequently does occur. One should predict gradual improvement with probably minimal residuals rather than predicting complete memory recovery.

Sometimes there is a profound clouding of sensorium. This is very rare with the short series of treatments used for depressions. It is more frequent with long series or when treatments are given daily or more often.

Most clinicians regard memory impairment as not contributing to the benefits from shock (it is not to make the patient forget symptoms); hence, treatments are likely to be spaced further apart if much memory loss is noted.

Physicians are sometimes reluctant to recommend shock because of a feeling that it is a drastic procedure and something painful or even punitive to a patient. Persons observing shock usually find it unpleasant to watch, possibly because of associations to the idea of a convulsion. Patients do not remember the actual administration of the treatment and do not recall pain in connection with it. If an insufficient dose of current is given and is not followed by one that produces a tonic and clonic reaction, pain may be recalled. Apprehension and discomfort are associated with using muscle relaxants unless sedation is also employed because the patient experiences air hunger if awake.

The degree of patient cooperation and the amount of apprehension concerning treatment depend in part on the doctor-patient relationship. Nursing routines are also important. Patients should know what to expect. They should be comfortable before treatment. Any post-treatment symptoms (e.g., headache; muscle aches; nausea) should be relieved by appropriate medication. The patient should have someone to talk with as he or she awakens, and patience and reassurance during the immediate post-treatment confusion are important.

Electroconvulsive therapy is usually given on an inpatient basis, since nowadays it is used mainly for seriously ill patients who require full-time hospitalization and nursing care. However, it can be given to day patients whose condition otherwise warrants day hospital care. Outpatient treatment is practical unless otherwise contraindicated if the patient can be accompanied to and from treatment and if the patient either does not have much post-treatment confusion or will have enough assistance from relatives and friends to keep it from being a problem.

Indications for Electroconvulsive Therapy

Indications for electroconvulsive therapy can be discussed in terms of the symptoms it relieves, the syndromes in which it is most effective, and its relative merits in comparison to other treatments.

Shock treatment is effective in the treatment of most types of depression (including depressions associated with Organic Mental Disorders), especially if the depression is accompanied by agitation or psychomotor retardation. It also tends to relieve excitement and hyperactivity. It is effective in Bipolar Affective Disorders, both for depressed and, to a lesser extent, for manic phases. It is beneficial in depressed periods in Cyclothymic Disorder if the depression is severe enough to warrant its use. It is less likely to be helpful in Dysthymic Disorder. It is helpful in Schizoaffective Disorder and in some types of Schizophrenia in which there are depressive elements. It is sometimes helpful in the catatonic type of Schizophrenic Disorder. Authorities differ as to whether it is helpful, and to what extent, in other types of Schizophrenic Disorder. Though it may be used in chronic cases, best results are reported when it is used in the first six months of illness, the Schizophreniform phase.

Since all of the conditions in which electroconvulsive therapy is helpful may now be treated in other ways, these must be taken into account in evaluating indications. At present, shock is recommended in:

1. Major depressions in which suicidal tendencies are present, and in which prompt clinical response is deemed necessary (results are faster and more certain than with antidepressant medication).
2. Those depressions in which there is a relative or absolute contraindication to the use of tricyclic antidepressants (e.g., glaucoma; prostatic hypertrophy; cardiovascular problems) or MAO Inhibitors (e.g., liver disease).
3. Other depressions, except Dysthymic Disorders, which fail to respond to an adequate trial of antidepressant medication. Shock should be considered for patients not responding in thirty days and seriously considered in all not in remission in sixty to ninety days.
4. Schizophreniform Disorders with depressive or catatonic manifestations in which medication and psychotherapy have been ineffective. If the patient is not responding adequately to other treatments, consideration of the use of shock therapy should not be postponed beyond the first six months of illness in acute cases.

The use of shock is also to be considered for some manics. Most patients respond to medications; shock can be tried for those who do not. If may also be used in preference to medication in some very acute cases in which hyperactivity is leading to exhaustion. It may be used in selected cases of Dysthymic Disorder which fail to respond to psychotherapy and likewise fail to benefit from medication.

Many would still advocate a trial of shock treatment in schizophrenic patients without depressive or catatonic features if all other treatment methods appear to be failing. This is in a way a "last resort," not that it is so dangerous or harmful, but because other approaches are preferred first. The only absolute contraindication for ECT is increased intracranial pressure from any cause.

Insulin Therapy is not widely used in the United States at present, although it is in other parts of the world (e.g., the People's Republic of China). Insulin was recognized to have a calming effect, and of course to stimulate appetite, soon after its discovery. Before the introduction of antianxiety agents, it was used in small, subcoma doses for that purpose for psychoneurotic patients and for some alcoholics and addicts during withdrawal. Sakel found the hypoglycemic coma produced by larger doses helpful in cases of Schizophrenic Disorder, and he developed an elaborate technique including not only a long series of comas but also a rehabilitative program. There are more dangers and complications than with electroconvulsive treatment; the treatment requires a skilled clinical team, and necessitates a great deal of nursing care. In many hospitals it is now deemed impractical. It is "statistically" less effective than the use of antipsychotic medications. However, when it can be used, it might still be considered for schizophrenics, perhaps especially those of the paranoid type, who fail to respond to other therapies.

Psychosurgery is also infrequently used, though some studies are still being reported. In many cases, the possibility of symptomatic relief from prefrontal lobotomy and similar procedures is negated by risks, complications, and side effects (including loss of some desirable components in the personality). Newer techniques have reduced the risk of these side effects, but the procedures are somewhat controversial, and concern over potential legal problems limits their use. At present, most clinicians restrict psychosurgery to intractable cases manifested by severe chronic agitation and/or dangerously aggressive tendencies in which the patient's prolonged and apparently incurable suffering, together with a persistent danger to oneself and others justifies it. A valid, informed consent for any such procedure is imperative (cf. Chapter 23).

Some other somatic therapies include several procedures in which convulsions are produced [e.g., Metrazol shock; Indoklon (flurothyl) inhalations], and others in which brief periods of unconsciousness are produced (e.g., carbon dioxide treatment), and some which employ long periods of coma (e.g., continuous sleep therapy with barbiturates). None of these are frequently used now. Some are obsolete but may still have occasional usefulness; others are still under investigation.

REVIEW QUESTIONS

1. What drugs are effective in the treatment of panic attacks? What are the advantages and disadvantages of each?
2. Discuss the indications for electroconvulsive therapy.
3. If you were recommending shock treatment to a depressed patient, what would you tell him or her about the procedure?
4. A drug study shows that two antipsychotics, A and B, are similar save that A is much more potent. A 1-mg dose of A is equivalent to 20 mg of B. Does this mean that A is a better drug? What advantages and/or disadvantages are there to using the more potent drug?
5. What is serotonin? Norepinephrine?
6. Discuss the side effects of the phenothiazines. How frequently does Tardive Dyskinesia occur? What can be done to reduce its incidence?
7. Look up some recent clinical research studies on the efficacy of various psychotropic drugs. Choose the study that you believe demonstrates the best research design and explain the reasons for your choice.
8. Compare the indications for use of: amitriptyline, methylphenidate, and phenelzine.
9. Construct a table showing the various types and degrees of depression and the therapies which might be most likely to be helpful for each.
10. What is meant by the catecholamine hypothesis of affective disorders? What relevance does it have for the selection of drugs and drug combinations for psychiatric disorders?

11. What are the indications for, toxic effects of, and contraindications of lithium carbonate?

SELECTED REFERENCES

1. American Psychiatric Association Task Force Report on Electroconvulsive Therapy: *Electroconvulsive Therapy.* Washington, D.C., American Psychiatric Association, 1978.

2. Babigian, Haroutun M., and Laurence B. Guttmacher: Epidemiologic considerations in electroconvulsive therapy. *Arch Gen Psychiatry* 41(3):246-253, 1984.

3. Bassuk, Ellen L., Stephen C. Schoonover, and Alan J. Gelenberg: *The Practitioner's Guide to Psychoactive Drugs.* 2nd ed. New York, Plenum, 1983.

4. Chu, Chung-Chou, Stephen E. Williams, James E. Wilson, and Stephen L. Ruedrich: The rational use of antianxiety agents. *Nebraska Med J* 68(8): 256-260, 1983.

5. Cole, Jonathan O.: New antidepressant drugs. *McLean Hosp J* 8(1):62-77, 1983.

6. Cole, Jonathan O.: Psychopharmacology update: Antipsychotic drugs: Is more better? *McLean Hosp J* 7(1):61-87, 1982.

7. Dietch, James: The nature and extent of benzodiazepine abuse: An overview of recent literature. *Hosp Community Psychiatry* 34(12):1139-1145, 1983.

8. Gaby, Nancy S., David S. Lefkowitz, and J. Ray Israel: Treatment of lithium tremor with metoprolol. *Am J Psychiatry* 140(5):593-595, 1983.

9. Hollister, Leo E.: *Clinical Pharmacology of Psychotherapeutic Drugs.* 2nd ed. Vol. 1 in *Monographs in Clinical Pharmacology.* Daniel L. Azarnoff (Ed.). New York, Churchill Livingstone, 1983.

10. Ingram, Nicholas A.W., and David B. Newgreen: The use of tacrine for tardive dyskinesia. *Am J Psychiatry* 140(12):1629-1631, 1983.

11. Kalinowsky, L.B.: Psychosurgery: The past twenty years. *Psychiatr J Univ Ottawa* 4(1):111-113, 1979.

12. Kane, John M., and James M. Smith: Tardive dyskinesia: Prevalence and risk factors, 1959 to 1979. *Arch Gen Psychiatry* 39(4):473-481, 1982.

13. Klett, James C., and Eugene Caffey, Jr.: Evaluating the long-term need for antiparkinson drugs by chronic schizophrenics. *Arch Gen Psychiatry* 26(4): 374-379, 1972.

14. Lieberman, Jeffrey A., John M. Kane, Dominick Gadaleta, Ronald Brenner, Michael S. Lesser, and Bruce Kinon: Methylphenidate challenge as a predictor of relapse in schizophrenia. *Am J Psychiatry* 141(5):633-638, 1984.

15. Linden, Robert, John M. Davis, and Joan Rubinstein: High vs. low dose treatment with antipsychotic agents. *Psychiatr Ann* 12(8):769-771, 775, 778-781, 1982.

16. Litovitz, Toby L., and William G. Troutman: Amoxapine overdose. *JAMA* 250(8):1069-1071, 1983.

17. May, David C., Stephan W. Morris, R. Malcolm Stewart, Barry J. Fenton, and F. Andrew Gaffney: Neuroleptic malignant syndrome: Response to dantrolene sodium. *Ann Intern Med* 98(2):183-184, 1983.

18. McCabe, Beverly, and Ming T. Tsuang: Dietary consideration in MAO inhibitor regimens. *J Clin Psychiatry* 43(5):178-181, 1982.

19. McGrath, Patrick J., Frederic M. Quitkin, Wilma Harrison, and Jonathan W. Stewart: Treatment of melancholia with tranylcypromine. *Am J Psychiatry* 141(2):228-289, 1984.

20. Mellinger, Glen D., Mitchell B. Balter, and Eberhard H. Uhlenhuth: Prevalence and correlates of the long-term regular use of anxiolytics. *JAMA* 251(3):375-379, 1984.

21. Mellman, Lisa A., and Jack M. Gormon: Successful treatment of obsessive-compulsive disorder with ECT. *Am J Psychiatry* 141(4):596-597, 1984.

22. Mueller, Peter S., John W. Vester, and Joseph Fermaglich: Neuroleptic malignant syndrome. *JAMA* 249(3):386-388, 1983.

23. Noyes, Russell, Dorothy J. Anderson, John Clancy, Raymond R. Crowe, Donald J. Slymen, Mohamed M. Ghoneim, and James V. Hinrichs: Diazepam and propranolol in panic disorder and agoraphobia. *Arch Gen Psychiatry* 41(3):287-292, 1984.

24. Quitkin, Frederic M., Judith G. Rabkin, Donald Ross, and Patrick J. McGrath: Duration of antidepressant drug treatment. *Arch Gen Psychiatry* 41(3):238-245, 1984.

25. Ramsey, T. Alan, and Malcolm Cox: Lithium and the kidney: A review. *Am J Psychiatry* 139(4):443-449, 1982.

26. Razani, J., Kerrin L. White, Judith White, George Simpson, Bruce Sloane, Ronald Rebal, and Ruby Palmer: The safety and efficacy of combined amitriptyline and tranylcypromine antidepressant treatment. *Arch Gen Psychiatry* 40(6):657-661, 1983.

27. Rickels, Karl, George Case, Robert W. Downing, and Andrew Winokur: Long-term diazepam therapy and clinical outcome. *JAMA* 250(6):767-771, 1983.

28. Tippin, Jon, and Fritz A. Henn: Modified leukotomy in the treatment of intractable obsessional neurosis. *Am J Psychiatry* 139(12):1601-1603, 1982.

29. Van Putten, Theodore, Philip R. A. May, and Stephen R. Marder: Response to antipsychotic medication: The doctor's and the consumer's view. *Am J Psychiatry* 141(1):16-19, 1984.

30.   Wilson, James E., Chung-Chou Chu, Stephen E. Williams, and Stephen L. Ruedrich: Clinical use of antidepressant medications. *Nebraska Med J* 69(5):148–153, 1984.

Chapter 21

COMMUNITY PSYCHIATRIC FACILITIES

AVAILABLE MENTAL HEALTH SERVICES

Though the majority of persons with psychiatric disorders are, and should be, treated by primary practitioners, there are some who require the service of specialists. For some of these, specialized facilities are also needed. There are currently over 28,000 psychiatrists in the United States, but the Graduate Medical Education National Advisory Committee (GMENAC) has estimated that by 1990 approximately 47,500 will be needed. About half of the psychiatrists are in private practice. Approximately 10 percent specialize in child and adolescent psychiatry. Some others limit their practices to the treatment of certain disorders or to the use of particular treatment modalities.

For patients requiring hospitalization, many general hospitals have psychiatric services. These serve more inpatient admissions than any other type of psychiatric facility, but they offer only short-term care. Many of these have special facilities for psychiatric patients; however, most patients can be cared for in general medical areas. If there is not a psychiatric unit, it may be impossible to care for disturbed or acutely suicidal patients.

Private psychiatric hospitals are available in most but not all states. The number of such hospitals is growing. In 1970 there were 160 psychiatric hospitals; by 1984 there were 210. About 70 percent of these are operated for profit. The majority of these are owned by corporate chains. There are about 15 chains operating psychiatric hospitals, but five of them operate the majority of the chain-owned facilities. Like the services in general hospitals, a number of the psychiatric hospitals primarily serve patients who need short-term hospitalization. A few provide long-term treatment, and some provide custodial or domiciliary care. Types of patients accepted and modes of therapy offered vary.

Additional psychiatric facilities include public mental hospitals and freestanding outpatient clinics. There are about 1000 of the latter in the United States.

In addition to available psychiatric services, psychotherapy or counseling is provided by a variety of other licensed (and unlicensed) practitioners both in private practice and in community agencies. Under the current standards of the Joint Commission on the Accreditation of Hospitals (JCAH) some of the licensed practitioners may have hospital staff privileges. Staff privileges for nonphysicians are governed by state laws and by hospital bylaws. Bylaws must provide for adequate medical examination and medical care, if needed, for patients of these practitioners. An increase in the number of nonphysicians having staff privileges is likely in the next few years.

The physician should be familiar with the work of the psychiatrists and other mental health practitioners in his or her community, with the clinics and agencies serving the mentally ill, and with the available inpatient facilities. One should be familiar with the type, quality, and cost of care provided. In regard to public clinics and hospitals, one should know eligibility requirements and intake or admission procedures. One needs to make appropriate referrals and prepare patients for what they will experience.

One's knowledge should not be limited to clinical facilities as such. Mental illness creates a number of problems for patients and their families. One must know what types of help are available from social agencies in one's community. One must be familiar with rehabilitation services. One needs to be aware of self-help groups, know how they operate, and know how to make referrals to them.

PROBLEMS IN OBTAINING CARE

Though it would appear, despite a projected shortage of psychiatrists, that the person with a psychiatric disorder has numerous options for obtaining care, there are some gaps in the system. Many public and private services are geared primarily to meet the needs of persons requiring short-term care. Chronic patients, and those with acute disorders needing extended care, may encounter problems in access to and financing of treatment. Two factors have influenced this in recent years.

First, there is the impact on psychiatric care from the efforts of government agencies and the insurance industry to control health care costs generally. Third-party payers tend to limit the number of outpatient visits covered and the number of days of hospitalization allowed. These restrictions are applied somewhat disproportionately to psychiatric patients. One reason for limited insurance coverage is lack of demand (as differentiated from need). In spite of the high incidence and prevalence of psychiatric disorders, and the fact that most families are likely to need mental health services at one time or another, a person is likely to deny the possibility. Another factor is concern on the part of insurers and the operators of prepaid medical plans, such as health maintenance organizations, about potential overutilization of mental health benefits. There is some, albeit not much, basis in reality for the concerns. There are studies that show that providing "free" care for psychiatric patients does not result in any more increased use than for any other medical care, and that mental health care costs are only a small percentage of total yearly health costs. There are other studies that show that patients who receive psychiatric treatment make less use of other health services. On the other hand, there is a tendency for some people to seek long-term psychotherapy for enhancement of the quality of life rather than for the treatment, or even prevention, of illness. Also, some patients consult psychiatrists, as they do other physicians, about personal problems that are not associated with any disorder.

Second, the number of chronic psychiatric patients in the community has increased greatly as a result of changing public policies regarding the institutional care of the mentally handicapped. As a matter of public policy, deinstitutionalization since 1960 has been achieved by discharging patients from state mental

hospitals and limiting admissions to them. The state hospital population has declined from over a half million to slightly over 100,000. The ethical basis for this
lies in offering greater freedom and autonomy to the chronically mentally ill person. A corollary assumption of the advocates of deinstitutionalization has been
that equally effective, or even better, treatment for these patients could be provided in their home communities. Unfortunately, adequate community facilities
for the chronically mentally ill have not been provided in most communities.
While the most obvious failures of deinstitutionalization are to be found among
the homeless "street people," there are many other chronically mentally ill people
who have unsatisfactory living arrangements and lack of access to treatment. Finally, in regard to deinstitutionalization, one must note that the term is partially
a misnomer. Dehospitalization is what has actually occurred. The state hospital
population has been vastly reduced. The number of people living in an institutional
setting has not been materially reduced. Increased numbers are to be found in cor-
rectional institutions, nursing homes, and board-and-care facilities.

There are probably three-quarters of a million chronic psychiatric patients in
nursing homes; half or more of these are geriatric. Nursing home care accounts
for more than a fourth of the total national expenditure for direct services to the
mentally ill. The quality of care in nursing homes is variable. Hospitals tend to
be overregulated, a factor in increasing health costs, but in some states nursing
homes may be underregulated. The amount of medical care available may be limited. Programs for psychiatric patients may be lacking. On the other hand, high-
quality programs can be found.

Some board-and-care homes offer long-term domicilliary care. Others are
primarily transitional living facilities and play a part in rehabilitation programs.

THE COMMUNITY MENTAL HEALTH CENTER MOVEMENT

In order to replace the state mental hospitals as the principal resource for the
care of chronic psychiatric patients government planners envisioned a nationwide
network of community mental health centers. The Community Mental Health Centers Act of 1963 provided for federal grants for the construction of community
mental health centers. Subsequent legislation provided funds to assist in the initial staffing of the centers.

The Community Mental Health Centers Act provided for state plans which

> shall provide for adequate community mental health facilities for the pro-
> vision of programs of comprehensive mental health services to all per-
> sons residing in the state and for furnishing such services to persons un-
> able to pay therefor, taking into account the population necessary to
> maintain and operate efficient facilities and for the financial resources
> available therefor.

It should be noted that while these facilities were to furnish services to persons
unable to pay, they were not limited to serving the medically indigent, but were
to provide services to all persons in the catchment area, including transients.
The law went on to provide for accessibility of services and said that the state
plan was to provide that every community mental health center shall "serve a population of not less than 75,000 and not more than 200,000 persons."

Comprehensive community mental health centers were mandated to provide
certain essential services. These services included inpatient care, outpatient care,
emergency service, consultation and education, court screening, followup care,

partial hospitalization, transitional care facilities (halfway houses), specialized services for children, specialized services for the elderly, programs for alcoholics, and programs for drug dependent patients and other drug misusers.

While federal funds were provided for part of the initial cost of staffing the centers, it was envisioned that they would ultimately be partially self-supporting and partially supported by their communities.

It is obvious that the program as a whole has been less than a complete success. It is less easy to evaluate the contribution of individual centers. Some have become valuable components of the mental health care delivery systems; others have not. Many have encountered financial difficulties. Some of the mandated services, if properly rendered to all comers, are expensive and are not likely to generate enough income to be self-supporting. Adequate community support has not always been available.

Staffing problems have existed and have affected the types of services rendered by the centers. There has been a tendency for the number of physicians on the staffs of these centers to decrease and the number of other mental health professionals to increase. Between 1970 and 1976 the average number of full-time psychiatrists per center dropped from 6.9 to 4.0, and this trend continues. This has been accompanied by a shift from a medical treatment model to a social rehabilitation model in many centers. However, an appreciable number of patients continue to receive medication. Some centers have failed to take a very active role in the care of chronic patients, but instead have developed a new clientele of persons who would have been served in the past by social agencies rather than medical facilities.

The future of community mental health centers remains uncertain, but many of the concepts involved in their development are sound and deserve further study, implementation, and evaluation. Ideally, small facilities offer certain advantages over large ones. Small facilities should enable patients to obtain greater individual attention. A location of services within the community, near the patients' homes and places of work, also offers advantages for some (though perhaps not all) patients.

The community mental health center with a wide range of services it must provide or at least coordinate is ideally situated to provide continuity of care. This is desirable for a variety of reasons, not the least of which is the fact that patients discharged from hospitals and referred for outpatient treatment or aftercare frequently fail to make and keep appointments. A clinic case manager can assist patients in following recommendations for further care. Continuity can be achieved in other settings. A practitioner can serve a patient throughout an illness, or if a transfer is needed, can make an appointment for the patient. When there is a transfer, a patient is more likely to keep appointments after hospitalization if he or she has actually met the new therapist before discharge.

The emphasis on preventive services, including emergency service and consultation and education, is potentially worthwhile as is the role of partial hospitalization and transitional care facilities.

PREVENTIVE SERVICES

In psychiatry, primary prevention is intended to keep illness from occurring. Secondary prevention decreases its prevalence by providing prompt treatment and shortening its course. Tertiary prevention reduces the residual impairment of the chronically ill through continued treatment and rehabilitation.

There are only a few psychiatric disorders for which effective methods of primary prevention are well established. Other interventions require validation through further research.

Public education, as a preventive tool, has been utilized by community mental health centers and other psychiatric facilities. Theoretically, educating people about the use of alcohol and drugs, beginning by teaching school children about them, ought to reduce the incidence of Substance Use Disorders. Sex education ought to reduce the incidence of Psychosexual Disorders. General instruction in mental hygiene might reduce the incidence of a variety of disorders. More research is necessary to determine how much benefit can be derived from such programs, what features of the programs are most likely to contribute to their being effective, and what features may be ineffective or even harmful.

Programs for early identification of persons "at risk" and the provision of treatment or counseling for such persons also merit further research. There is, of course, concern that labeling such persons, especially children, may evoke discriminatory attitudes toward them and increase rather than decrease risks of maladaptation. Designating someone as being at risk could be a self-fulfilling prophecy. On the other hand, there is a good rationale for giving persons at risk for psychiatric disorder, just as for other illnesses, special attention.

Consultative programs also have a preventive function. Consulting activities are not limited to case-oriented or therapist-oriented services, but include programmatic consultation. Program-oriented consultation to school systems and to employers designed to reduce environmental stress may contribute to primary prevention. Likewise, various social action programs to improve the quality of life have been advocated.

Community mental health centers have also attempted to teach primary caretakers techniques of crisis intervention, emotional first aid, and counseling. People who are in a position to help others (e.g., teachers; police; administrators) ought to be able to help people with personal problems before these problems lead to Adjustment Disorders or precipitate other psychiatric illnesses. Similarly, the availability of prompt crisis intervention by professionals to help people in stress situations should be valuable.

While there may be doubt about the efficacy of certain strategies for primary prevention, the efficacy of secondary prevention is less controversial. There is little doubt that early case identification and prompt treatment reduces the extent of psychiatric disability.

Tertiary prevention is essential, if the chronic mental patient is to function adequately in the community. If there is a need for continued treatment, as is often the case, the patient must not only have *access* to professional service, but also may require encouragement and help to utilize it. He or she may need the services of various community agencies and may need help from a social worker, a visiting nurse, or a case manager at a community mental health center in order to find and take advantage of available help. Many chronic patients need vocational training or vocational rehabilitation. Sheltered workshops are needed for some. Some need supervised living arrangements, and others who can live on their own need help with various problems in daily living. Social skills training and training in self-care are needed by others.

PARTIAL HOSPITALIZATION

Most communities do not have adequate partial hospitalization services for the mentally ill. Though partial hospitalization services were mandated for the comprehensive community mental health services, they can also be offered by other hospitals and clinics. One reason that they have not been more widely offered has been the reluctance of third-party payers to cover these services. Partial hospitalization services should be effective in cost containment. Partial hospitalization is less expensive than full hospitalization. It can be used for both acute and chronic cases.

Many patients do not need to be in the hospital around the clock for diagnostic studies and nursing observation. Many treatments that require more observation than is possible on an outpatient basis still do not require full-time hospitalization. Part-time hospitalization may be sufficient to remove a patient from stressful elements in the environment. It gives the person an opportunity to benefit from the therapeutic milieu. Even a relative danger to the self may not require complete hospitalization (e.g., a person with some suicidal tendencies may be in greater danger when family members are away during the day than when they are home at night).

The most common partial hospital facility is the day hospital. It enables the patient to have observation and treatment during the day, but it allows him or her to be alone with the family in the evening. The night hospital allows some patients to work during the day and to have treatment in the evenings. It may be particularly helpful to patients who function well while at work but have difficulty during leisure time (e.g., some alcoholics). The weekend hospital offers milieu therapy together with more intensive observation and treatment than is possible in an outpatient setting. It may be especially helpful to patients who live at a distance from treatment centers.

CHOOSING BETWEEN COMMUNITY AND INSTITUTIONAL CARE

Sometimes the practitioner must help a patient and family decide between community care and institutionalization. Indications for short-term hospitalization have been discussed in Chapter 18. Decisions about long-term hospitalization, especially when one is considering custodial or domiciliary care rather than extended treatment, represent a different type of problem.

In some cases the decision is relatively easy. Though a patient may have many psychiatric symptoms that have failed to respond to treatment, if he or she is not dangerous to the self or others, can take care of his or her own needs, is able to live with family members or alone, and prefers to remain in the community there is little reason to consider institutionalization. On the other hand, there is no question that a helpless, profoundly retarded patient or a severely brain damaged person may have to have a lifetime of institutional care.

For other cases the decision is more difficult. Examples: (1) A young adult woman has been known to be mentally retarded since early childhood. For a time she was cared for at home and placed in special classes at school, but she was never able to learn to read and write. She learned to feed herself, to bathe, and to dress. During adolescence she was sent to a residential treatment center and efforts were made to teach her a trade. These failed. Her behavior in public is sometimes peculiar, but she has never harmed anyone or attempted to harm anyone. Her family can no longer make a home for her. Should she be placed on welfare, given some supervision by a social agency, mental health center, or board-and-care home and allowed to remain in the community? Or should she be sent to live in an institution? (2) A schizophrenic man of 35 has had multiple hospitalizations over a 3-year period. There was some improvement during his first hospitalization, but there has been no change since. He has had several different types of treatment. He still has delusions and hallucinations. Rehabilitation counselors feel that he is unemployable. He is not aggressive. Should he be cared for in a state hospital, a nursing home, a board-and-care home, or should he simply be left on his own in the community?

Decisions in cases like these should not be based on an a priori assumption that all community care is good and all institutional care is bad. Before the development of the state hospitals in the nineteenth century, mental patients were cared for in the community (often in jails and almshouses). The "village idiot" remained in the community, but under less than desirable circumstances. For a look at community care in Elizabethan times we have Shakespeare's description of the Bedlam beggars (cf. *King Lear,* Act II, Scene II, and Act III, Scene IV, especially Edgar's speech that begins, "Poor Tom, that eats the swimming frog...." Is modern community care any better? Certainly not, for the homeless derelict. Often not for the patient who is living in a "tranquilizer ghetto," and is experiencing unsanitary and sometimes dangerous living conditions as well as possible exploitation. Possibly not, for the person in a substandard nursing home lacking treatment and rehabilitation programs and offering few activities aside from watching television.

If it is *possible* for the patient to receive long-term care in a public institution, or if long-term private hospital care can be afforded, is this a better option? To answer the question one first has to know what available facilities have to offer. One needs to know what the patient's living condition will be like in the institution, how much freedom he or she will have (are the wards open or are patients locked up?), and what treatment, rehabilitation, and activity programs are available. One needs to know the same sorts of things about the quality of life and the availability of care in the community.

The decision will often rest not on whether community care in general is better than institutional care, but on whether available community programs are better than available institutions. One has to assess carefully the patient's relative ability to provide for his or her needs and one must carefully ascertain the patient's actual preference. Many deinstitutionalized patients are happier and better satisfied with community living; some are not. Some patients reject the idea of institutional care because of unrealistic fears or misinformation about it, and sometimes these concerns are dispelled by a visit to the facility.

As a physician caring for an individual patient one's recommendations are based on the patient's needs and preferences, but are limited by the options actually available. As a concerned citizen, one should know what ought to be available.

REVIEW QUESTIONS

1. What is a day hospital? What are the indications for day hospital care?
2. Discuss primary, secondary, and tertiary prevention of disability from mental illness.
3. The alcoholism treatment program of a state hospital routinely refers patients to an aftercare clinic at the time they are discharged from the hospital. Only 25 percent of patients referred actually keep regular appointments at the clinic. Speculate as to possible reasons. Based on the reason(s) you think most probable, suggest ways of increasing the number of patients receiving aftercare.
4. Look in the yellow pages of your telephone directory for psychotherapists and for marriage and family counselors. What professional disciplines are represented? How do the services provided by these therapists and counselors differ from those provided by psychiatrists and other physicians?

5. How do you account for the growth in the number of investor-owned psychiatric hospitals? Do you expect it to continue? If so, why?
6. To what extent are chronic mental patients being cared for in nursing homes? What do you know about the type and quality of care for such patients in nursing homes in your community?
7. What were the reasons that led to the deinstitutionalization of the chronically mentally ill? How successful has deinstitutionalization been? How could it be made more successful?
8. Name three self-help groups that are available for psychiatric patients in your community. Describe the way each functions.

SELECTED REFERENCES

1. American Psychiatric Association: *Economic Fact Book for Psychiatry.* Washington, D.C., American Psychiatric Press, 1983.

2. Bachrach, Leona L.: General hospital psychiatry: Overview from a sociological perspective. *Am J Psychiatry* 138(7):879-887, 1981.

3. Caplan, Gerald, and Henry Grunebaum: Perspectives on primary prevention. *Arch Gen Psychiatry* 17(3):331-346, 1967.

4. Dunham, H. Warren: *Social Realities and Community Psychiatry.* New York, Behavioral Publications, 1975.

5. Eaton, Merrill T.: The future of the public mental hospital. *The American Handbook of Psychiatry,* Vol. 6. New York, Basic Books, 1975, 780-790.

6. Geller, Jeffrey: Arson: An unforeseen sequela of deinstitutionalization. *Am J Psychiatry* 141(4):504-508, 1984.

7. Goldman, Howard H., Neal H. Adams, and Carl A. Taube: Deinstitutionalization: The data demythologized. *Hosp Community Psychiatry* 34(2):129-134, 1983.

8. Goldman, Howard H., Antoinette A. Gattozzi, and Carl A. Taube: Defining and counting the chronically mentally ill. *Hosp Community Psychiatry* 32(1):21-27, 1981.

9. Joint Commission on Mental Illness and Health: *Action for Mental Health.* Final Report, 1961. New York, Basic Books, 1961.

10. Jones, Maxwell: The concept of a therapeutic community. *Am J Psychiatry* 112(8):647-650, 1956.

11. Kaplan, Harold I., and Benjamin J. Sadock (Eds.): *Modern Synopsis of Comprehensive Textbook of Psychiatry/III.* 3rd ed. Baltimore, Williams & Wilkins, 1981, pp. 1010-1016.

12. Kinard, E. Milling: Discharged patients who desire to return to the hospital. *Hosp Community Psychiatry* 32(3):194-197, 1981.

13. Langsley, Donald G., and James T. Barter: Psychiatric roles in the community mental health center. *Hosp Community Psychiatry* 34(8):729-733, 1983.

14. Lehman, Anthony F., Nancy C. Ward, and Lawrence S. Linn: Chronic mental patients: The quality of life issue. *Am J Psychiatry* 139(10):1271-1276, 1982.

15. Levenson, Alan I.: The growth of investor-owned psychiatric hospitals. *Am J Psychiatry* 139(7):902-907, 1982.

16. Levin, Bruce Lubotsky, and Jay H. Glasser: A national survey of prepaid mental health services. *Hosp Community Psychiatry* 35(4):350-355, 1984.

17. Mollica, Richard F.: From asylum to community: The threatened disintegration of public psychiatry. *New Engl J Med* 308:367-373, 1983.

18. Schulberg, Herbert C.: *The Treatment of Psychiatric Patients in General Hospitals: A Research Agenda and Annotated Bibliography.* Rockville, Maryland, National Institute of Mental Health, Division of Biometry and Epidemiology, 1984.

19. Talbott, John A. (Ed.): *Unified Mental Health Systems: Utopia Unrealized.* Number 18 of the series *New Directions for Mental Health Services.* H. Richard Lamb (Ed.). San Francisco, Jossey-Bass, 1983.

Chapter 22

PSYCHIATRY IN PRIMARY CARE MEDICINE

PSYCHIATRIC SKILLS IN PRIMARY PRACTICE

The primary practitioner's knowledge of psychiatry and the behavioral sciences is useful in the care of patients with nonpsychiatric illnesses. It is used not only in managing those disorders discussed in Chapter 9 in which psychological factors contribute to the cause of illness, but also in dealing with the reactions of other patients to illness and its consequences. To deal effectively with sick people, one must understand their fears, realistic and otherwise; their anxieties; and their feelings of depression. One must be aware of the mental mechanisms used in controlling those feelings. One recognizes emotional needs, including dependent needs and needs to remain in control. One is aware of the effect of handicaps and limitations imposed by illness on the self-image.

This knowledge helps one put patients at ease and offer them appropriate reassurance. It also keeps one aware of situations in which symptomatic treatment for emotional distress may be needed. It enables the physician to win the patient's confidence and to establish a collaborative relationship in which the patient will report symptoms and problems promptly and follow medical advice.

PRIMARY CARE PHYSICIANS
TREAT PSYCHIATRIC PATIENTS

Many more psychiatric patients are under the care of primary physicians (internists, family physicians, and pediatricians) than are treated by psychiatrists. The National Institute of Mental Health estimates that 60 percent of Americans suffering from psychiatric/psychological disorders are treated by nonpsychiatric physicians. Also, the referral by the nonpsychiatric physician to mental health professionals is low, ranging from somewhere below 1 to 8 percent of all patients seen having a psychiatric/psychological disorder. Since between 5 and 43 percent of patients seen by primary physicians have predominantly emotional problems, depending upon the setting in which they are initially seen (e.g., inpatient general medical wards have a frequency of depression as high as 50 percent, while outpatient pediatric facilities would have an incidence as low as 5 percent), primary physicians are treating the majority of psychiatric problems themselves. The family physician is usually the first person consulted by psychiatric patients whose illnesses are primarily manifested by symptoms. He or she is also the first person consulted by many patients whose main complaints are of *problems,* though a large number of others first seek the help of clergymen.

Accurate diagnosis and proper treatment of these patients is a major responsibility of the primary physician. There are not enough psychiatrists to do the job. There will not be enough in the foreseeable future. Even if there were enough psychiatrists, the generalist's role in mental health care would not be eliminated. Does having enough cardiologists in town relieve the family doctor from having to listen to hearts?

Some patients bypass the primary physician to seek psychiatric aid directly for nervousness or depression, but it is rare for a patient with a Somatoform Disorder or a psychosomatic disease to do this. Those who finally recognize a need for psychiatric attention independently have often lost some viscera before coming to that conclusion. If they are to be diagnosed promptly and accurately, the primary care physician must make the diagnosis.

Those patients who take their problems and symptoms first to the family doctor usually want him or her to treat them. They have good reasons, and these are an asset to the primary physician in his or her psychiatric practice. The family doctor is someone the patient knows and trusts. He or she can establish rapport quicker than the stranger-specialist, knows a great deal about the patient from previous office visits, and usually knows other members of the family. House calls may have furnished a picture of the patient's home life. All this information helps in understanding the patient and grasping the nature of the problem.

Failure to diagnose and to offer proper treatment or appropriate referral often leads patients to "shop" for a doctor who can and will understand them. It may lead them to cultists. If many physicians were to decline to care for psychiatric patients, the unmet needs would promote the development of new healing professions. Like too great an emphasis on specialization, this would be a move away from family medicine, from comprehensive integrated care, from treatment of the person rather than the parts. Fortunately, most primary physicians are doing effective psychiatric work.

THE PSYCHIATRIC PRACTICE OF THE PRIMARY PHYSICIAN

The psychiatric activities of the primary practitioner include:

1. Examination and diagnosis
2. Treatment
3. Referral of selected cases
4. Prophylaxis
5. Social and community psychiatry

Examination and Diagnosis

No medical examination is complete without psychiatric evaluation. Psychiatric examination should not be limited to those patients who present chief complaints suggestive of emotional disorder (e.g., anxiety; nervousness; depression) or who show obvious signs of psychiatric distress. Patients fail to mention psychiatric symptoms for a variety of reasons:

1. Lack of awareness of the symptoms or of their significance
2. Belief that symptoms are secondary to some other disorder which is mentioned as a chief complaint
3. Supposition that the physician will recognize the difficulty without being told
4. Embarrassment
5. Fear of disapproval or ridicule
6. Intentional concealment (e.g., in examinations for insurance; employment; military service)
7. A combination of some of the above factors

A depressed patient will sometimes consult a physician a few days before committing suicide, but make no mention of feeling depressed (though he or she may already have talked of suicide at home or procured the means for the attempt). Fortunately, psychiatric examination is not time consuming. During the time that a medical history is being taken and a physical examination completed, the necessary observations can be made. One has only to keep the mental examination in mind, look for the findings, and organize them. Only a few specific questions are needed unless there are positive findings which require more detailed investigation.

In addition to but not in lieu of mental examination, some primary physicians who do a comprehensive examination of new patients or for annual physicals include a health questionnaire containing psychiatric items. When signs of psychiatric disorder are found, enough must be learned about the case to make an accurate diagnosis. Recognizing that there is a disorder is not enough, even for referral. Classification; estimation of disability and discomfort; recognition of dangers to life, health, or well-being if untreated; knowledge of duration and progress; and measures of motivation, intelligence, and ego strength are all necessary for the clinician if he or she is to decide whether treatment is strongly indicated, elective, or unnecessary; whether it is needed *immediately;* and whether hospitalization needs to be considered. Obviously, if the primary physician is going to treat the patient, an accurate diagnosis is necessary. Even if he or she is certain that referral to a specialist will be made, it is necessary to decide to whom, and how quickly an appointment is necessary. Evaluation is necessary not only for those patients who come because of a psychiatric disorder, or other symptoms secondary to emotional disease, but also for those who have unrelated illnesses. When the psychiatric disorder is an incidental finding, one still must determine if treatment is needed. Also a knowledge of the mental status, character structure, and defense mechanisms of the patient will help the physician manage other illnesses.

Even in the absence of psychiatric disease, mental examination findings can be useful to the physician in general medical management. The better one understands the personality structure of the patient, the more clearly one can comprehend the patient's feelings and communications. At times, specific decisions are made on the basis of personality factors. Examples: (1) A woman brings a sick child to the doctor. The child can be treated at home but complicated instructions must be followed faithfully. The clinician estimates the woman's intelligence as in the dull normal or borderline range. She has, however, good ego strength and strong superego values. He feels that she can give adequate care, so he does not hospitalize the child; he explains the instructions in simple terms, makes sure the mother understands them, arranges for a visiting nurse to assist, and gives written instructions to the woman along with the verbal ones. If he knows that the father is capable of helping, he may also enlist his cooperation. (2) A patient has a painful lesion. The clinician recognizes that the patient has strong unmet dependency needs; she believes that these might add a risk of addiction. She does not prescribe a narcotic which she would otherwise prescribe, but gives other analgesics and arranges for special nursing care (as much because of the dependent needs as because of the lesion). (3) A man has a relatively minor injury. The physician believes that radiological studies can be safely deferred. He knows the patient has projective tendencies. He does not postpone the x-rays pending observation, but has them done at once, not only because of the added medicolegal risk but also because he knows that the patient would otherwise be dissatisfied and suspicious and that this would cause unnecessary anxiety. (4) An obstetrical patient is nearing term. She has moderate anxiety, some reaction formation against dependency needs, and an underlying, largely unconscious fear of abandonment. On the basis of the patient's personality, a decision is made to induce labor at term rather than run the risk of having her go into labor at a time when she might be alone at home and/or when the physician could not be in immediate attendance.

In the foregoing examples, none of the patients is mentally ill. None needs psychiatric treatment. They might, if improperly managed. Patients who do have diagnosable disorders, even mild ones not requiring treatment, present even more marked problems in general medical care. Examples: (1) A mildly passive-aggressive patient is obese and hypertensive. He can be expected to resist passively any attempts to order him to lose weight. The physician discusses the weight problem in a way that the patient feels that he is making his own decision to reduce; a struggle between patient and physician (always a losing battle) is avoided. (2) A patient with an Hysterical Personality has neurological symptoms and requires a spinal fluid examination. The physician usually does the procedure on an outpatient basis. She recognizes the risk of conversion paralysis following spinal tap and hospitalizes the patient for the procedure. (3) A physician is caring for the infant of a mildly obsessive-compulsive mother. The mother's case is chronic and not disabling. Treatment is elective. However, it is recognized that usual instruction concerning routine child care will be overdone. Special instructions are prepared which take into account the compulsivity. (4) A patient has a mild chronic duodenal ulcer. He has dependency problems and is a heavy smoker. The physician has felt that limiting smoking might lead to perforation of the ulcer and has not urged it. The patient develops another condition which requires that smoking be stopped. The physician decides that the patient must be supplied with another way of meeting oral dependent needs before this can be done.

The primary physician prescribing medication for various diseases often assumes that nearly all patients will take the medicines as directed. This is not the case. Some patients do not have prescriptions filled at all and an appreciable number of other patients fail to follow directions. Up to half of the patients for whom medication is prescribed fail to adhere to treatment sufficiently to obtain full benefit. Many factors account for this, ranging from failure of the physician to give adequate instruction to the patient to unpleasant side effects of the medications prescribed. However, application of a knowledge of the emotional makeup of the patient and that person's attitude toward taking medicine when discussing treatment with a patient will help reduce the incidence of treatment failures resulting from poor patient cooperation in taking prescribed medication.

Refusal of recommended diagnostic or treatment procedures also occurs in nearly 10 percent of hospitalized patients. Some refusals of elective procedures are reasonable choices. Others reflect problems in the doctor/patient relationship or failures to understand the patients' concerns.

Psychiatric Treatment in Primary Care Medicine

Informal Psychotherapy

Informal psychotherapy is used in:

1. Treatment of some Adjustment Disorders
2. Symptomatic and expectant treatment of some acute Anxiety Disorders
3. Supportive treatment of Personality Disorders and some chronic neuroses
4. Maintenance therapy of selected chronic psychotics

The Adjustment Disorder is the commonest cause of anxiety seen in general practice. Most cases are readily treatable. Often only a few appointments are necessary and these need not be of fixed duration. The situation is discussed and clarified. Alternatives to coping with it are discussed. Symptomatic medication is used as indicated (cf. Chapter 6).

Acute Generalized Anxiety Disorders, especially when there is fair ego strength and some external contributing stress, are often self-limited. Brief discussions of personal problems, some opportunity for catharsis and ventilation, a reassuring attitude, and appropriate medication often suffice.

The Personality Disorders may be influenced greatly by consistent efforts of the physician, incidental to other contacts with the patient, to support (show an interest in; encourage) adaptive behavior, healthful activities and interests, and effective ego defenses (e.g., the family physician of a woman with a Compulsive Personality who is rigid, meticulous, and rarely enjoys life asks the patient about recreational activities whenever he sees her for routine examinations and general medical care. He takes a few minutes to discuss what she has done; but he does not attempt to prescribe recreation as he knows it would be undertaken, in that case, as a duty not as fun. Though her house is usually quite neat, she apologizes for its untidiness whenever he makes a house call. He supports some of her rationalizations about being too busy with other things by indicating that they are more important than housework. He also comments on preferring a home that is "lived in"). The same methods are sometimes used for chronic neuroses when the prognosis for definitive therapy is poor and disability is not marked.

Some chronic psychotic patients, especially schizophrenics, who have had the maximum benefit of hospital treatment, and others who have not required hospitalization but are not candidates for definitive therapy (cf. Chapter 11) do require follow-up care to prevent acute exacerbations. Medication is helpful to some. Many can benefit from brief appointments at monthly or less frequent intervals. Only a few minutes need be scheduled; a longer appointment can be given subsequently if the patient has problems to discuss. In these appointments, the physician notes any tendency toward relapse or exacerbation. The patient has an opportunity to talk briefly about problems in daily living, and gains a feeling of security and a great deal of general ego support from the physician's continued interest in her or his well-being. If the patient is on medication, to look at these visits only as medication checks is to miss an important therapeutic component.

Formal Psychotherapy

Formal psychotherapy may be used by the primary physician. One can schedule regular appointments of fixed duration. One can use any of several psychotherapeutic techniques, including the method described in Chapter 19, other analytically oriented therapies, and nondirective therapies. One can use adjunctive medications.

There are some techniques of psychotherapy (e.g., psychoanalysis) that are too complex and require too much time to learn to be practical for someone who does not intend to specialize in their application. Some somatic therapies, while not being so difficult to master, are relatively impractical, since they require a hospital setting and a trained clinical team. Objection is sometimes made that definitive psychotherapy is too time consuming for the primary physician. This objection is readily answerable. In the first place, one is not thinking of psychoanalysis, which indeed is time consuming (several hundred hours, usually). One is thinking of brief psychotherapy. The average number of visits per patient to psychiatric clinics is four to six. Some of these patients are seen for consultation only, and some are actually drop-outs; so, perhaps a more realistic estimate of the number of appointments required by the average patient might range from six to eight or 20 to 30, depending on the type of cases accepted and the techniques used. True, even this takes time. However, giving the distressed patient regular appointments may eliminate a number of unscheduled visits, telephone calls, and house calls.

Formal psychotherapy usually requires appointments of a fixed duration and frequency. Holding these during regular office hours when patients are waiting their turns or when several patients are in stages of undress in various consulting rooms could be disruptive. However, time can be set aside for patients who prefer, or need, to be seen by appointment. There are patients other than the psychiatric who are better managed if they do not have to wait or be rushed. There are patients who much prefer to go to a doctor who will, barring surgical and obstetrical emergencies, see them on time. A person who must take time from work to go to the doctor may save money by paying a higher fee to a physician who works by specific appointment and in whose office one will not have to spend most of an afternoon.

Family practitioners average 12 to 18 minutes per patient; general psychiatrists average 20 to 30 minutes; psychiatrists who do primarily investigative psychotherapy often use 45- or 50-minute appointments. These differences deserve some study. In a particular technique, is a 45-minute appointment three times as good as a 15-minute one? Is it any better or worse than three 15-minute appointments? Evidence is scanty. Brief contact therapy has been shown to be effective. Perhaps the usual psychotherapeutic "hour" is more a matter of convenience and tradition than necessity. Certainly, investigative therapy takes time; there is a lot to talk about before a patient is understood. Some patients need time to relax and start talking. Some cannot maintain continuity from one appointment to another. On the other hand, some patients use short appointments more efficiently. If the patient needs longer appointments than the physician would normally schedule for the usual consulting fee, psychotherapy may be impractical from an economic point of view. There is a simple solution. Charge for the time required to do the work properly. Make sure the patient understands.

What patients should the primary physician treat? One's first answer is, as many as possible. Of course, this depends in part on skill and interest. It depends on the availability of specialists and the practicality of making referrals. It depends on whether one can admit psychiatric patients to the general hospital and whether it has adequate staff and facilities for their care. Certainly, the family physician should treat most Adjustment Disorders and many acute Anxiety Disorders, including those needing formal rather than informal psychotherapy. The primary physician utilizes psychotherapeutic techniques to treat patients with nonpsychiatric diseases in which psychological factors definitely affect the disorder.

If available, psychiatric consultation should be obtained before treating depressed patients who have a high suicide risk. Likewise, consultation is desirable before attempting an investigative therapy for a borderline psychotic patient because of the risk of precipitating a Psychosis. The primary physician should refer patients who need therapies she or he does not employ (e.g., electric shock; psychoanalysis). Perhaps the most important consideration is not deciding whom to treat, but for how long. Whether informal or formal psychotherapy is used, a patient who has an acute, presumably treatable condition should not be allowed to become chronic. If the patient is not responding to brief outpatient psychotherapy, consultation is indicated to decide whether the patient should be referred for specialized treatment, hospitalized, or continued on the treatment program with or without modification. Referral of the patient who has developed a dependent transference can be traumatic, antitherapeutic, and interpreted as a rejection. It must be done with tact. Perhaps at the beginning when a series of appointments is agreed upon, a decision as to how long to continue in the absence of progress can be made with an understanding that at the end of the period, a consultation will be arranged. Otherwise, the possibility of referral can be introduced at the time progress is reviewed, as something that can be offered since improvement is apparently too slow. One can indicate a continued interest in the patient, even a continued willingness to work with the patient after consultation if one prefers.

In addition to mastering one or more techniques of individual psychotherapy, the primary doctor might consider learning a method of group therapy. This is not as yet common in family medicine, but it probably should be. Group therapy is no harder to master than individual therapy. It is a potentially useful technique in family practice. The primary physician, because of the volume of practice, may find organizing groups easier than does the solo specialist. It is of interest that group therapy was introduced in this country by an internist, Joseph Pratt, who first used the method with tubercular patients. He believed that he could save time and work more efficiently by giving patients advice and instruction in groups. This was essentially a classroom method, a didactic technique of group treatment. Later, in the evolution of his work, he applied his method to psychiatric patients. The family practitioner of today might well recapitulate Pratt's experience, though one would use somewhat different techniques. One could use group methods for expectant mothers, for example, as well as for patients with emotional disorders.

Maintenance Therapy

Psychoactive medication, alone or as an adjunct to psychotherapy, is widely used by primary physicians in the treatment of psychiatric patients and for symptomatic purposes in treating other patients. About four-fifths of the prescriptions for anxiolytics and two-thirds of prescriptions for antidepressants are written by nonpsychiatrists. Such medications are among the most widely prescribed drugs in this country. They are powerful agents and the clinician using them must be thoroughly familiar with their indications, contraindications, and side effects (cf. Chapter 20) so as to avoid underutilization, overutilization, and inappropriate use.

Referral of Psychiatric Patients

Primary doctors make three types of referral of psychiatric patients:

1. Referral for consultation. The referring physician is willing and expects to continue treating the patient unless the psychiatrist recommends to the contrary. There are specific reasons for wanting an opinion (e.g., confirmation of diagnosis; evaluation of suicide risk; suggestion concerning treatment plan). It is important that the consultant know that the referring physician is

prepared to continue treating the case. The psychiatrist must also know exactly what is wanted. Otherwise, the report may not answer the questions that give rise to the request.

2.   Referral to a psychiatrist for diagnosis and treatment, if indicated. Again, the purpose of referral must be clear to the psychiatrist.

3.   Referral to a nonpsychiatrist for counseling or adjunctive therapy. Referrals are sometimes made to psychologists, social workers, vocational counselors, school counselors, and ministers. Patients referred are usually those who have personal problems about which the counselor is especially qualified to advise. Many such patients do not have a diagnosable illness; however, some patients with Adjustment Disorders and others with Personality Disorders may be referred. In making these referrals the physician usually should plan to continue regular contacts with the patient for ongoing attention to differential diagnosis, use of symptomatic medication when indicated, and evaluation of progress.

To make an appropriate referral, the physician must know the resources of the community. One needs to know who the qualified psychiatrists are. One should know what kind of patients they treat and what methods they use. Most psychiatrists restrict practice to some degree. One should know how promptly appointments can be given. Psychiatrists who do intensive psychotherapy often have waiting lists. However, many reserve some time for emergency consultations and urgent treatment cases. It is helpful to know the psychiatrist's way of handling telephone calls. Formal psychotherapeutic interviews should not be interrupted. Some therapists leave time between appointments when they can be reached by phone and/or can return phone calls from their patients and from physicians. Others prefer to handle telephone calls at certain hours during the day when they are doing work that can tolerate interruption.

The family doctor should be thoroughly familiar with hospital facilities. This includes knowing the types of patients accepted, treatments used, usual duration and cost of hospitalization, admission procedures, and the probable delay (if any) in obtaining admission. He or she should also be able to describe the hospital facilities and routines to patients and their families. One should know the fears and concerns a patient may have about care in a psychiatric facility and be able to correct misapprehensions. Though the way that a given patient will perceive psychiatric care is an individual matter and must be ascertained directly from the patient, a general appreciation of patients' feelings about illness and treatment may be obtained from fictional and autobiographical accounts of psychiatric care (cf. Selected References 13, 17, 18).

One should also know the nonmedical counseling services available. One should know the types of patients accepted and the qualifications and skills of the counselors.

Referring patients who recognize a need for psychiatric treatment is relatively easy. Referring others requires skill and tact. The physician rightfully hesitates to tell the patient abruptly, "I think you ought to see a psychiatrist." For the unsophisticated patient this may be frightening. One may wonder about his or her sanity and may fear hospitalization "in some snake pit." She or he may think the physician is not taking the complaint seriously, or saying, "it is all in your head." The physician should take time to clarify and define the problem and then use the patient's own words in expressing the need for consultation. It is best not to try to convince a patient that a symptom is psychogenic if the patient has already rejected that possibility. It is possible, however, to recommend consultation as part of a complete study. At the same time, the patient's attitude can be respected and acknowledged (a patient complains of headaches. After careful study, the physician believes they are tension headaches associated with an Anxiety Disorder. The patient has made it clear that he does not accept the diagnosis. The physician grants that there are many other causes for headache, indicates that headaches like those which the patient has can sometimes be produced by tension, and suggests that a consultant's opinion would be helpful — "even though you don't feel that nervousness plays an important role in your case"). Patients who lack insight are more likely to accept the possibility of an emotional factor or stresses and worries making a disease worse than they are to consider emotional distress as the cause of illness.

Prophylaxis

There are a number of ways in which the primary physician can help prevent mental illness. These include:

1.   Attention to the emotional development of infants and children. Instruction in child care during the early stages of psychosexual development is given to mothers. Their practices in child care are observed. Errors resulting from ignorance or misinformation are corrected. Stress to the child resulting from emotional problems of parents, including those related to marital difficulties, are also noted and, when necessary, family counseling or psychotherapy for one or both parents may be recommended.

2.   Evaluation and counseling of the healthy adolescent. Among the problems of all adolescents are those related to the acquisition of social skills, vocational choice, and career planning, and the development of healthy attitudes toward sexuality. The shy, timid, withdrawn youth who is not making a satisfactory social adjustment may or may not be preschizophrenic. In any case, he or she needs help. The physician can learn something of the adolescent's plans for the future. Making allowance for changeability and for occasional unrealistic fantasies that are not really taken seriously, one should make certain the patient is making workable future plans and not ones that will lead to almost certain disappointment, failure, and frustration. In dealing with sexual attitudes, the physician avoids probing personal questions and should also avoid giving a stereotyped "sex talk." One does ask questions about sexual development as part of a history by systems in connection with physical examinations. In doing this, one may identify areas of concern or, at least, open the topic in a way that permits the patient to ask questions.

3.   Helping patients modify character traits that add to susceptibility to emotional illness (e.g., reducing the rigidity often associated with the premorbid personality of persons who develop major depressions in late middle age; dealing with dependency problems that might later lead to psychosomatic disorders; helping patients find healthy outlets for aggression).

4.   Recognizing and dealing with prodromal symptoms of mental illness (e.g., helping patients recognize and modify unhealthy drinking habits before Alcoholism develops; this is done by more sophisticated techniques than issuing a warning or prescribing a quota).

5.   Seeing that patients are prepared for life's stresses so as to prevent Adjustment Disorders and their sequelae (e.g., premarital counseling; counseling expectant mothers; preretirement counseling).

6.   Seeing that patients have adequate support in times of crisis. This can be done only if the ego strength of the patients and their probable abilities to tolerate stress are known. It requires a relationship in which the patient lets the doctor know when he or she is under stress.

Social and Community Psychiatry

The medical practitioner occupies an important role in the community. He or she has prestige; with it goes responsibility. Most physicians are active community leaders. Despite busy schedules they join service clubs; they serve on boards and committees. Directly or indirectly, they do much to mold public opinion.

The physician can help reduce the incidence of mental disorder and its impact on the community by:

1. Taking an active role in community efforts to reduce unhealthy stresses; poverty, unemployment (and insecurity in employment), vocational stresses, unnecessarily stressful practices in the school systems, etc.
2. Acting when possible to reduce interpersonal tensions and conflict between groups in the community (e.g., active promotion of improved interracial relations).
3. Encouraging opportunities for the realization of human potential. Encouraging educational facilities for the young and for adults.
4. Disseminating information on mental hygiene and mental health. Instruction of lay groups. Instruction of groups who may need to recognize and cope with emotional disorder (e.g., policemen; teachers).
5. Encouraging the development of mental health facilities. While the family physician can treat most psychiatric patients and usually does not need special facilities, there is a need for psychiatrists and psychiatric hospital beds. Services should be available both for those who can afford private care and for the indigent.

There is one especially important aspect of the development of mental health facilities. The physicians of the community have a responsibility to see that these facilities are for real; that they maintain adequate standards of care. A well-meaning lay group in the community may organize a clinic, rent offices, and hire personnel without achieving the desired results. They need guidance and support from an informed group of practitioners. At times, they and the community can profit from a withdrawal of support until standards of care are adequately met.

CONTINUING EDUCATION IN PSYCHIATRY

Most medical schools of today offer an adequate, basic preparation in psychiatry to the student. However, like other specialties, psychiatry changes. New diagnostic methods are developed, new techniques of therapy are introduced and old ones are modified, and new drugs come into use. To some extent the physician can keep up by reading books and journals. Interviewing techniques can be learned by experience. Experience includes a critical study of what one does and its results; otherwise, experience is only repetition of mistakes. After studying a case, if a consultation is found necessary, questions may be asked of the consultant beyond those necessary for the main purpose of the consultation to confirm clinical impressions. However, many physicians find that postgraduate courses for continuing education are desirable. Lectures, short courses, seminars, and workshops are sponsored by medical centers and by various professional organizations, including the American Academy of Family Physicians and the American Psychiatric Association.

When short courses are planned the primary physicians and psychiatrists doing the planning should study the needs and preferences of the practitioners carefully.

Often doctors indicate a preference for lectures or clinical demonstrations rather than seminars or group discussions. Care should be given in deciding what subjects can best be presented by the various methods, and how methods can be combined. A frequent complaint about short courses is that they are superficial, repetitive, and sometimes more exhortations than instructive lectures. The fault often lies in the selection of topics that cannot be covered other than superficially in the allotted time.

Instruction in diagnostic or therapeutic interviewing technique, beyond offering a few elementary suggestions and in discussions helping the development of constructive attitudes, almost requires supervised experience. This is rarely practical in a short course. Courses extending over a period of time with monthly or even weekly meetings have been used. For the physician who does not have access to such programs, an alternative approach is to arrange to work, under supervision, on a part-time basis (a half-day a week, perhaps) in a psychiatric hospital or community mental health clinic.

REVIEW QUESTIONS

1. What percentage of the patients seen by the average family physician are primarily psychiatric cases? What percent have some emotional problems but have other needs for medical care? In what percent of cases are psychiatric factors negligible? On what did you base your estimate? Can you find references on the subject? Have you asked practitioners about the impressions gained from their own clinical practices?
2. Whom do emotionally disturbed people consult first about their difficulties? Why?
3. How does a physician's experience in treating a patient for another illness help in the evaluation and treatment of the patient if he or she develops an acute psychiatric disorder?
4. What information should a primary physician have from a state mental hospital from which a patient has been recently discharged in order to give adequate follow-up care?
5. An adolescent boy who has been generally well-adjusted develops tension headaches. The family doctor believes they are symptomatic of an Adjustment Disorder. She believes they are related to the boy's inability to cope with pressure from parents and teachers for academic achievement and participation in extracurricular activities beyond his capacities. Assuming the patient is willing, to what extent should the physician discuss her findings and recommendations with the parents? With teachers? Should the physician treat the patient? Refer him and his parents to a social agency for family counseling? Refer him to a school counselor? Refer him to a psychiatrist? Why? What factors might alter your recommendation?
6. In the case described in question 5, if the physician elects to treat the patient herself, should she use informal psychotherapy? Medication as a main method of treatment? Medication as an adjunctive treatment? Why? What factors would alter the decision?
7. If the patient described in question 5 is referred to a nonphysician counselor, should the family doctor continue to see the patient for this complaint? Why?
8. It has been estimated that the average physician sees six suicidal patients yearly. How does one recognize these patients? How can the primary physician reduce the incidence of suicide among his or her patients?
9. Discuss possible uses for group therapy in family practice.

10. A patient is hospitalized for abdominal pain. The physician suspects a Somatization Disorder and wishes a consultation. He arranges for a psychiatrist to see the patient the following day. What should he tell the patient about the reason for the consultation?

SELECTED REFERENCES

1. Aldrich, C. Knight, and Samuel E. Miller: Early teaching of family medicine. *Family Practice Recertification* 5(11):25-27, 31, 159-164, 1983.

2. Burdick, Bruce M., Cooper B. Holmes, and Ronald F. Waln: Recognition of suicide signs by physicians in different areas of specialization. *J Med Ed* 58(9):716-721, 1983.

3. Castelnuovo-Tedesco, Pietro: The twenty-minute hour: An approach to the postgraduate teaching of psychiatry. *Am J Psychiatry* 123(7):786-791, 1967.

4. Eaton, Merrill, T., Jr.: Investigative psychotherapy in general practice. *Med Times* 91:942-947, 1963.

5. Eraker, Stephen A., John P. Kirscht, and Marshall H. Becker: Understanding and improving patient compliance. *Ann Intern Med* 100(2):258-268, 1984.

6. Fauman, Michael A.: Psychiatric components of medical and surgical practice: A survey of general hospital physicians. *Am J Psychiatry* 138(10):1298-1301, 1981.

7. Fauman, Michael A.: Psychiatric components of medical and surgical practice. II: Referral and treatment of psychiatric disorders. *Am J Psychiatry* 140(6):760-763, 1983.

8. Goldberg, David, Jane J. Steele, Alan Johnson, and Charles Smith: Ability of primary care physicians to make accurate ratings of psychiatric symptoms. *Arch Gen Psychiatry* 39(7):829-833, 1982.

9. Karasu, Toksoz B.: Psychotherapy of the medically ill. *Am J Psychiatry* 136(1):1-11, 1979.

10. Popkin, Michael K., Thomas B. Mackenzie, Allan L. Callies, and Richard C. W. Hall: Yield of psychiatric consultants' recommendations for diagnostic action. *Arch Gen Psychiatry* 39(7):843-845, 1982.

11. Regier, Darrel A., Irving D. Goldberg, Barbara J. Burns, Janet Hankin, Edwin W. Hoeper, and Gregory R. Nycz: Specialist/generalist division of responsibility for patients with mental disorders. *Arch Gen Psychiatry* 39(2):219-224, 1982.

12. Rynearson, Edward K.: The helpful physician and the unhelpable patient. *Postgrad Med* 58(2):145-150, 1975.

13. Smith, Nancy Covert: *Journey Out of Nowhere.* Waco, Texas, Word Books, 1974.

14. Strain, James J.: Needs for psychiatry in the general hospital. *Hosp Community Psychiatry* 33(12):996-1001, 1982.

15. Thompson, Troy L., Alan Stoudemire, Wayne D. Mitchell, and Richard L. Grant: Underrecognition of patients' psychosocial distress in a university hospital medical clinic. *Am J Psychiatry* 140(2):158-161, 1983.

16. Usdin, Gene, and J. Lewis: *Psychiatry in General Medical Practice.* New York, McGraw-Hill, 1979.

17. Ward, Mary Jane: *Counter Clockwise.* Chicago, Regency, 1969.

18. Ward, Mary Jane: *The Snake Pit.* New York, Random House, 1946.

Part IV

FORENSIC PSYCHIATRY, HISTORY,
AND BOARD EXAMINATION REVIEW

Chapter 23

PSYCHIATRY AND THE LAW

LAWYERS AND PSYCHIATRISTS

The lawyer and the psychiatrist have much in common. In fact, their scores on vocational aptitude and interest tests show a striking similarity. They are both in
professions dedicated to service to others. Both deal with human problems. Both
are bound by a professional code of ethics which carries with it responsibilities beyond those of a person engaged in a trade and often outweighing pecuniary considerations. Both spend much of their time seeking truth. There are some dissimilar-
ities. The lawyer deals in absolutes (answer the question, Yes or No; the accused
is guilty or not guilty, never partly to blame.) The psychiatrist, like other scientists, thinks largely in relative terms. The lawyer sees the human being as rational,
capable of making conscious choices and exercising free will. The psychiatrist
views much of human behavior as irrational and occurring under the influence of
unconscious forces and/or conditioning (learning) which has taken place outside of
conscious awareness. Psychiatric theory is based on determinism (the concept that
psychological phenomena and acts of will are determined by antecedent causes).
The lawyer, having had little if any experience in working with the mentally ill,
and possibly having been influenced by authors critical of the "medical model," is
likely not to view the mentally ill person as sick but simply as deviant, and to view
deviance as a right based upon free choice as long as deviant behavior does not
harm others.

The physician seeking to benefit a patient focuses upon that person's needs,
and on ways to contribute to his or her health and welfare; while the lawyer emphasize rights and liberties, viewing them as having priority over or being necessary for health and welfare. The physician may see certain interventions as bene-
ficent and desirable that the lawyer views as paternalistic and undesirable.

In the courtroom, the lawyer seeks truth through use of the adversary method;
sides are taken and debated, with each side seeking facts and expert opinions which
support its viewpoint as strongly as possible. The method is an unfamiliar and uncomfortable one for the psychiatrist who is more used to resolving contradictions
than disputing them.

A value judgment on these differences is irrelevant in most interactions between physician and attorney; the important thing is a mutual understanding which

permits meaningful communication. As well as understanding lawyers, the psychiatrist must understand laws. He or she must understand not only legal responsibilities to patients but also many laws that affect the activities of those patients.

Each state has its own laws, so a discussion of laws relating to the practice of psychiatry and to the rights of mental patients must be general rather than specific. The topics discussed in this chapter can do little more than raise a question for each practitioner; what are the laws on this matter in your state? Some laws should be known as soon as practice is started; others can be studied as need arises. It is desirable to read the laws and know their exact language. However, the physician should stop short of trying to interpret them; this is the task of the attorney. Even if one is in compliance with state laws, and an issue is raised, for example, one concerning patient rights, legal advice may be needed, since the constitutionality of a state law may be challenged.

Every practitioner should have an attorney who can be consulted when legal questions arise in his or her practice. Often, questions concerning laws and legal definitions can be answered by telephone, and if suitable advance arrangements are made, the cost is nominal. When the psychiatrist testifies in court, one should know the laws relevant to the subject on which one is testifying, the legal definitions of the terms employed, the basic questions that one is likely to be asked, and how best to phrase one's answers so as to communicate the needed medical information clearly.

THE PSYCHIATRIST'S LEGAL
RESPONSIBILITIES TO PATIENTS

Many of the laws applying to patient care have much the same application to psychiatry as to other branches of medicine.

Malpractice, negligence, and abandonment are prohibited. Most definitions of malpractice give some weight to the standards of the community. On going into practice in a new community, the psychiatrist should become familiar with the methods used by the recognized, qualified specialists already in the area (e.g., how often are blood levels obtained for patients on lithium maintenance?). If there are not enough practitioners in the community to establish a standard, a knowledge of the practices and teaching of departments of psychiatry in the nearest medical schools might be helpful. Certainly, the practitioner may depart from local custom without being guilty of bad practice. One may have a routine procedure that is different from one's colleagues. One should know that it is different and be prepared to defend it. It is better to look for references and other data to validate and justify a procedure before something goes wrong than after. If one departs from local custom not routinely, but in a specific case, the records should clearly show the reasons. If the change in methods involves a major calculated risk, or if it involves anything unusual, inadequately tested, or experimental, consultation is desirable, and informed consent is imperative.

Proving malpractice or negligence requires essentially the same proof as any other negligence action, with a preponderance of evidence to establish:

1. The physician had a duty to conform to a particular standard of practice.
2. The physician failed to adhere to that standard through some act of commission or omission.
3. That act was the direct or proximate cause of harm (damage) to the patient.

Some examples of situations in which the issue of negligence might arise in psychiatric practice include: (1) A psychiatrist's usual practice in evaluating certain types of patients includes a physical examination which he records on a form. After the heading Pelvic Examination he writes deferred; he does not subsequently perform that examination and does not include his reason for not doing it in his progress notes. A few weeks later, another physician discovers that the patient has an advanced carcinoma of the cervix. The psychiatrist is not supposed to be an expert in gynecology, but a review of the situation might suggest that he had carelessly overlooked something that was part of his own usual procedure. Had he not routinely done physicals or had he written omitted instead of deferred, and preferably added a few words of explanation, an inspection of the records would still show an unfortunate decision, but not, in all probability, a negligent one. (2) A patient taking a phenothiazine has a routine blood count which shows a marked leukopenia. The physician orders no other tests, does not stop medication, and does not apparently make any effort to account for or treat the leukopenia. Agranulocytosis follows and the patient dies. In inspecting the records, one might suspect that she failed to read the laboratory report. Negligence. A progress note stating that she did not regard the leukopenia as severe enough to warrant stopping the drug might not absolve her of bad judgment, or even of malpractice, but would remove one suspicion of carelessness. (3) A patient threatens suicide. The clinician records this in a progress note. He offers no explanation of why he did not take the threat seriously or why he did nothing about it. The patient kills himself. Was the psychiatrist negligent? Probably not, but it might be difficult to establish this. Certainly bad practice occurs; so does negligence. However, a bad outcome does not prove malpractice or negligence. The principle of res ipsa loquitur (the facts speak for themselves) applies only to a bad outcome which could only occur as a result of negligence or bad practice, and when it applies expert testimony is not required to establish malpractice. An error or a wrong decision is not necessarily a result of bad practice or carelessness. The physician who is sued for malpractice, though he or she has practiced properly and carefully, has as his or her best defense good and complete records. Another protection includes the use of consultants when major calculated risks must be taken, or when patients or their families express dissatisfaction with or reluctance to follow recommendations.

Once a physician undertakes the care of a patient, other than in a situation in which patient and physician both understand the relationship to be limited to an evaluation or consultation, he or she has an ongoing responsibility to the patient until the patient recovers, formally dismisses the doctor, or is dismissed. The issue of abandonment might arise in certain circumstances.

1.   The physician is not available when needed (e.g., is away on vacation) and has failed to make arrangements for the care of patients. One should have someone of equal competence available to take calls.

2.   The physician dismisses a patient (e.g., for failure to follow medical advice; because the physician no longer has time to care for him or her) without adequate notice. Adequate notice should represent sufficient time for the patient to make other arrangements for care. The amount of time necessary depends on the available facilities of the community.

3.   The doctor fails to respond to an emergency call. Certainly, the therapist is not obliged to make a house call or even offer an extra appointment every time a manipulative patient claims to be in a panic; to do so would be antitherapeutic as well as a trifle masochistic. This is a matter of clinical judgment; if the patient really needs help, she or he should have it. Likewise, the physician is not obliged to give care that is outside of his or her area of competence or requires facilities

which are unavailable (e.g., a patient has made a suicide attempt and needs a surgeon, not a psychiatrist; a patient is developing acute psychotic symptoms and needs hospitalization, but there are no beds available in the hospitals where the therapist has staff privileges). However, the therapist cannot evade responsibility by simply suggesting that another physician be called. One may help make arrangements or may simply suggest them; but if one does the latter, one should either recontact the patient to make sure that care has been obtained or should have an understanding with the patient that he or she will be notified if there are difficulties in making necessary arrangements for care. If the physician can be available only during office hours, offers outpatient care only, and expects patients to make other arrangements if hospitalization is desired, or does not make house calls under any circumstances, it is probably necessary for the patient to know this from the beginning of the doctor-patient relationship.

A *promise of cure* renders a physician liable if recovery does not take place. The psychiatrist should not make or imply such a promise in an attempt to be reassuring. A physician's attitude has more value in reassuring a patient than the content of what is said, but it is possible to give an encouraging prognosis without promising cure, and at the same time without alarming the patient by the way reassuring statements are qualified.

It is possible that in some uses of hypnosis, suggestion, or persuasion, the physician might want to make statements which could be interpreted as promising cure. If these cannot be altered without impairing the treatment program, legal consultation might be desirable.

Taking advantage of information obtained from the patient in the course of treatment, or taking advantage of the patient's dependence upon the psychiatrist is unethical, and it may be illegal for the psychiatrist as it would be for any other physician. Because of this, as well as for technical reasons related to therapy, the psychiatrist keeps his or her business affairs entirely separate from practice and avoids business transactions with patients. Social contacts with patients are also minimized.

Sexual activity with patients, and under most circumstances with former patients, is unethical. It may lead to malpractice suits for improper treatment. Criminal charges are likely if the patient does not consent or is under age. Criminal charges may also result if there is reason to believe that the patient was not mentally competent at the time, either because of serious mental illness or because of a treatment that interfered with the patient's ability to exercise will power and judgment, such as hypnosis or the administration of intravenous sedation.

Charges of unethical conduct, or damage suits, alleging sexual activity with former patients are based on the ongoing effects of unresolved transference and dependence on the physician, and in some instances on the physician's misuse of his or her knowledge of the patient's vulnerability.

Not all accusations of improper sexual conduct are true. The physician may be placed in a compromising position by the frankly seductive patient (sometimes hostilely motivated and trying, consciously or unconsciously, to embarrass the doctor). Accusations may stem from the delusions of a paranoid patient or the fantasies of an hysterical one. To reduce the risk of accusations of improper conduct, the physician:

1. Minimizes social contacts with patients while they are in treatment and for a reasonable period afterward.
2. Maintains adequate records. These would include any record of previous tendencies to make similar accusations together with other factors in the patient's personality which might account for them. Records also show what actually occurs during appointments.

3. Avoids excessive privacy during interviews. The fact that a secretary or office nurse is in an adjoining room, that doors are not locked, and that blinds are not drawn in the office tend to make any such accusation less plausible. When the patient's behavior, or mental content, creates a special problem in this area, the physician may even want to arrange to have someone enter the treatment room unexpectedly now and then, as if to deliver a message or bring in papers, though these interruptions would usually be avoided during therapy.

4. Has a nurse or some other chaperone present when patients are disrobed, under the influence of heavy sedation, or hypnotized. In selected cases it may also be advisable to have someone along if one is to make a house call or see a patient after hours.

5. Obtains formal consultation in cases in which erotic transference (or counter-transference) becomes a problem.

It should be remembered that accusations of homosexual misconduct are as likely to occur as are those of heterosexual misconduct.

Informed consent is a rapidly evolving legal issue, and one must be alert to changing requirements. The case of Slater vs. Baker and Stapleton in England in 1767 concerning an orthopedic procedure established the precedent that a patient has the right to be informed of a proposed procedure. Though it became customary to obtained signed, witnessed consent for surgical procedures, experimental treatments, and later such psychiatric treatments as electroconvulsive therapy, it was not until 1960 (Natanson vs. Kline; Mitchell vs. Robinson) that the validity of such consent was legally challenged and the necessity for informing patients of possible serious hazards of treatment was established.

In order to give informed consent, a rational person must know not only what treatment is being proposed and its possible consequences, favorable and unfavorable, but also what other courses of action are available (including not treating the condition at all) and what consequences these may have. It sounds simple, albeit time consuming, for the physician to give the patient this information in order to obtain consent and document having done so. However, studies have shown that even when care is taken to inform patients adequately, many of them fail to grasp the significance of what they have been told.

Exceptions to the requirement for informed consent include emergency situations in which there is not time to obtain it and circumstances in which the patient waives the right, for example, by clearly indicating a desire not to be told of risks and possible undesirable consequences.

Giving information about risks and side effects requires tact, lest the patient be unnecessarily upset. However, if one wishes to withhold information because of concern that furnishing it would be harmful to the patient one would be wise to obtain:

1. Professional consultation
2. Legal advice
3. The consent of the patient's family

In addition to tact, one also uses common sense. If a neuroleptic has multiple side effects, and the patient is shown the list of all that have been reported, discussion should focus on those that are (a) likely to occur, and (b) consequential. One does not warn of the dangers of angioneurotic edema every time one gives an aspirin.

Treating an involuntary patient presents special problems. First, the fact that the patient is involuntary may raise the issue of coercion and casts doubt on the patient's ability to give a truly voluntary consent. Second, if state law allows the use of certain somatic treatments without consent in such cases, one must recognize that constitutional issues could be raised based on the reasoning that a procedure that affects the mind (this includes giving psychoactive drugs) may infringe upon one's rights under the first amendment.

Finally, for both voluntary and involuntary patients, one has the question of whether the patient is mentally able, i.e., competent to give consent even if he or she is willing to do so. There is no simple or established test of such competence. One has to take into account the general ability of the patient to think logically and make rational decisions, the specific ability to understand and make decisions about proposed treatment, and the freedom from delusions or irrational ideas that may lead to an unreasonable choice. In regard to evaluating a choice as unreasonable, one must be sure that one could establish its lack of reasonableness to an intelligent lay person. It is not unreasonable, necessarily, to disagree with one's doctor's advice!

Since one is open to suits for malpractice and for charges of battery if one treats a person without having proper informed consent, it is suggested that competent voluntary patients always have the treatment plan explained to them, including an explanation of its risks and of the other options available, and that this be documented and witnessed. Some question that this is always necessary when one uses psychoactive drugs. It has been suggested that with drugs that may cause Tardive Dyskinesia an interval between instituting therapy and discussing this risk is appropriate, since drugs that may cause Tardive Dyskinesia are unlikely to do so if used in small doses for a short period of time. Nevertheless, it is likely that the advantages of obtaining and documenting consent routinely outweigh the disadvantages.

Though it is generally legally presumed that one is competent until adjudged otherwise, if a physician seriously doubts a voluntary patient's competence to give consent, it may be desirable to recommend guardianship before using treatments with appreciable risks and to obtain the guardian's consent as well as the patient's.

For involuntary patients, one obtains consent if possible. If one's state law allows some treatments to be given to involuntary patients without consent, and a patient who is able to indicate a choice objects to a proposed treatment, he or she should have the opportunity to seek legal counsel except in emergencies. Treatment of the involuntary incompetent patient is facilitated by having a guardian who can consent or a legal mechanism through which some person may act in the patient's behalf in consenting or withholding consent. A system that requires a hearing each time a treatment plan is changed is unnecessarily cumbersome.

A parent's consent is usually necessary and sometimes sufficient for procedures affecting persons under legal age. This may not apply to the emancipated minor, the married girl in her teens, nor the adolescent who has *permanently* left home and is earning his or her own living. Even when parents consent, the minor's own consent is desirable; he or she might otherwise wish to take action against the physician on reaching maturity.

A person who has given informed consent is free to withdraw that consent at any time.

Involuntary Hospitalization and Patients' Rights

Sometimes a person with a serious mental illness does not have sufficient insight to recognize that he or she is ill and in need of treatment. For such a person, involuntary hospitalization may be considered, but it is possible only if certain legal criteria are met. The legal criteria have changed markedly in recent years, and are still subject to change both through the enactment of new laws and as a result of court decisions on the constitutionality of these and of existing ones.

In early times, laws governing the care of the mentally ill focused more on their property rights than their personal rights or needs for treatment (after all, there was not much available by way of treatment). As early as the thirteenth century, English law recognized the need for the government to assume custody of the property of natural fools (persons mentally retarded from birth) and persons who become non compos mentis (persons with serious acquired mental disorders). Property of congenitally retarded persons was to be kept for their heirs, and that of persons with acquired mental illness was to be returned to them when they recovered. Care was the responsibility of the family, though some hospitals and "asylums" were available. Patients who created a disturbance in the community were jailed.

When a system of state mental hospitals was developed in the United States in the nineteenth century in order to rescue the mentally ill from almshouses and jails (cf. Chapter 24) admission procedures were relatively informal. Later complaints arose of some patients being deprived of liberty unnecessarily by being committed for mild disorders, and accusations were made that some people were placed in mental hospitals even though they were not mentally ill. In the 1860s a Mrs. Packard was committed to an Illinois State Hospital by her husband, a minister. She felt that her husband had put her in the hospital to get rid of her (though the hospital superintendent disagreed) and after several attempts secured her release. She later wrote a book, *Modern Persecution, or Insane Asylums Unveiled,* which so impressed the Illinois legislators that a law was enacted requiring a jury trial prior to commitment to a mental institution.

Around this time other states enacted commitment laws, though most did not require jury trial. Generally, the laws sought only to establish the presence of mental illness, insanity, and the fact that the person was a proper subject for hospital treatment. Testimony or certification by physicians, usually two, was generally required to establish this.

Additional major changes in commitment laws did not occur until the 1970s. Various groups that were concerned about the civil liberties of the mentally ill successfully urged enactment of laws that would prevent a person being hospitalized, and accordingly deprived of freedom, solely because he or she had a mental illness. Impetus for these changes was provided by the Supreme Court decision in 1975 in the Donaldson case, discussed later in this chapter. However, many states made more extensive changes in their laws than were required by that decision.

Though laws vary from state to state, most of them require that a person, in order to be hospitalized involuntarily, in addition to being mentally ill, must be:

1. Dangerous to the self
2. Dangerous to others
3. Gravely disabled

Dangerousness to self is usually defined so as to mean an immediate suicide risk manifested by attempts at suicide, threats of it, or overt acts that clearly indicate suicidal intent. The fact that a person with a certain disorder has a statistical probability of suicide several times that of the average person would not be sufficient to establish the immediate dangerousness to the self required for commitment. Likewise, conduct that would in the long run be detrimental to one's health or that would jeopardize one's career does not meet this criteria.

Dangerousness to others is also evaluated on the basis of overt behavior or threats. Grave disability implies an inability to care for one's own needs that is so great that one could not survive outside an institution. The criteria for determining grave disability are quite specific and rigid in some states, but in others are less narrow and allow the exercise of clinical judgment and common sense in evaluating a patient's needs.

While dangerousness and grave disability are required for involuntary hospitalization in most states, some permit commitment when care and treatment is essential to a person's welfare and the patient is unable to understand the need for hospitalization.

Commitment laws require adversarial hearings and periodic review of the continued need for hospitalization. They usually require that treatment be given in the least restrictive setting possible.

Most laws permit some form of temporary or emergency admission on the certification of law enforcement officers (or sometimes physicians). Usually only a few days hospitalization is allowed on this type of certification. It is intended to give time for the patient to be examined and for arrangements to be made for a hearing if commitment is deemed necessary.

There has been concern over the hospitalization of children at the request of their parents. It has been contended that children should have due process hearings, since parents do not *always* act in the best interest of the child. However, the Supreme Court has upheld laws in two states, Georgia and Pennsylvania, that do not require preconfinement hearings in all cases of parental request for hospitalization. The court held that parents retain a substantial role in such a decision, absent a finding of neglect or abuse. Parental right is not absolute but is subject to medical judgment. Need is noted for a neutral fact finder, but a medical decision-making process can qualify. As in the case of consent to treatment, the child's consent to hospitalization should also be obtained if possible, and the child has the right to an adversarial hearing if he or she desires it.

A Uniform Alcoholism and Intoxication Treatment Act, now enacted in a majority of states, identifies Alcoholism as an illness and makes it a health, not a criminal, issue. Along with this, separate procedures for involuntary hospitalization of persons with Alcoholism and other forms of Chemical Dependence may exist and may have criteria different from those required for the involuntary hospitalization of persons with other forms of mental illness.

Sometimes there are separate laws for the legal commitment of sexual psychopaths. Some sexual psychopath laws are intended to protect sick offenders and see that they get treatment. Others are intended to protect society by providing prolonged confinement. The latter have two disadvantages: they may, in effect, give an individual an indeterminate sentence for a minor offense; on the other hand, they may send a dangerous offender to an institution without adequate security provisions.

In legal actions generally, there are three standards of proof:

1. Preponderance of evidence
2. Clear and convincing evidence
3. Proof beyond a reasonable doubt

For involuntary commitment, the second, clear and convincing evidence, is the level required (Addington vs. Texas).

Current commitment laws in most states do not adequately address the needs of all mentally ill persons. A patient who does not recognize that he or she is ill and is incompetent to make a decision regarding treatment may greatly impair his or her well-being and do great harm to a future life situation without at any point representing an immediate danger of grave bodily harm to the self or others or being gravely disabled in the usual sense of helplessness (e.g., a manic patient may bankrupt himself and his family; a person who is not eating whether because of Schizophrenia, depression, or Anorexia Nervosa may reach a level of malnutrition which will have a permanent effect on health long before impending starvation makes a threat to life immediate). The right of such persons to receive care must be legally established, too. There should be provision for involuntary hospitalization and treatment, at least for a reasonable period of time, based upon (1) mental illness, and (2) incompetence for making decisions about treatment. Such incompetence is surely easier to establish on the basis of medical evidence, and to explain to a board of mental health or a court, than is danger. It is hoped that in the next few years laws will be modified for meeting the needs of the patient whose illness has robbed him or her of the ability to make rational treatment decisions. It is recognized that such modifications must protect the individual's rights. Modification could take the form of providing additional bases for commitment or could develop appropriate mechanisms for establishing incompetency and providing for effective guardianship.

Whatever the laws are concerning involuntary hospitalization, the alternative of voluntary hospitalization should be used whenever possible. A voluntary admission may be formal or informal. An informal voluntary admission is appropriate for the vast majority of patients. The patient simply enters the mental hospital as one would enter any other hospital of one's own free will and leaves when one chooses. A more formal voluntary admission procedure requires the patient to sign a consent for hospitalization and usually requires giving a certain number of days notice in writing if one wishes to leave. The voluntary agreement is more likely to be necessary in the closed ward psychiatric hospital than in the open hospital. The staff of the closed hospital may wish evidence of the patient's consent to be confined. The provision for written notice may be of value to the hospital which wishes to discourage a misuse of facilities (e.g., an alcoholic patient not actually desiring treatment who wants to use the hospital as a hotel on a cold night). It can also be used to give the hospital time to notify relatives to come for a patient or to arrange for involuntary admission if this appears necessary. Because of the effect on the morale of other patients, however, many psychiatrists prefer to avoid having a patient's status changed from voluntary to involuntary unless this is absolutely necessary. In cases of reasonable doubt, it is often better to discharge the voluntary patient on request, if he or she cannot be persuaded to the contrary, and if further hospitalization is needed to have it begin on an involuntary basis.

Responsibilities to hospitalized patients are much the same as those to the voluntary outpatient, though the physician may become responsible for the standards of care (or negligence) of a number of hospital employees who may be viewed as his or her agents in the treatment of the patient. There may be times at which one will wish a legal opinion as to the responsibility for certain hospital policies and procedures. The staff physician directly responsible for a patient may be the person named in a damage suit even though the complaint results from a hospital policy or procedure over which he or she had no control. There may be times when a physician must insist on a change in hospital policies, and if the physician is unsuccessful in obtaining such a change, he or she must take patients elsewhere if in private practice, or seek another job if employed.

Since legal commitment is becoming less common, some of the problems that it created are less serious for the contemporary psychiatrist than they were for our predecessors. An underlying, though usually at least partly erroneous, assumption concerning the committed patient was that of total irresponsibility. The fact that a patient needs treatment per se, does not necessarily imply an inability to judge the nature and consequences of his or her acts, assess the motives of other people, and protect his or her own interests by normally prudent decisions. Even a patient who is irresponsible in some respects, and is not capable of making some decisions, may be responsible in other areas. However, the idea of total irresponsibility would imply that the physician, or the hospital superintendent, must constantly guard and protect the helpless person. Following this reasoning, if the patient destroys or loses valuable property, it is the superintendent's fault (lock valuables in a safe); if the patient spends money foolishly or gambles it away, the superintendent is to blame (do not let the patients carry money); if the patient gets hurt in any way, there is a presumption of negligence (do not let the patients handle sharp objects); if a woman patient gets pregnant, the superintendent may not be to blame personally, but she or he is responsible for not having taken adequate precautions (keep women patients segregated from men). Obviously, the facetious parenthetical solutions to these problems are for the protection of the superintendent and staff, not the patient. Nevertheless, while the suggestions are facetious, they were standard practices in many mental hospitals in the past. For example, many a state hospital superintendent took a far more restrictive outlook on the sex life of women patients than might the dean of the most strict of girls' schools. In fact, it was virtually impossible in some state hospitals for any woman of child-bearing age with intact reproductive organs to gain permission to take a walk on the hospital campus or go into community unaccompanied, no matter how mild her mental condition or how beneficial it might have been for her to have some privileges.

Depriving patients of belongings, money, and liberty in the interest of careful guardianship was both dehumanizing and antitherapeutic. Fortunately, it is no longer necessary as a matter of hospital policy. However, there are certain patients whose condition genuinely requires special protection. While special protection may be necessary, overprotection is not. Sometimes a failure to utilize some safeguards involves a calculated risk. When calculated risks are taken, they should usually be discussed in staff meetings or with consultants, and adequate records should be maintained to indicate that the risks were undertaken on the basis of careful medical judgment, not negligence.

Patients, especially those too sick to complain, must be protected from any abuse, mishandling, or roughness by hospital employees. In some states battered child laws are extended to cover certain incompetent patients and make failure to report any possible abuse a misdemeanor.

In attempting to provide the least restrictive possible setting for treating a potentially assaultive patient, one must also take into account one's responsibility for protecting other patients.

The degree to which legal commitment, and in some states other types of admission to a state mental hospital, affects the patient's civil rights (voting; obtaining a driver's license; etc.) varies. Ideally, no rights should be lost as a result of hospitalization itself.

A hospitalized patient may have certain specific rights (e.g., the right to have visitors; the right to make telephone calls) which for involuntary patients may be explicitly described in commitment laws, or which may simply be a matter of hospital policy. In either case, the physician must be familiar with these rights and see that they are observed. If a particular legal right is inappropriate for a specific patient (free access to the telephone is not desirable for a paraphilic patient who uses it to make obscene phone calls) one may need legal consultation about the handling of the situation.

Steps may be necessary to have conservators appointed in cases in which involuntarily hospitalized patients are unable to handle financial affairs. Other patients may need guardians to protect their interests.

Ethically, the right of the hospitalized patient to appropriate treatment is assumed. In a 1966 decision by Judge David L. Bazelon in a case against the superintendent of St. Elizabeth's Hospital in the District of Columbia (Rouse vs. Cameron) gave indication that for involuntary patients courts may enforce the right to treatment. Judge Bazelon held that if there is no treatment, the rationale for commitment disappears and the individual should be released. The more recent (June, 1975) United States Supreme Court decision in the Donaldson case (Donaldson vs. O'Connor) held in effect that if patients are capable of surviving outside an institution, are not dangerous, and are not receiving treatment, then there is no justification for their detention. The role of the mental hospital, therefore, is seen as a treatment facility, not a custodial one.

Another aspect of the right to treatment was involved in the case against one of the Alabama state hospitals (Wyatt vs. Stickney) in which the issue was the adequacy of treatment and living conditions within the facility. The court set minimum standards for care, including staffing patterns as well as physical facilities and other things related to living conditions.

Issues concerning the right to refuse treatment have been touched upon earlier in this chapter in the discussion of informed consent. Though some state laws specifically permit giving involuntary patients treatment without their consent under certain circumstances, the constitutionality of some of these laws is in question. In Utah, patients are deemed to have no right to refuse treatment for an illness that led to commitment, since a judicial determination of competency to refuse treatment is an integral part of the commitment procedure.

Since 1975 there have been several cases involving the right to refuse treatment that have gone to appellate courts. These include Rogers vs. Okin in Massachusetts, Rennie vs. Klein in New Jersey, A.E. & R.R. vs. Mitchell in Utah, and the United States vs. Leatherman in Washington, D.C. Widely different conclusions have been reached thus far. The scope of the right to refuse treatment and the procedure to override it remains unclear in most jurisdictions. In Massachusetts a complicated and time-consuming legal procedure is required and only a judge, using the standard of substituted judgment, can authorize administration of antipsychotic medication to a patient who refuses it in the absence of an emergency. In Utah, as indicated above, no special procedure is needed, as incompetence is established at the time of commitment. In New Jersey and in the District of Columbia, pending further litigation, authorization can be made on the basis of the in-hospital medical review.

In jurisdictions where there is no legal precedent, the physician treating involuntary patients should secure consent when possible, conform to state laws (and hope they prove to be constitutional), and work with the hospital staff and administration to establish review procedures that safeguard patients' rights.

There are some problems to be foreseen if courts or legislatures attempt to select the types of treatment suitable and appropriate for specific patients. The precedent set by some of the new commitment laws and by court decisions related to the right to treatment and the right to refuse treatment may have disturbing implications for medicine as a whole.

Confidentiality is an important responsibility to both inpatients and outpatients. It is important from the clinical point of view, for diagnosis and successful treatment often depend on the patient's candor. The patient can be candid in revealing damaging personal information only if he or she can be sure that it is confidential. From the legal point of view, revealing any information about a patient, even the fact that she or he is in treatment, may be libel. A libel is not, as is popularly supposed, something false and defamatory; it is the "publication" of anything damaging a person's reputation. While in an enlightened society it should not harm anyone's reputation to have it known that one has the good sense to seek professional help for personal problems, it might. For example, some employer might fail to promote a person to a responsible position on learning that the employee was in therapy. A political career can be damaged by publicity about previous psychiatric treatment even if complete recovery has taken place.

In the treatment of mildly ill voluntary outpatients, this responsibility creates no problems. The physician does not talk about persons under treatment (including questions about whether someone is being seen). No reports are furnished without the patient's signed consent. If a spouse or parent wants information, the need for confidentiality can be explained and cooperation is usually obtained.

In the care of more seriously ill patients, the physician may feel it imperative to maintain liaison with the family or, in some instances, the employer. For this one can usually obtain the patient's written permission. However, if the patient refuses permission, the psychiatrist may need to verify the legal responsibilities, which may in some instances override the responsibility for confidentiality. For example, if a married person's behavior endangers his or her life, the physician may be required to inform the spouse. If good relationships are maintained with patients, consent for reports that the doctor feels are indicated are usually obtained and exceptions are so rare that it is not unreasonable to suggest legal consultation when they occur.

A similar problem exists when a patient is threatening violence to someone. If the physician does not believe that there is real and immediate danger, as is often the case, records must clearly indicate this. If there is an immediate danger and the patient is unwilling to accept hospitalization, legal consultation may be desirable concerning possible involuntary hospitalization and/or warning to the intended victim. The Supreme Court of California ruled in 1974 (Tarasoff vs. Regents of the University of California) that in cases of danger a physician is legally obligated to warn the potential victim.

This ruling applies when the potential victim is known, not when the danger may be to any one of a large group of potential targets. In other words, if a paranoid patient has threatened to seek revenge against the legal profession by killing "some lawyer or other," one is not obligated to notify all members of the bar association. On the other hand, release of such a patient in disregard of the danger, could be a basis for a malpractice suit.

The Tarasoff decision creates some problems because of its likelihood of discouraging some people who need treatment from getting it and/or from being candid with their physicians. One obviously wants to prevent a patient's harming another person. This is not simply a duty to society, but is a duty to the patient as well since the patient, as well as the victim, suffers disastrous consequences from such an act.

Sometimes, a signed consent initiated by a third party should be viewed with some caution. A student, for example, may feel obligated or may even be under some pressure to furnish a report of psychiatric treatment to the dean. One may sign a consent and yet not really want a report sent. Usually, it is possible to furnish reports which satisfy the legitimate needs leading to the request without revealing information that the patient would rather keep confidential. However, in some situations, psychiatrists feel it best to decline to send a report even though the patient does consent in writing.

In many states the patient's talks with the psychiatrist are privileged communications. That is, the psychiatrist cannot be required to answer questions about them in court unless the patient waives privilege. As in general medicine, privileged communication is limited to those things revealed in connection with illness, but if a patient is treated with an expressive psychotherapy, everything disclosed is disclosed in connection with the illness. If the patient waives privilege, it usually must be waived completely. In a state in which privileged communication applies to the psychiatric interview, the following situation might arise: A divorced woman is in treatment. Her husband instituted legal proceedings to obtain custody of children, charging among other things that his wife's mental condition makes her unfit to care for them. The therapist's testimony might be sought by either husband or wife:

1. If the husband seeks it, the physician probably cannot be required (or even permitted) to testify unless the wife, acting on her lawyer's advice, elects to allow it.
2. If the wife requests testimony and the psychiatrist believes that her mental condition does not interfere with her ability to care for her children, she may waive privilege and have him or her called as a witness. In that case, however, questions may be asked in cross-examination about other things that she has discussed, some of which might be embarrassing. The psychiatrist could, with the patient's permission, confer with her lawyer and bring those things which might be disadvantageous or embarrassing to her to the attorney's attention. The lawyer would be able to advise the psychiatrist and the client of the probability of these things having to be discussed, and a decision could be reached as to whether it would actually be in the patient's best interest to waive privilege and call the psychiatrist as a witness.
3. If the wife wants the psychiatrist's testimony, but the psychiatrist cannot conscientiously testify in her behalf, it is unlikely that her attorney will want the therapist as a witness. A conference with the lawyer, with the patient's permission, would lead to a withdrawal of the request. Any exception to this would suggest a serious breakdown in communications (e.g., the lawyer might feel that the psychiatrist merely wished to avoid appearing in court, and if subpoenaed, could be forced to give information favorable to the client).

In the Lifschutz case in California (1970), though the defendant had waived privilege and asked the psychiatrist to disclose information, the psychiatrist, feeling that the disclosure would be harmful to the patient, refused and was held in contempt. The California Supreme Court ruled that there was no need for absolute confidentiality and gave the judge the right to decide what information was necessary.

The claim of privilege may be challenged if a communication is not made in private. This can create a problem in cases of patients in group or family therapy.

If the psychiatrist practices in a state in which the interviews are not regarded as privileged communication, if there are any exceptions, or if the records can be subpoenaed by a party hostile to the patient, one should know exactly under what circumstances one might be forced to testify about one's patients and under what circumstances one's records would cease to be confidential. In other cases, one may weigh more carefully the need for certain data and avoid particular lines of questioning (or keep the patient from introducing some types of information) unless it is absolutely necessary clinically. One must remember that patients asked to think aloud report fantasies as well as facts. In keeping records, because of the possible exceptions to confidentiality noted, and also because of the need to share a certain amount of information with third-party payers and peer review organizations, the physician must consider carefully what types of data are actually necessary and relevant, and avoid recording unnecessary anecdotal material.

The psychiatrist examining patients for a third party (an employer; the court; an insurance company) should not only have the patient's consent for the report but should be sure that both understand the purpose of the examination and the psychiatrist's role.

In some states, doing a procedure at the request of law enforcement authorities (e.g., obtaining a blood sample for a blood alcohol determination; performing a test for narcotic addiction; doing a diagnostic interview under intravenous sedation) may constitute an assault unless the patient freely consents. In other states, certain such procedures are permitted under the laws when properly requested by officials.

The responsibilities of nonmedical therapists are as yet not well defined. The nonphysician doing therapy in private practice needs legal advice to avoid violations of licensing laws and to determine what are the legal responsibilities to patients or clients. If the nonmedical therapist is an employee of the physician or works under the physician's direction, the physician is responsible; the therapist is the physician's agent. Referral for treatment by a nonmedical therapist not employed by the physician does not in itself terminate the doctor-patient relationship or free the physician from responsibility for the patient's care.

THE PSYCHIATRIST'S RESPONSIBILITIES AS AN EXPERT WITNESS

The physician may be asked to testify as an expert witness about the mental health of a patient, usually with specific reference to the patient's competence to discharge certain responsibilities as a citizen. Sometimes the patient involved is one whom the psychiatrist is treating or has treated (and the question of privileged communication arises). More often, the physician is asked to examine the patient by the court or by an attorney. Sometimes one is asked to testify on the basis of records concerning the patient or to give an opinion on a hypothetical question without having examined the patient. In legal proceedings a hypothetical question is assembled from material that has been introduced as evidence.

In a trial, the psychiatrist often is asked to testify by one side or the other. This leads to the "battle of experts" so often misunderstood by the layman. The differences in opinion brought out by the adversary method are usually related to legal definitions and requirements, not to medical diagnosis.

The ability of a mentally ill person to stand trial for a crime must sometimes be determined by the court, and a psychiatrist may be asked to examine the patient and testify on this point. This type of pretrial examination is intended to determine the accused person's condition at the time of examination rather than at the time of the alleged offense. In most states, a mentally ill person can be tried if:

1. He or she is capable of understanding the charges that have been made. This point is not always as simple as it may seem. The person might be able to name the crime with which he or she is charged and have no real idea of what is meant.
2. He or she is able to participate in his or her own defense. It may be difficult to determine whether a person who does not cooperate with an attorney is unable or merely unwilling to do so. An example of inability to participate in one's own defense: A patient with Dementia has gross defects in memory. Because of these, he is not able to furnish his attorney information about his activities at the time of an alleged offense.

If a patient is found unable to stand trial for a relatively minor offense, it is possible for him or her to be referred for voluntary or involuntary psychiatric treatment, if the condition is treatable, and the charges may be dropped. However, if the offense is serious, the charges usually will not be dropped and the patient will have to stand trial on becoming well enough to do so. This can lead to unfortunate situations. Suppose that the patient is innocent; in treatment, each time there is improvement he or she is faced with the stress of impending trial and may relapse. Likewise, in the case of an untreatable patient, this sort of situation could lead to a long period of institutional confinement which would not otherwise have occurred. However, in the case of Jackson vs. Indiana it was ruled that the defendant could be held for only a reasonable time in order to reach a degree of mental competence to permit standing trial. On this basis, if a defendant did not get well enough to stand trial in a reasonable length of time, charges would have to be dropped and some other disposition such as an ordinary legal commitment considered.

Determination of criminal responsibility is an entirely different matter from determining the ability to stand trial. It is concerned with the defendant's condition at the time of an alleged offense and might be utilized in a defense of not guilty by reason of insanity. The basic idea is a humanitarian one. There would be a general concurrence in our society that a person is not to be blamed if one does not know what one is doing or cannot help it. The implementation of this rather simple humanitarian principle in a way that prevents abuse has perplexed lawyers and psychiatrists for generations. Four basic formulas have influenced the development of legal requirements for the determination of criminal responsibility:

1.   The M'Naghten Rules
2.   The concept of irresistible impulse
3.   The Durham Rule
4.   The American Law Institute Formula

M'Naghten Rules

The M'Naghten Rules have been the basis for the statutes governing criminal responsibility in many states. They come to us from England where, in 1843, M'Naghten shot a Mr. Edward Drummond, the private secretary of Sir Robert Peel, the Prime Minister. There is little question that M'Naghten was mentally ill. He had apparently long harbored delusions about Sir Robert, for whom his bullet was actually intended. The jury found him not guilty by reason of insanity. In part because the case involved a prominent person, it achieved considerable notoriety and was the subject of much discussion. The House of Lords attempted to formulate rules by which in the future the defense of not guilty by reason of insanity would be regulated. In essence, these rules provide that a person is not guilty if he or she meets any of the following three criteria:

1.   He or she does not understand the nature and consequences of the act. Examples: (1) A patient in a delirium struggles with someone who is trying to put him to bed. He strikes the person and inflicts a serious injury. He is at the time disoriented for time, place, and person. He has no idea what he is doing. (2) A severe mental retardate picks up a gun and shoots someone. He knows that it is a gun "like in the movies," but he has no concept of death and no realization that what he has done is more than what healthy children might do with toy guns in a game.

2.   He or she does not know that the act is wrong. This is not a matter of ignorance of the law, but of inability to tell right from wrong.
3.   The act is the result of a delusion which would justify it. For example, if a paranoid patient believes that someone is spreading lies about him, depriving him of rightful property, or trifling with his wife, and he takes the law into his own hands and kills his supposed persecutor, he is *not* absolved from blame under this rule, since even if his beliefs had been true rather than delusional he should have sought legal redress instead of killing. However, if he believes he is killing someone in self-defense, or if he imagines that he is a soldier attacking the enemy he may be absolved from blame.

There is room for some difference of opinion as to how these rules are to be interpreted. A knowledge of the nature and consequences of acts or of right and wrong may be relative. However, by any interpretation of the M'Naghten Rules, it is obvious that many patients who are very sick mentally would be held responsible for criminal acts. These rules are intended to determine responsibility, not degree of illness.

The rules are usually not applicable if irresponsibility results from use of alcohol or drugs taken voluntarily and with a knowledge of the possible consequences. However, in those states which have enacted the Uniform Alcoholism and Intoxication Treatment Act and identify Alcoholism as an illness, it is quite possible that an alcoholic (or drug-dependent) person might be regarded as irresponsible when intoxicated.

Irresistible Impulse

Irresistible impulse has been recognized as a defense in some states. To establish that an act stems from an irresistible impulse it is usually necessary to show a lack of premeditation or preparation and to show that the urge to perform the act was so strong that it would be carried out whatever the circumstances (would he do it if there were a policeman standing at his shoulder?).

The concept of irresistible impulse would appear to be quite applicable to the compulsive behavior patterns which sometimes play a part in shoplifting, arson, some sex offenses, etc. (even auto theft, usually for "joy riding," may be compulsive), but more often it is invoked as a defense for a sudden outburst of violent behavior under stress, a type of temporary insanity which, if medically diagnosable at all, would perhaps fall in the classification of Adjustment Disorder, Impulse Control Disorder, or possibly some form of Personality Disorder. A catathymic crisis may lead to irresistible impulse.

Durham Rule

The Durham Rule, no longer in use, was based on a decision by Judge David L. Bazelon in the District of Columbia in 1954. The defendant's attorney cited an earlier precedent from the New Hampshire courts. The rule is, simply, that the accused is not criminally responsible if the unlawful act was the product of mental disease or mental defect. The word product here is an important one, and at times difficult to evaluate, since one cannot assume that all criminal acts of a mentally ill person result from the illness.

The American Law Institute Formula

In 1972 a new precedent superseded the Durham Rule in the District of Columbia as a result of the decision in the Brawner case (United States vs. Brawner). The Brawner decision utilized recommendations of the American Law Institute proposed in the Model Penal Code. This is essentially a "modified M'Naghten" and the definition of criminal responsibility includes the phrase "lacks substantial capacity either to appreciate the criminality (wrongfulness) of his conduct or conform ... to the law." The American Law Institute's recommendation excluded abnormalities manifested only by repeated criminal or antisocial conduct. It differs from the M'Naghten Rule in two ways. The word substantial adds some flexibility. Reference to the ability to conform to the law introduces a volitional element which incorporates the concept of irresistible impulse.

Proposed Changes in the Insanity Defense

In the past, when capital punishment was more widely used, the insanity defense was employed primarily to spare the offender's life. A patient found not guilty by reason of insanity was likely to be committed to a hospital for the criminally insane or to a state hospital with a maximum security unit, and in the absence of a recovery was likely to remain in such a facility for life. In the 1970s changes in laws governing involuntary hospitalization led to some concern about an increased probability of early release for offenders found not guilty by reason of insanity. It was felt that some such patients might not display dangerousness by threats or overt acts while in the hospital, but might still be dangerous to others if discharged. For example, a patient who is asymptomatic and not dangerous while taking medication might discontinue medication and relapse.

An impetus to reinspection of the insanity defense was provided by John Hinckley's acquittal by reason of insanity on charges of attempting to assassinate President Reagan. Some states have changed their laws and a number of others have considered or are considering changes.

Both the American Psychiatric Association and the American Bar association have endorsed the elimination of the volitional component (capacity to conform conduct to the requirements of law) from the American Law Institute Formula. The American Medical Association has recommended abolition of the insanity defense. However, it recommends statutes providing for acquittal when a defendant as a result of mental disease lacks the state of mind (mens rea) required as an element of the offense charged. This may represent a distinction, but little real difference, from the cognitive portion of the M'Naghten Rule.

Some states (e.g., Arizona) have placed the burden of proof on the defendant. This requires the defendant to prove that he is not guilty, by reason of insanity, by clear and convincing evidence. This departs from the basic concept that one is innocent until proven guilty and that prosecution has the responsibility for proof.

The American Medical Association recommendations include, for defendants who do not satisfy criteria for acquittal under mens rea provisions, considering mental illness as a factor in mitigation of sentence. There is reasonable doubt that this would provide treatment not otherwise available for prisoners and some likelihood that it would lead to plea bargaining. While possibly advantageous in some cases, in others it could lead to premature release of dangerous persons.

This concept of diminished responsibility is somewhat similar to proposals for a possible sentence of guilty but mentally ill for persons who do not meet the criteria for not guilty by reason of insanity. This has been criticized as being likely to confuse juries that might see it as a compromise between guilty and not guilty by reason of insanity, though it would not really change the significance of a guilty verdict.

Despite its problems, caution should be used in advocating the elimination of the insanity defense. The entire body of law relating to responsibility, civil and criminal, takes into account intent and understanding. Perhaps the solution to the problem of the insanity defense lies in furnishing juries better bases for evaluating that defense, and in modifying commitment laws to provide better safeguards against the premature release of the mentally ill dangerous offender, while at the same time not preventing the release of the mentally ill offender who has recovered and is no longer a danger to society. Only thus can there be an adequate balance between considerations relating to the rights of the individual, whatever he or she may have done, and those relating to the rights, including the safety, of the public.

In 1983 the Supreme Court ruled that persons found not guilty by reason of insanity can be held in a mental hospital under a less rigorous standard of proof (of continuing danger, for example) than is required for civilly committed patients (Jones vs. United States). This can be taken into account in revising state commitment laws.

The ability to make a will (testamentary capacity) is another legal question on which psychiatric testimony may be sought. When this does not concern one of the physician's own patients, one must sometimes testify in response to a hypothetical question based upon evidence concerning a deceased person. Sometimes the psychiatrist is asked to examine a person about to make a will. To make a valid will, a person must know that he or she is making a will and the person's mental state must be such that he or she:

1.   Knows the value of the estate (not necessarily to the penny)
2.   Is capable of knowing who might logically be among the heirs
3.   Is not turned against any possible heir by a delusion
4.   Is not pathologically suggestible or abnormally susceptible to persuasion

To make a contract, a person must be able to understand the significance of making such an agreement; he or she must be able to deliberate upon it (not necessarily being able to understand all technicalities, but being able to recognize points on which he or she may require information or professional advice) and must be able to give consent (i.e., a delusional belief that one was acting under duress might impair the capacity to consent).

Marriage requires an ability to understand the nature of that contract and the responsibilities it involves. It is usually invalid if the person consents because of a delusional belief. Concealment of mental illness is usually a basis for annulment. The mentally ill person, having grounds, can usually seek a divorce (there are exceptions in the case of committed patients in some states). Mental illness does not, in itself, excuse a patient who has given the spouse other grounds for divorce if the patient is capable of contesting the action (able to understand it, and able to cooperate with the attorney). Mental illness itself is usually a basis for divorce only if it has required a set number of years of hospitalization and is incurable.

Patients are sometimes afraid (and sometimes threatened by a spouse seeking divorce) that being under psychiatric treatment or having a history of mental hospital care will be a reason for denial of custody of children. This is unlikely. Usually, the evidence concerning the type of care given the children, their emotional growth and development, and the patient's behavior around them is more relevant to the capacity to be a good parent than is the existence of emotional disorder and personal problems, past or present.

The ability to testify in court (an issue, for example, if a mentally ill or retarded person witnesses a crime) usually depends on the ability to observe and render a correct account, together with the ability to understand the meaning of an oath or affirmation.

Mental health prior to suicide is occasionally an issue. Sometimes an insurance policy can be paid only if the suicide is "while insane," and, in some cases, suicide "while insane" offers increased indemnity comparable to accident. Unless there are specific legal rules to the contrary, evidence of a psychosis (with depressive elements or with other features that might account for suicide) is adequate.

Obtaining compensation for emotional illness caused by another's negligence (e.g., mental illness following an industrial accident; an automobile accident) is subject to rapidly changing legal precedents. At one time it was often necessary to establish that brain damage resulted from the accident. This led to a great deal of attention being paid to precise differential diagnosis between mild Organic Brain Syndromes with post-traumatic neurotic manifestations and neuroses precipitated by trauma. Often, cases showed a mixture of findings, and conflicting testimony was frequent. The distinction, to the extent that it can be made, is useful in planning treatment and in arriving at a prognosis, but now it is less often legally necessary, since the neurosis itself is usually compensable if liability can be established. Even a horrifying experience with no injury to the body itself can be compensable if it results in mental illness.

The physician may be asked to testify as to the existence of the illness, the degree of suffering, the amount of disability for gainful occupation, the prognosis, and the possible cost of medical care. These can usually be determined clinically.

The cause and effect relationship between injury, or traumatic experience, and illness may present more of a problem. The probability that the experience could cause the illness or make an existing illness worse can be estimated. However, the question of possible onset prior to, or subsequent and unrelated to, a trauma depends on history. History from the patient, not under oath, during mental examination, is not adequate evidence. The examining physician must sometimes advise the attorney what information is needed in evidence for one to form an opinion from the history.

Proof of malingering is more a job for a detective than a psychiatrist, but the psychiatrist, if he or she cannot form an opinion, may be able to advise about what data would be necessary as evidence to form one. The existence of, and even some abuse of, secondary gain does not establish malingering (most of us have managed to enjoy a fringe benefit or two when we've been sick or injured, if nothing more than a little unneeded attention from a friendly nurse). Being able to engage in recreational activities does not necessarily mean that one is able to work. More precise proof that fraudulent claims are being made is necessary.

The physician caring for the person who has a mental illness following trauma must take into account in advising the patient and the attorney the effect of the stress of prolonged litigation or court appearances on the patient. Sometimes a settlement is preferable from a medical standpoint. However, the popular notion that lump sum compensation as opposed to continued benefits shortens illness lacks scientific proof.

CODES OF ETHICS

The physician should be familiar with the codes of conduct of the professional organizations to which he or she belongs. For the psychiatrist, the Principles of

Medical Ethics with Annotations Especially Applicable to Psychiatry is required reading. Penalties for violation of such codes of conduct range from admonition to expulsion. The significance of being disciplined by a professional organization is not that one is prevented from attending meetings and receiving publications, but that it may influence one's ability to secure licenses and hospital staff privileges. If one is accused of unethical conduct, one should seek legal advice.

PSYCHIATRISTS AND LAWYERS

The psychiatrist can help lawyers, their clients, and the community by sharing knowledge with the legal profession. The psychiatrist who can devote some time to teaching in law schools or who is willing to conduct seminars for groups of lawyers can help them do a better job of protecting the interests of the mentally ill. Medical organizations should make themselves heard when new laws relating to mental illness are under consideration.

In some cases a psychiatrist may be of more value to a lawyer, and serve the ends of justice better, as a consultant than as a witness. Helping the lawyer understand a client's condition, or helping him or her know what facts are medically relevant, should be sought as evidence, or brought out in direct or cross-examination, can be highly useful.

The psychiatrist who is asked to examine a patient as a possible medical witness should have a clear idea of the problem to be solved by the examination (if he or she is able to form an opinion) and of the legal definitions of sanity, responsibility, competence, etc., involved. One should get some impression of whether testimony will be required or if a report will be sufficient, though often the lawyer cannot be sure. One may want to know, insofar as the lawyer can predict, when the testimony will be required, about how long he or she will be away from the office, and the likelihood of arranging a convenient time. In planning the time commitment, one should usually discuss the probability of a pretrial conference. The lawyer should, but may not, request this. The physician should be sure the lawyer understands the report and its implications. One should know what questions are likely to be asked.

Financial arrangements should be clearly understood. Local medical societies may have policies concerning these. Usually, one charges a basic consultation fee and an hourly charge for additional time involved. If a fixed fee is offered, or preferred, it should be adequate to compensate for time that may be used in addition to the examination and actual court appearance. Time used in conferences and in reviewing records or medical literature should be considered. The offer of a fee based on the contingency of the patient's obtaining a judgment is usually rejected on ethical grounds. One should know who will pay the fee and when. Some law firms will pay for consultations themselves; others pass the bill on to the client, who may not be a good credit risk (especially if the lawyer decides she or he cannot use the testimony, or if the client loses the case). When the court has authorized consultation (e.g., for an indigent), payment may not take place until the case is settled.

Some psychiatrists, in a wish to help an unfortunate person, set unreasonably low fees, and when they encounter greater time expenditures than were expected, difficulties in collection, and some unpleasantness in court become resistive to court work. There are times when one wants to, and should, donate time and effort. Also, there is a place for organized medicine to provide panels of experts to serve those who cannot afford consultation and to encourage the development of court clinics.

On the witness stand, the physician must understand his or her role and that of the lawyers if justice is to be served. One is there not to take sides, but to furnish information, to answer questions asked. One should know the legal situation and anticipate the questions asked. One should plan to answer in language understandable to the layman and should be prepared to explain how he or she arrived at the professional opinion, if this is requested. One should know if asked to answer a question "Yes or No" that one may go on and qualify one's answer. If a lawyer attempts to prevent this, and the other attorney does not object, one may ask the judge if one may have leeway to amplify. If something relative must be put in absolute terms, one must understand the degrees involved. In psychiatric research, a measure of probability that allows one chance in a thousand for error may not be convincing enough to warrant a positive statement. In some legal situations one can allow an even greater possibility of error or chance and still give definite testimony.

A witness should address, look at, the judge and speak loudly enough that the court reporter can hear distinctly. One can best maintain dignity during cross-examination if one recognizes the nature of the adversary method and realizes that what may appear to be an attack on professional ability, if not character as well, is impersonal and part of the job. One should let it serve to help bring out truth, not temper, or even irony. If an attorney asks a question that causes one to say something that is in apparent contradiction to previous testimony, one should be calm (and not act trapped, though one may be at the moment treated as if "caught"), and usually should wait to be asked (perhaps by the other lawyer, later) for an explanation of the seeming ambiguity. One should not hesitate to say, "I don't know," or to admit a failure to understand a question.

Do not hesitate to ask to have a question repeated or clarified; one should never try to answer a question that one does not understand. If asked what one is being paid for one's testimony, one should remember that payment is not for the testimony but for one's time. The reply is phrased accordingly.

It is usually possible if asked about charts and records to ask to look at them to refresh one's recollection. Sometimes one is asked if he or she read a certain book. Often this is a reference book that no one in his or her right mind, except possibly the author and the publisher, has actually read. Say No unless you have read it word for word (the same edition). You may be read passages from it anyway to help bring out medical facts. Often a lawyer will ask if someone is an authority; this generally means he or she will quote something out of context from that authority that sounds contrary to something you are expected to say so that you will apparently be proved wrong by someone you acknowledge as an authority. No one is an authority on every aspect of medicine, and even a person who is an authority on similar cases would not expect generalizations to apply to all cases automatically and without individual study. He or she may know the subject, but no one can be an authority on a particular case without having examined the patient (or at least studied the patient's records). If this sort of use of "authorities" is likely in cross-examination, one might get some guidance as to how to handle the situation in pretrial conference in order to avoid a discussion of a textbook rather than the case in point.

When a lawyer wishes to see the psychiatrist about one of the doctor's patients, the first thing to do is to ascertain the purpose. If it deals with the patient's hospitalization, treatment program, or rights, it is important to remember the lawyer's role as an adversary. Though one does not think of oneself as the patient's adversary, that will probably be the way that the lawyer structures the situation. One may see the lawyer privately to discuss the purpose of his or her intervention, and if the lawyer's wishes can be accommodated or a reasonable compromise seems achievable, one may discuss the problem. However, if the lawyer brings up an issue that is not readily resolved, one avoids comment until one has consulted one's own attorney. Arguments are to be avoided; not only are they unlikely to accomplish anything, but they may create additional problems.

Health law in general, and mental health law in particular, are growing legal subspecialties. If one accepts this fact and attempts to understand the role and viewpoint of the legal profession, one can deal with it effectively.

REVIEW QUESTIONS

1. What are the laws in your state governing the involuntary admission of patients to psychiatric hospitals? What improvements would you suggest in them? Why?

2. What is meant by informed consent? What should a patient be told about electroconvulsive therapy before agreeing to it? Should the patient's spouse be given the same information? Why?

3. A patient in therapy says that he has stolen valuable tools from his employer. Should this be reported to the employer? To the police? What else should be done?

4. A political figure is arrested during a riot. Though there is apparently a great deal of evidence against her, she claims innocence. She claims the charge is nonsense and that she is framed by political opponents. You are asked to examine her before her trial. She has no wish to plead not guilty by reason of insanity. What should you try to establish during your examination?

5. Discuss the history of the insanity defense, including recent changes and proposed changes. What are the laws in your state? What changes, if any, would you recommend in them?

6. Discuss the right to refuse treatment. Under what circumstances do you feel that it should be overridden? Are your opinions compatible with laws and court decisions affecting practice in your community?

7. A newspaper reporter asks you about the mental health of a prominent person who has made some revealing statements about himself on television. You have not examined the person and do not have his consent for making a statement about him. Is it ethical for you to offer an opinion? Is it legal?

8. A voluntary patient refuses to take medication. He is told that if he does not take it, he will be committed to a state hospital. He then consents. Is his consent valid? How should the situation have been handled?

9. A nurse reports that a hospitalized patient is writing crazy letters to a number of public officials, and asks if they should be read by someone on the staff before they are sent. What is your reply? Why?

10. An elderly gentleman asks you to examine him at the request of his attorney. He wishes to leave the bulk of his estate to a housekeeper and feels that his children may contest his will. Describe the examination you would perform. What specific facts should you include in your records?

SELECTED REFERENCES

1. American Medical Association Committee on Medicolegal Problems Board of Trustees: Insanity defense in criminal trials and limitation of psychiatric testimony. *JAMA* 251(22):2967-2981, 1984.

2. American Psychiatric Association: *The Principles of Medical Ethics: With Annotations Especially Applicable to Psychiatry.* 1981 Edition Revised. Washington, D.C., American Psychiatric Association, 1982.

3. American Psychiatric Association Insanity Defense Work Group: American Psychiatric Association statement on the insanity defense. *Am J Psychiatry* 140(6):681-688, 1983.

4. Appelbaum, Paul S.: Do the mentally disabled have the right to be physicians? *Hosp Community Psychiatry* 33(5):351-352, 1982.

5. Appelbaum, Paul S.: Refusing treatment: The uncertainty continues. *Hosp Community Psychiatry* 34(1):11-12, 1983.

6. Cooper, Almeta E.: Duty to warn third parties. *JAMA* 248(4):431-432, 1982.

7. Deveaugh-Geiss, Joseph: Informed consent for neuroleptic therapy. *Am J Psychiatry* 136(7):959-962, 1979.

8. Ennis, Bruce, and Loren Siegel: *The Rights of Mental Patients.* New York, Avon Books, 1973.

9. Hiday, Virginia Aldige: Are lawyers enemies of psychiatrists? A survey of civil commitment counsel and judges. *Am J Psychiatry* 140(3):323-326, 1983.

10. Horan, Dennis J., and Robert J. Milligan: Recent developments in psychiatric malpractice. *Behavioral Sciences and the Law* 1(1):23-37, 1983.

11. Knapp, Samuel, and Leon Vandecreek: Malpractice risks with suicidal patients. *Psychotherapy: Theory, Research and Practice* 20(3):274-280, 1983.

12. Lebegue, Breck, and Lincoln D. Clark: Incompetence to refuse treatment: A necessary condition for civil commitment. *Am J Psychiatry* 138(8):1075-1077, 1981.

13. Mills, Mark J., Thomas G. Gutheil, Mary Ann Igneri, and Lester Grinspoon: Mental patients' knowledge of in-hospital rights. *Am J Psychiatry* 140(2):225-228, 1983.

14. Mills, Mark J., Jerome A. Yesavage, and Thomas G. Gutheil: Continuing case law development in the right to refuse treatment. *Am J Psychiatry* 140(6):715-719, 1983.

15. Neugebauer, Richard: Medieval and early modern theories of mental illness. *Arch Gen Psychiatry* 36(4):477-483, 1979.

16. Perr, Irwin N.: The insanity defense: A tale of two cities. *Am J Psychiatry* 140(7):873-876, 1983.

17. Rachlin, Stephen, Abraham L. Halpern, and Stanley L. Portnow: The volitional rule, personality disorders and the insanity defense. *Psychiatr Ann* 14(2):139-147, 1984.

18. Roth, Loren H., Alan Meisel, and Charles W. Lidz: Tests of competency to consent to treatment. *Am J Psychiatry* 134(3):279-284, 1977.

19. Schetky, Diane H., and James L. Cavanaugh: Child psychiatry perspective: Psychiatric malpractice. *J Am Acad Child Psychiatry* 21(5):521-526, 1982.

20. Slovenko, Ralph: Commentaries on psychiatry and law: "Guilty but mentally ill." *J of Psychiatry and Law* 10(4):541-555, 1982.

21. Slovenko, Ralph: The hazards of writing or disclosing information in psychiatry. *Behavioral Sciences and the Law* 1(1):109-127, 1983.

22. Stickney, Stonewall: Wyatt v. Stickney: The right to treatment. *Psychiatr Ann* 4(8):32-45, 1974.

23. Stone, Alan A.: Informed consent: Special problems for psychiatry. *Hosp Community Psychiatry* 30(5):321-327, 1979.

24. Wettstein, Robert M.: Tardive dyskinesia and malpractice. *Behavioral Sciences and the Law* 1(1):85-107, 1983.

25. Wickware, D. M.: The insanity defense -- Should it be revised? *Psychiatr J Univ Ottawa* 8(4):198-201, 1983.

26. Yesavage, Jerome A.: A study of mandatory review of civil commitment. *Arch Gen Psychiatry* 41(3):305-308, 1984.

Chapter 24

THE HISTORY OF PSYCHIATRY

ANCIENT MEDICINE

People in primitive cultures considered illnesses of all kinds to be manifestations of the supernatural. Mental illness particularly was thought to result from posession by evil spirits and demons or as a consequence of incurring the disfavor of the gods. Diagnosis and treatment were, therefore, functions of priests, medicine men, or witch doctors. Records of such medical practices can be found in the earliest of recorded history. For example, one of the early priest-physicians was Imhotep of Egypt. He was an advisor to the Pharoah's family in about 5000 B.C. and was later deified. References to mental disorders occur in the Old Testament. Ancient Hindu writings contain observations on mental disorders similar to those recorded by the early Greek physicians and philosophers.

GRECO-ROMAN MEDICINE

In ancient Greece, the healing arts were practiced in temples dedicated to Aesculapius. People went to the temples to be cured of their sicknesses through purification (by bathing, sacrifice, herbs, and religious ceremonies) and incubation (sleep in which the person was to dream of the illness and awaken cured). Aesculapius was a chieftain and physician who had a talent for healing. He practiced with his sons around 1200 B.C. and was considered to be half god.

During the sixth century B.C. emotions and emotional problems, as well as many physical disorders, were considered to be in the domain, not of the physicians, but of the philosophers such as Heraclitus, Empedocles, and Protagoras. In the fourth century B.C. Hippocrates, a physician, observed and described several mental disorders. From his descriptions these would now be recognized as delirium (his term was phrenites), Mania, postpartum psychoses, Melancholia, Paranoia, and epilepsy. He observed these disorders and described them with remarkable accuracy; he explained them by the humoral theory, which was originated by Pythagorus two centuries previously.

Plato, and later Aristotle, described several mental disorders. Plato considered the brain to be the seat of the soul and the sense receptors, but Aristotle thought these functions lay in the heart.

In Alexandria, at about the same time (300 B.C.), Herophilus and Erasistratus investigated the brain and peripheral nerves by dissection.

One of the earliest Roman physicians was Asclepiades, in the second century B.C. He was a capable clinician who devised treatments utilizing diet, pleasant surroundings, and some forms of hydrotherapy. He described hallucinations, illusions, and delusions, and although he did not use these terms, he distinguished among them. He also differentiated the clinical features of acute and chronic disorders.

Celsus compiled the medical knowledge up to the first century A.D., including the views of Hippocrates and Asclepiades. He described many of the prevailing methods of treatment, including restraint in chains, bloodletting, purging, starvation, and beatings for mental patients.

Aretaeus of Cappadocia was also a historian. He is credited with the observation that Mania and Melancholia were phases of the same disorder. He described the clinical manifestations of Senile Dementia, Hysteria, and the aura phenomenon of epilepsy.

The writings of Caelius Aurelianus presented a summary of treatment practices recommended by the physician Soranus and critically reviewed the treatments in vogue during his time. Soranus was opposed to inhumane treatment methods and suggested that patients be treated according to their individual needs and backgrounds. He did not believe in using the purges and hypnotics common to the treatment practices of his time; instead, he suggested proper food, comfortable surroundings, and freedom from irritating or exciting contacts.

In the second century A.D., Galen described several neurological disorders, but wrote little about psychiatric illness except to comment on amnesia and migraine. However, his awareness of emotional factors of disease was evident in his clinical work. Galen collected the medical knowledge of the past and added his own observations. His work was to influence medical thought for the next 16 centuries. After Galen's time, medicine, especially psychiatry, was appropriated by religion, superstition, and magic. Until the fourth century A.D., little provision had been made for care of the mentally ill in hospitals. Wards to care for people suffering from mental disorders were established in a few of the general hospitals founded in the fourth century A.D. A hospital for the mentally ill was built in Jerusalem in the fifth century A.D.

THE DARK AGES

As Western medicine declined, progress in investigation, description, and treatment continued in the Near East until about the eleventh century, by men such as Aetius of Mesopotamia and Alexander Thralles in the sixth century; Paul of Aegina in the seventh; Rhazes of Bagdad in the ninth; and Avicenna of Persia in the eleventh century. Mental illnesses were described in detail and treatment was more humane than that of the European countries.

Astrology, alchemy, demonology, and sorcery were prevalent in the Dark Ages. Some treatments of mental illness were by exorcism, by the influence of saintly relics employed by the religious leaders, or by the incantations and magic of the sorcerers. The belief in witchcraft and demonology spread throughout Europe and remained long after the coming of the Renaissance. Seeking out, torturing, and burning accused witches was common practice for several centuries. Some accused witches were no doubt mentally ill; others were simply peculiar, and some were accused for political reasons or out of enmity. Two monks, Sprenger and Kraemer, wrote a book, *Malleus Maleficarum,* the *Witches Hammer,* in the fifteenth century. This document, which served as a basis for the investigation and prosecution of witches by the Church for three centuries, argued that anyone could be bewitched, outlined the forms that bewitching could take, related clinical histories of persons convicted of being witches, described means of identifying witches, and set forth the proceedings for sentencing and executing them.

Though demonology was a prevalent theory of madness during medieval times, it was not universally accepted. There were rational physicians and scholars who believed that mental illness had natural causes. Barotholomaeus, a thirteenth century monk, was among these.

It is difficult to evaluate the impact of opponents of superstition and demonology or to know just how widely demonology was actually believed.

Evidence of the more enlightened views of madness is found in the fact that many hospitals were founded during this period. In Fez, Bagdad, and Cairo in the eighth century, and in Damascus and Aleppo in the thirteenth century, hospitals were established which made provisions for treatment of the mentally ill. In Europe, mental hospitals were founded in Metz and Braunschweiger in the twelfth and thirteenth centuries, and the people of the village of Gheel in Belgium began caring for the mentally ill in their homes in the twelfth century. The Hotel Dieu in Paris was built in 652 as a hostel for aged clergy and was not used for the care of the insane until 1660, the year the famous Bicetre of Paris was built. In England, the priory of St. Mary of Bethlehem, better known as Bedlam, was built in the thirteenth century and has a history of continuous service for the treatment of the insane since the fourteenth century. The first mental hospital on the American continent was built at San Hipolito in Mexico in the sixteenth century.

THE SIXTEENTH CENTURY

In the sixteenth century, a few men opposed the mainstream of thought on witchcraft and possession. Among them were three contemporaries: Vives, Paracelsus, and Agrippa. Juan Vives, a Spanish philosopher who formulated principles of human psychology, emphasized the need to understand the workings of the mind and the importance of the emotions in the processes of remembering and forgetting. His descriptions of the drives of men were similar to the formulations of Sigmund Freud three centuries later. Vives recommended kindly treatment of the mentally ill. Paracelsus (Theophrastus Bombastus von Hohenheim) was an argumentative rebellious physician who rejected demonology. He emphasized treatment more than theory and utilized alchemy, astrology, and mysticism. In his writings were the beginnings of a formulation of the unconscious motivation of the Neuroses. Cornelius Agrippa was also a physician, a restless, brilliant inventor, who was disliked and persecuted for his opposition to the torture of suspected witches. His dog, a black French poodle, named Monsieur, was rumored to be an incarnation of the devil. For 3 years prior to his death he taught a young student who was destined to make great contributions to Renaissance psychiatry, Johan Weyer. After studying with Agrippa, Weyer became a physician. He was a serious student, a careful observer, and an able clinician. Although he made several contributions to medicine, among them the invention of a vaginal speculum and a description of scurvy, his major interest was in mental diseases. He opposed the popular beliefs in demonology and attacked them with simple logical reasoning. In his *De Praestigiis Daemonum,* he pointed out that the majority of men and women who were accused of witchcraft were sick people who should be treated by physicians.

He spoke out against the monks who used torture to obtain confessions from suspected witches. He observed that some of the manifestations of possession could result from ingestion of drugs such as belladonna or opium. He noted that those thought to be bewitched were suggestible and that mass contagion of hysterical illness could be avoided or ended by separation of the afflicted ones. In his clinical records there were accurate descriptions of many clinical entities, among them the condition now called Schizophrenia.

Jean Bodin, a lawyer, opposed Weyer. He held to the traditional views and protested Weyer's interference in areas which Bodin thought were rightfully legal and theological, not medical. A few years later, Paul Zacchias, a physician who devoted himself to medicolegal matters, also opposed Weyer's views. As Weyer is often called the first clinical psychiatrist, Zacchias has been called the founder of legal medicine.

Soon after Weyer published *De Praestigiis Daemonum,* Reginald Scot, in England, published *Discovery of Witchcraft.* He denied that witches existed and called them imaginary conceptions. His views were immediately countered by King James I in *Demonology.*

Belief in witchcraft prevailed in colonial America, reaching a peak in the Salem witch trials of 1692.

THE SEVENTEENTH CENTURY

Felix Plater, late in the sixteenth and early in the seventeenth century, went into the dungeons where the mentally ill were housed, studied the people he found there, and evolved a classification of mental disorders. He divided mental illness into acquired, congenital, and hereditary types.

In the seventeenth century the course of psychiatric thinking was influenced primarily by philosophers such as Francis Bacon, and by neurologists and neuro-anatomists such as Thomas Sydenham and Thomas Willis. Willis advocated harsh treatment of the mentally ill. Treatment had remained the same for centuries and was essentially restraint in chains, bloodletting, and purgatives. Willis observed material from his dissections of cerebral pathology and described clinical conditions such as apoplexy, idiocy, Melancholia, and Mania, which he, too, proposed were different stages of the same illness. He recognized general paralysis of the insane as a disease entity.

Hysteria had been attributed to the wanderings of the uterus and this etiology had been accepted for centuries. Charles Lepois proposed that the cause of Hysteria was to be found in the brain and emotions, not the uterus.

THE EIGHTEENTH CENTURY

George Ernest Stahl, early in the eighteenth century, emphasized the relationship of the mind and the body. He divided mental illnesses into those of mental or emotional origin, and those of physical origin. He observed the interaction between mind and body, citing as an example vomiting from emotional causes.

Classification became attractive to scholars of the eighteenth century. Francois deSauvages, in France, published a systematic disease classification, including over 300 pages devoted to mental illnesses. Others interested in devising classifications of mental diseases were William Cullen, Erasmus Darwin, and Immanuel Kant. Cullen, in Scotland, is thought to have originated the term Neurosis.

General hospitals and jails had housed the mentally ill for centuries, along with paupers and other prisoners. Treatment was rare and inmates were chained, starved, beaten, and bled. However, it should not be assumed that all mentally ill people were institutionalized, locked up for life, and tortured. Many remained with their families or elsewhere in the community. Those that were confined were often confined for relatively short periods of time.

Jean Columbiere, physician in charge of the Hotel Dieu prior to the French Revolution, was disturbed by the lack of public interest in the mentally ill. He protested the vile living conditions and lack of treatment in the hospitals. Physicians in other countries began to demand humane treatment of the insane about the same time. One of these was Vincenzo Chiarugi in Italy. In England, William Tuke, a Quaker layman, founded the York Retreat, a model hospital providing humane care. Tuke insisted that the patients should have personal attention, work or other occupations, good living conditions, and freedom from mechanical restraints.

Johann Reil, a neurologist, contributed not only to knowledge of the anatomy of the cerebellum, but also described emotional disorders. He is credited with originating the term psychiatry. He advocated psychological treatment of the insane by what he called noninjurious torture, throwing patients suddenly into water, firing cannons, and arousing such emotions as anger and disgust.

Joseph Daquin, in France, believed that the mental hospital was a place for treatment and research, not for confinement alone. He encouraged attention to moral treatment of the insane. His views were similar to those of a somewhat younger French physician, Philippe Pinel. Pinel was physician-in-chief of the Bicêtre and Salpêtrière in Paris during the French Revolution, under both Napoleon and the Bourbons. He was shocked by the conditions in the hospitals at the time he took charge and obtained permission to free the inmates from their chains, no small accomplishment during the political turmoil of the revolutionary days. Although Pinel wrote extensively on psychiatric illness, he is remembered for his contributions to hospital reforms.

Anton Mesmer arrived in Paris in the same year as Pinel. He became famous for his animal magnetism, also known as mesmerism, a treatment by touch and trance induction which produced somnambulism, convulsions, and anesthesia. His methods found favor with Neurotics of the time and he was popular with the public, but his theory and practices were questioned by reputable physicians. His greatest successes were in curing hysterical illness. Interest in hypnotism, as the surgeon, James Braid, renamed Mesmer's animal magnetism, increased; it became more widely used as a therapeutic tool when Charcot, the neurologist who described tabes, amyotrophic lateral sclerosis, and multiple sclerosis, established his Salpêtrière School of Hypnosis. Charcot used hypnosis primarily as a tool in the investigation of Hysteria. Its therapeutic use was boosted by A. A. Liebeault and Hippolyte Bernheim, who together founded the Nancy School of Hypnosis. They used hypnosis to investigate and treat the Neuroses. Charcot proposed that only Hysterics could be hypnotized, but Bernheim claimed that nearly all people are susceptible to suggestion.

The French physician, Benedict Morel, was a clinician and a scholar. His particular interests were medicolegal problems and historical studies of the medical literature of several European countries and the United States. His orientation was largely organic, with his first studies being confined to goiter and cretinism and his later ones to degenerative disorders. He described Dementia precoce, which he considered to be precursor of what is now called Schizophrenia.

Francis J. Gall, a neuroanatomist and neurophysiologist, devised a system for character reading which he called phrenology. He attempted to relate conformation of the surface of the skull to character traits, on the theory that these traits were the product of under- or overdevelopment of certain areas of the brain, and that this was reflected in changes in the surface of the skull.

In colonial America, no hospital facilities were available for the care of the insane until 1752, when the Pennsylvania Hospital was built, and a ward was designated for the care of the mentally ill. Until that time the insane were housed in poorhouses, blockhouses, and jails. The first American mental hospital was the Eastern Lunatic Hospital at Williamsburg, Virginia, founded in 1773.

One of the early members of the staff on the Pennsylvania Hospital was a Quaker physician who had signed the Declaration of Independence, Benjamin Rush. He has been called the Father of American Psychiatry. He treated patients kindly and insisted upon clean living conditions. However, he advocated surprise baths, restraint, some forms of punishment, and the use of mechanical devices such as a gyrator and tranquilizer chair which he invented. He introduced important reforms into the hospital such as the use of work, exercise, and amusement, and he advocated segregation of the mildly ill from the severely ill. He classified mental disease into two groups, general and partial intellectual derangement. He wrote the first treatise on psychiatry published in America.

THE NINETEENTH CENTURY

Progress in psychiatry was rapid in Europe, especially in France, during the nineteenth century. Pinel's reforms were continued by his pupil, Esquirol, who was an able teacher and administrator. Esquirol was one of the first to apply statistical methods in hospital administration. He called attention to psychological factors in the etiology of mental illness and is said to be the first to introduce the term hallucination. He was interested in criminal psychology, but prison reform and the criminally insane were the primary focus of another of Pinel's pupils, Ferrus. Ferrus initiated what was later to be called occupational therapy by establishing a farm where the patients could work. He disagreed strongly with the Englishman, John Conolly, on the matter of what Conolly called nonrestraint. Conolly urged the abolition of all mechanical restraints, a concept which stirred a great deal of controversy in Europe and America. He was supported by a fellow Englishman, Robert Hill, who demonstrated the value of nonrestraint at the Lincoln Asylum, and was opposed by Isaac Ray in America, who preferred mechanical restraints to manual restraint by attendants. From Conolly and Hill's campaign to remove restraints came the beginning of the "open door" system which gave patients freedom to move around in the hospital and, later, in the community.

Jean Falret was one of Esquirol's students. He was especially interested in depression and suicidal drives. He noted the relationship of periods of elation and depression and called this disorder the circular insanity.

Although the French psychiatrists emphasized the psychological aspects of mental illness, they held to the idea that mental disease was the product of specific lesions of the brain or meninges. In keeping with this neurophysiological orientation, Falret and others such as Baillarger, Bayle, and Calmeil contributed to the establishment of criteria for the diagnosis of general paralysis, which John Haslam had previously described. Although syphilitic infection was suspected to be involved in the etiology of general paresis during the early and middle nineteenth century, the spirochetes of *Treponema pallidum* were not demonstrated in primary syphilitic lesions until the early twentieth century. Spirochetes were found in the cerebral cortex by Noguchi and Moore in 1913, and in 1917, Wagner-Jauregg cured two Italian soldiers of paresis by inoculating them with malaria to induce a high fever.

Classification and clinical descriptions occupied the attention of German psychiatrists of the nineteenth century. Griesinger attributed all mental disorders to physiological dysfunction of the nervous system and considered psychological reactions to be reflexes. Kraepelin's writings extended into the twentieth century. He followed Moebius in dividing mental illness into endogenous and exogenous disorders. His clinical orientation included a prognostic approach to the Psychoses, in which he termed those which resulted in recovery as Manic Depressive Psychoses and those which led to deterioration as Dementia Praecox.

Karl Kahlbaum stressed observation of abnormal behavior and described symptom complexes. He introduced terms such as catatonia and cyclothymia. Another German, Ewald Hecker, described hebephrenia. Krafft-Ebing, Stark, and Schule added their classification systems to those of Heinroth, Wernicke, and others.

In England, Daniel Hack Tuke, great-grandson of William Tuke, continued the family tradition of enlightened treatment of patients, but English psychiatrists generally were concerned more with medicolegal matters. D.H. Tuke was the first physician in the Tuke family and contributed much to the psychiatry of his time. He, too, devised a classification system and wrote a history of mental illness in the British Isles.

Pavlov and Bechterew, in Russia, began their work on biological conditioning during the nineteenth century and influenced the future course of Russian psychiatric thought. Bechterew was also interested in hypnotism and used it for a time. Korsakoff studied Alcoholism and described some of the results of chronic Alcoholism.

An American schoolteacher, Dorothea Lynde Dix, met Daniel Hack Tuke in England, where she had gone to recover from a lung disorder, and she became interested in the mentally ill. When she returned to America she discovered shocking conditions in the almshouses and jails housing the mentally ill. She spent her life campaigning for reform in the care of the insane and was influential in the founding of over 30 mental hospitals in the United States.

The American Psychiatric Association, originally called the Association of Medical Superintendents of American Institutions for the Insane, was formed in 1844 when 13 superintendents of mental hospitals met to discuss their mutual problems. The first volume of the *American Journal of Insanity* was published by this group in the same year. The first volume of this journal, which was edited by Amariah Brigham, listed Samuel B. Woodward, Luther V. Bell, Thomas Kirkbride, Pliny Earl, John Gray, John Galt, and Isaac Ray among the superintendents and resident physicians of lunatic asylums in the United States. George Beard introduced the concept of neurasthenia in the middle of the nineteenth century and Silar Wier Mitchell proposed his famous rest cure. Somewhat later, Morton Prince described the multiple personality.

THE TWENTIETH CENTURY

Developments in psychiatry at the close of the nineteenth century continued to influence the psychiatric theory and practice of the twentieth century. Neuropathologists and neuroanatomists emphasized the physiological elements of mental disorders. The use of hypnosis of Charcot and Bernheim and their schools of hypnosis led to new concepts of investigation and treatment of mental disease.

Physical approaches to treatment changed very little until 1933 when Manfred Sakel introduced insulin coma treatment of Schizophrenia. The technique of inducing convulsions by Metrazol (pentylenetetrazol) was developed by von Meduna of Budapest in 1935, shortly to be supplanted by Cerletti and Bini's electroconvulsive treatment method. Psychosurgery was originated by Moniz and Lima in Portugal, and it was introduced into the United States by Walter Freeman.

Pharmacological treatments, including barbiturates and bromides, were used with varying success. These agents were largely replaced by newer sedative and tranquilizing agents after chlorpromazine became available in 1954.

Two theories which attempted to correlate physical conformation with personality were devised. Ernest Kretschmer described the asthenic, athletic, pyknic, and dysplastic body types and attempted to relate body type to personality characteristics, especially those associated with Cyclothymic Disorders and Schizoid Personalities. Sheldon's work on somatotypes appeared later. He grouped people into endomorphs, who had round soft bodies and pleasant personalities, mesomorphs, who were muscular and aggressive, and ectomorphs, who were tall, slender, sensitive, and shy.

The foundations for psychoanalytic theory were laid late in the nineteenth century by some of the men who studied with Charcot and Bernheim. One of whom, Pierre Janet, developed many concepts which were similar in content but different in terminology from those of another physician who visited the Salpêtrière and Nancy Schools, Sigmund Freud, a neuropathologist from Vienna. Janet recognized the influence of the unconscious and of memories and emotional trauma in the production of mental symptoms, although he held to the idea that Hysteria resulted from a constitutional weakness. He described psychasthenia and spoke of dissociation. He was highly critical of Freud, and later referred to his own use of the word unconscious as a figure of speech.

Early in his career, Freud and Josef Breuer, a general practitioner, observed a hypnotized patient and collaborated to formulate theories regarding the unconscious motivation of behavior and the benefits of abreaction and catharsis in treatment of the Neuroses. Freud soon found that the patient was able to recall previously unremembered past events without hypnosis by means of what he termed "free association." Several of Freud's contributions were to continue to influence psychiatric thought, among them his theories of the instincts, the concepts of repression and resistance, the technique of dream interpretation, the concept of infantile sexuality, and the stages of psychosexual development. Freud named his new technique psychoanalysis. Others who became interested in psychoanalysis were Alfred Adler, Karl Abraham, Otto Rank, Sandor Ferenzi, Carl Jung, and Eugen Bleuler. Abraham and Ferenzi were early pupils of Freud; the former elaborated on the stages of psychosexual development, and the latter altered Freud's techniques to include more activity on the part of the therapist. Rank theorized that all anxiety was related to the anxiety of being born, that is, to birth trauma.

Adler's theories diverged rather markedly from Freud's, despite their early associations. Adler emphasized the importance of drives toward self-assertion and postulated that people attempt to compensate for feelings of inferiority by striving toward power, domination, and superiority. He believed that aggression, not sex, was the important drive in motivating people to action. Adler emphasized individual differences in goals and behavior. He is credited with originating the term inferiority complex.

Jung and Freud also viewed man and the unconscious somewhat differently. Jung believed that the unconscious has two parts: a personal unconscious and a racial or collective unconscious. Because of his views on human needs for religious experience and his interpretations of dream symbols, Jung has often been called a mystic. Jung developed the concepts of introversion and extroversion. He also developed and used a word association test. Jung was one of the first to point out the influence of the parent's neurotic problems on the developing child.

Eugen Bleuler had spent many years investigating Dementia Praecox and concluded that it did not always end in dementia as had previously been described. He was interested in applying psychoanalytic methods to the study and treatment of Psychosis. Bleuler introduced the term Schizophrenia, which he felt should be applied to what he considered to be a group of psychotic disorders having common characteristics. He divided the symptoms of Schizophrenia into primary and secondary symptoms.

Freud visited the United States only once, in 1909, when he was invited by Stanley Hall to lecture at Clark University in Worcester, Massachusetts. His writings were introduced into America largely through the work of a former pupil, A. A. Brill, who translated Freud's work into English.

Others who were influential in establishing the psychoanalytic movement in the United States were James J. Putnam of Harvard University, Smith Ely Jelliffe, William Alanson White, and Adolf Meyer. Jelliffe, who edited the *Journal of Nervous and Mental Diseases* and the *Psychoanalytic Review,* and his coeditor, William A. White, who was superintendent of St. Elizabeth's Hospital for over 30 years, were among the first prominent American psychiatrists to espouse psychoanalysis.

As director of the New York State Psychiatric Institute and then professor of psychiatry at Johns Hopkins University, Adolf Meyer was a leader in American psychiatry. His approach to mental illness was psychobiological; he recognized the influence of multiple forces, not only biological, but also social and psychological in the molding of personality. Emphasizing early experiences and parental reactions, he attributed disturbances to maladaptive habit patterns. He classified illness, not into rigid entities as previously had been done, but into reaction patterns. He believed that to understand and help the patient, the therapist must obtain a great deal of information about him or her. To aid in gathering and interpreting this material, Meyer developed a life chart combining numerous factors affecting the person's behavior. Although he did not accept all of Freud's theories, Meyer was one of the founders of the American Psychoanalytic Association.

Departures from psychoanalytic theory by Karen Horney, Erich Fromm, and Harry Stack Sullivan emphasized cultural and interpersonal aspects of behavior. These three, along with Abraham Kardiner, are often called the neo-Freudians.

In Europe, another form of analysis, existential analysis, developed from philosophical origins. In this treatment method, the therapist attempts to arouse feelings in himself or herself that make it possible to truly comprehend the patient's experiences. The roots of existential analysis were in the philosophical writings of Kierkegaard, and the theory has been developed by Jaspers, Heidegger, Binswanger, and Buber. Emphasis is on the experiencing of events, not upon the events themselves.

Two other developments in the first half of the twentieth century were the mental hygiene movement and the emergence of child psychiatry. The mental hygiene movement started in America with Clifford Beers' account of his own experiences as a mental patient. There had been previous publications dealing with the problems of mental hygiene, one of them written by Isaac Ray, but it was after Beers' story was published that the movement gained momentum.

William Healy established the first child guidance clinic to help the juvenile court deal with delinquent children. Interest in the psychiatric problems of children grew and the subspecialty of child psychiatry developed.

The history of psychiatric theory in the first half of the twentieth century was primarily that of psychoanalysis and the theories which grew out of psychoanalytic concepts and which still exert a profound influence on psychiatric practice (including the practice of those who do not use, or even who reject, psychoanalysis itself). However, developments in psychiatry have been rapid and numerous in all areas.

The contributions of biochemical, pharmacological, and neuropathological research and of sociology, anthropology, and experimental psychology have influenced psychiatric thought.

Since 1950 major developments in psychiatric practice have included an emphasis on community psychiatry which was, perhaps overoptimistically, described as a third psychiatric revolution (the first being the movement toward nonrestraint in the late eighteenth and early nineteenth centuries, and the second being the introduction of psychoanalytic theory and its influence on psychotherapeutic practice), and on the deinstitutionalization of the chronically mentally ill. Rapid advances in understanding of the biochemistry of mental illness and in pharmacology have made chemotherapy an increasingly important weapon against disability resulting from mental illness. Psychotherapeutic practice has been influenced by an emphasis on crisis intervention and brief psychotherapies; and there has been a proliferation of new therapeutic techniques (cf. Chapter 21) used by an increasing variety of therapists and counselors in addition to physicians. Increasing demands for psychiatric service together with changes in the delivery of health care and the health care system as a whole will shape future developments.

REVIEW QUESTIONS

1. What treatment methods were commonly used during the Greco-Roman period?
2. Who was Celsus and what were his contributions?
3. From your knowledge of the centuries during which the belief in witchcraft prevailed, identify and discuss the following people: Sprenger, Kraemer, Vives, Paracelsus, Agrippa, Weyer, Bodin.
4. Who was Phillippe Pinel? Anton Mesmer?
5. Trace the history of somatic therapies.
6. What names do you associate with the concept and practice of nonrestraint?
7. Identify and discuss the contributions of the following: Charcot, Janet, Freud, Bleuler, Rush, Meyer, D. H. Tuke, Adler, Jung.

SELECTED REFERENCES

1. Alexander, Franz G., and S. T. Selesnick: *The History of Psychiatry.* New York, Harper and Row, 1966.

2. Arieti, Silvano: *American Handbook of Psychiatry,* Vol. 1, Revised ed. New York, Basic Books, 1973, pp. 2-117.

3. Bleuler, Manfred: Some aspects of the history of Swiss psychiatry. *Am J Psychiatry* 130(9):991-994, 1973.

4. Davis, David: A chronology of seventy famous "named" cases in psychiatry. *J Oper Psychiatry* 5(2):17-23, 1974.

5. Freedman, Alfred M., Harold I. Kaplan, and Benjamin Sadock: *Comprehensive Textbook of Psychiatry.* 3rd ed. Baltimore, William & Wilkins, 1982, pp. 1-98.

6. Goshen, Charles E. (Ed.): *Documentary History of Psychiatry.* New York, Philosophical Library, 1967.

7. Havens, Leston L.: Twentieth-century psychiatry: A view from the sea. *Am J Psychiatry* 138(10):1279-1287, 1981.

8. Kolb, L. C., and H. Keith H. Brodie: *Modern Clinical Psychiatry.* 10th ed. Philadelphia, Saunders, 1982, pp. 1-26.

9. Neugebauer, Richard: Medieval and early modern theories of mental illness. *Arch Gen Psychiatry* 36:477-483, 1979.

10. Peterson, Dale (Ed.): *A Mad People's History of Madness.* Pittsburgh, Pennsylvania, Pittsburgh Press, 1982.

11. Rosenblatt, Aaron: Concepts of the asylum in the care of the mentally ill. *Hosp Community Psychiatry* 35(3):244-250, 1984.

12. Schoeneman, Thomas J.: Criticisms of the psychopathological interpretation of witch hunts: A review. *Am J Psychiatry* 139(8):1028-1032, 1982.

13. Sedler, Mark J. (translated by M. J. Sedler and Eric C. Dessain): Falret's discovery: The origin of the concept of bipolar affective illness. *Am J Psychiatry* 140(9):1127-1133, 1983.

14. Stone, Lawrence: Madness. *The New York Times Review of Books* 29(20):28-36, 1982.

15. Thompson, Clara: *Psychoanalysis, Evolution and Development.* New York, Hermitage House, 1950.

16. Whyte, L. L.: *Unconscious Before Freud (Classics in Psychiatry Series).* New York, St. Martin's Press, 1979.

17. Zilboorg, Gregory: *A History of Medical Psychology.* New York, Norton, 1941.

Chapter 25

PREPARING FOR WRITTEN AND ORAL EXAMINATIONS

APPROACHING A REVIEW

A review should be just that. It is a reinspection and reorganization of things that one has already learned. Even if it has been a long time since you have had the relevant courses, do not be alarmed by the prospect of an examination. Relearning is a rapid process. If you have been out of school or residency for several years, in addition to review you will need to learn some new material.

In reviewing, concentrate on fundamentals. If you can answer all of the very elementary basic questions well, you can afford to miss some of the esoteric and unusual ones. Not only are the majority of licensure examination questions quite basic, but even on the specialty boards at least half of the questions are fundamental ones.

For relearning it may help you to glance over the texts and notes you actually used in your initial learning, if they are still available. However, you will find that a review text will help you relearn the material it contains, will remind you of other things you have learned before, and will help bring your information up to date.

If you are reading this some time before you actually expect to take board examinations, you can simplify your review by remembering to learn as you go. You need a basic store of factual information. Modern education, quite properly, stresses understanding concepts more than memorizing facts, but tests, written and oral, call for a certain amount of factual data, much of which is not material that you are using in day-to-day practice. A little memorizing of factual material each week is better than a crash program. Classifications, names and dates, doses and formulas, and statistical information can be placed on cards posted where you see them daily. The inside of the bathroom door can serve as a good bulletin board for such things (if you have a tolerant spouse). Or you may want to make yourself some flash cards and spend a few minutes with them each day. If you are memorizing lists, remember to spend a little extra time on the middle of the list, as it is easier to remember the first and last items.

Another thing that will help is to remember references. You will multiply the value of your journal reading many times if when you come to interesting articles you will write down key points together with the name of the author, the title, and the journal, and spend a little extra time fixing these things in your memory.

Before taking any examination, get as much information about it as you can. Any information about the scope of an examination and the sources from which questions are drawn can help you plan your review. It helps also to know something of the style of questions, as you will review differently for objective (e.g., multiple choice) examinations than you will for essay examinations or oral examinations. Often, you get helpful information from the examining boards. Otherwise, you can get the information from people who have taken the examination in the recent past. When available, old examinations are very helpful in review. This is true even if no questions are ever repeated, since the old examinations help you familiarize yourself with the style of questions and the general areas covered.

HOW TO TAKE OBJECTIVE (e.g., MULTIPLE CHOICE) EXAMINATIONS AND MAINTAIN YOUR SANITY

For medical school graduates who have completed training since 1960, the importance of skill in taking objective examinations needs no emphasis. This skill is necessary not only for success in taking examinations in medical school, but also in taking the examinations of the National Board of Medical Examiners, the FLEX examination for licensure, and the first, written, part of the examination for certification by the American Board of Psychiatry and Neurology.

Most medical students and physicians must take objective examinations from time to time. For optimal performance on such examinations it is important not only to know the subject well, but also to understand how such questions are usually constructed, and to practice answering questions of this type. If the examination has a time limit, it is important to look it over as a whole and budget one's time so that one will finish. All instructions should be read carefully before answering questions. Each question should be read fully even if one believes one knows the correct answer without reading all of the possible responses. If unfamiliar words are encountered, think of possible Latin or Greek origins, or of similar words in English or other languages which may provide a clue to meaning. One should, of course, be familiar with all commonly used prefixes and suffixes. Sometimes if one is not sure of the answer to a question, one may have a hunch. Often this feeling is based on a not altogether conscious recollection, and for most people, following such hunches will yield better than chance results.

Even a well-prepared candidate will encounter some questions that seem altogether unfamiliar. If one has ever encountered the material, free association, when time permits, can be used to help recover the memory. Otherwise, one may be forced to guess. If one takes into account the design of objective questions, one may obtain better than chance results by guessing and can make a better score than one would make if one omitted these questions.

There are four general types of questions on objective examinations: (1) one best response, (2) standard matching, (3) comparison matching, (4) multiple true-false (Type K). Some authors expand this list, but these four are the basic types and other types are simply variants.

1.   *One Best Response* questions include the standard multiple choice style with which most people are familiar. These questions have become so much a part of the life of the average physician that jokes and cartoons have physicians asking

patients to "please rephrase those symptoms in the form of a multiple choice question." The directions state: The statement below is followed by five (sometimes four) suggested responses; select the one BEST response. The suggested answers are called foils, incorrect foils are called distractors. Variations of the one best response style of question include: select the least likely, most likely, true statement, false statement, etc.

Example: Which of the following is a Psychosis?
a.   Antisocial Personality Disorder
b.   Generalized Anxiety Disorder
c.   Schizophrenia
d.   Adjustment Disorder with Depressed Mood
e.   All of the above
     Answer: (c) Schizophrenia

How to Out-Fox the Fox:
a.   Foil (c) is more often correct than the others, so it is the best one to guess if you do not know the answer.
b.   If all the foils are short except one, choose the long statement.
c.   If (a) seems correct, read (d) and (e) carefully to avoid missing a more correct statement.
d.   If a series of numbers are presented, (a) and (e) are usually incorrect.
e.   If "all of the above" or "none of the above" is offered as a foil, it is correct more often than one would expect statistically.
f.   Foils with "always" or "never" are usually incorrect; most dogmatic statements are incorrect.
g.   You will score better if you guess the same foil on all questions on which you cannot rule out any distractors. (Obviously, each distractor you can rule out improves your guessing percentage.)

2.   *Standard Matching* questions are also familiar to most people. The directions state: Two lists are presented; match those items in the first column to those in the second column. Each item may be used once, more than once, or not at all.
Example:
     1. Freud
     2. Wolpe
     3. Berne
     4. Bob Dylan
     5. Benjamin Rush
a.   Transactional Analysis
b.   Psychoanalysis
c.   Father of American Psychiatry
d.   Systematic Desensitization
e.   None of the above
     Answers: 1. (b) 2. (d) 3. (a) 4. (e) 5. (c)

How to Out-Fox the Fox:
a.   Read each list and select the items you know (usually two or three of the five).
b.   With only two items remaining you have a 50-50 chance of guessing the correct answer. Most often all items are not used. Your odds are better to match all of the items rather than try and guess which item is omitted or used twice (granted, you usually miss one this way, but you also get one correct and, since the scores are curved, you fare better with a guaranteed four of five rather than risking three of five).

c.   Recently the National Board examinations Part I and II and the American Board of Psychiatry and Neurology written examination have had a tendency NOT to use all of the items on this type of question. Knowing that you may use one item twice or even three times and may not use one of the items at all will keep you thinking.

3.   *Comparison Matching* questions appear especially simple. Surprisingly, the scores on these questions are not as high as one would expect. The directions state: Choose (a) if the item is associated with (A) only; choose (b) if the item is associated with (B) only; choose (c) if the item is associated with both (A) and (B); choose (d) if the item is associated with neither (A) nor (B). Then one finds a list of statements labeled (A) and (B) and four statements numbered 1-4.
Example:
a.   (A) only
b.   (B) only
c.   Both
d.   Neither
      (A) Marijuana
      (B) LSD
1.   Causes euphoria
2.   Invariably produces an Organic Brain Syndrome with Psychosis
3.   Causes hallucinations even in low doses (100 µg)
4.   Has been used by an estimated 30 million Americans
      Answers: 1. (c) both, 2. (d) neither (the trick here is the word invariably), 3. (b) (B) only, 4. (a) (A) only.

How to Out-Fox the Fox:
a.   "Both" is usually the most common answer with "neither" second.
b.   "(A) only" and "(B) only" are rarely used more than once each per question, and sometimes not at all.

4.   *Multiple True-False (Type K)* questions separate the winners from the losers. First, they are relatively difficult. Second, they are time consuming and, since they are usually in the last portion of the examination, those who read slowly or obsess excessively in the beginning of the test will not have time to finish them all. Third, they usually comprise about one-half of the total number of questions; thus, they make or break you by sheer dint of numbers. The directions are easiest to explain by using an example.
Choose:
      a. If 1, 2, and 3 are correct
      b. If 1 and 3 are correct
      c. If 2 and 4 are correct
      d. If only 4 is correct
      e. If all are correct
Which of the following are primary symptoms of Schizophrenia?
1.   Autism
2.   Hallucinations
3.   Ambivalence
4.   Delusions
      Answer: (b) 1 and 3 are correct

How to Out-Fox the Fox:
      It is mandatory to practice this type of question until you love (hate) them

(Why penalize yourself because you lack such a simple skill as taking multiple true-false questions?) These questions are true-false and NEVER forget that. Beginning with the fourth foil and proceeding to the first, read each choice and mark it true or false.

If foil number four is *true* then: 1. (a), (1, 2, and 3) and (b) (1 and 3) are wrong, leaving (c) (2 and 4), (d) (4 only), and (e) All of the above as possible; 2. Next read item number two. If number two is false, then (c) and (e) are also and the answer is (d). If number two is true, (d) is wrong and (c) and (e) remain possible. 3. Lastly, read items number one and three. If either is true the answer is (e) (you do not need to know both answers); if neither one or three is true, the answer is (c).

If item number four is *false,* then: 1. (c) (2 and 4), (d) (4 only), and (e) All of the above are wrong; (a) (1, 2, and 3) and (b) (1 and 3) remain possible. 2. Items one and three have to be correct. 3. Proceed to item number two. If it is true, then the answer is (a); if it is false, the answer is (b).

If you *do not know* the answer to item four: Proceed to item number three. 1. If three is false (a), (b), and (e) are incorrect. Proceed to item number two. If number two is true, the answer is (c). If number two is false, the answer is (d). 2. If number three is true, (c) is incorrect. Read item number two; if two is false, then (a) and (e) are incorrect. If item two is true, (b) is incorrect. If numbers two and three are correct, number one has to be correct. For guessing purposes (a) is often used slightly more frequently than (e).

On most examinations you will have about 40 seconds for each question, but it is wise to calculate the actual amount of time available and pace yourself accordingly. As mentioned earlier, the multiple true-false questions are usually at the end of the examination, so there is no time to obsess in the early going. If you do not know the answer in the Best Choice or Matching Sections, guess and mark your booklet for future reference *if* you have time to return to it.

When returning to the harder questions, go ahead and change answers if the spirit moves you. Two different studies have shown that you have about a 3:1 chance in your favor of changing an answer from incorrect to correct. It is an old wives tale that you miss more questions by changing answers. It is possible that taking the examination triggers subliminal information or previous associations. Another possibility rests in the answer to one question being contained in another.

Ride the curve home.

How to Prepare For and Take Oral
Examinations in Psychiatry

In preparing for oral examinations, review aloud. During your review, ask someone to criticize your answers for style as well as content. It is extremely important to organize your answers, not only because there is not much time, but also because examiners have specific points in mind when they ask a question. Before responding to the examiner's question, it is a good idea to form an outline mentally for your answer. In an oral psychiatric examination you are likely to be asked to do a mental status examination on either a real or imaginary patient in case conference style. The mental status examination is a good place to practice the outline method of presentation. You should be able to present the mental status of Schizophrenia, an Adjustment Disorder, two or three types of Neurosis, Major Depression, Bipolar Affective Disorder, at least two Personality Disorders, and an Organic Mental Disorder. It should take no longer than 5 minutes for the presentation unless the case is extremely complicated. You are at risk to be interrupted during any oral presentation; an outline facilitates your picking up where you left off without sacrificing completeness and without repeating yourself.

When you go to take the examination your physical appearance should be a reflection of your profession. Your hair should be well groomed, your clothes clean and pressed. For a woman, a dress or skirted suit is appropriate; for a man, a suit and tie is preferred. Try to fit the usual image of the physician. Note the usual dress and grooming of successful physicians of your sex as observed during their working hours (but do not wear a white laboratory coat). Note also how other professionals and executives dress. Look as if you were a member of such a group at work; not as if you were going to a picnic or a cocktail party. One need not be concerned about conscious prejudice on the part of examiners, which is rare, but one should recognize that one's appearance may evoke an unconscious positive or negative reaction.

When you actually go to the examination, do not be concerned about nervousness. You are supposed to be anxious; after all, an examination is a stressful situation for most people. The examiners expect you to be anxious and will make some effort to put you at ease. The critical factor on this issue is to externalize your anxiety. If you feel like shaking, go ahead and shake. If you internalize your feelings they will likely surface as hostility, aloofness, cynicism, or facetiousness, any or all of which can cause you to do badly on an oral examination. If you are not aware of the way others perceive your usual behavior when anxious, ask your friends and colleagues how they think you might react under such circumstances so that you can better correct for any such tendencies.

If live patients are used, be certain to show them proper respect. Begin by introducing yourself. Unless the patient is a child, use his or her last name, and do not address the patient by the first name (even if the examiner introduces the patient to you that way). Observe the social amenities. Be pleasant and friendly, but not overly solicitous or pompous. In some clinical examinations (e.g., the oral examinations of the American Board of Psychiatry and Neurology) more failures are probably the result of not establishing rapport with the patient than any other single cause. One should sense the patient's reaction to one's behavior and make adjustments accordingly. If the patient and the examiner perceive one as distant, disinterested, hostile, supercilious, or a "smart-ass," failure is likely. Ask the patient if he or she has been told the purpose of the interview. If he or she says No, explain that you are taking an examination and your ability to interview and understand him or her will be graded.

It is reasonable to inquire whether the subject is a patient at the hospital or clinic where the examination is taking place, how long he or she has been a patient there, and the reason for initially seeking treatment. The patient may then be asked to tell you about his or her illness and the response is then supplemented by such questions as are needed to complete a history of the present illness, mental examination, and relevant past history. Questioning should make appropriate use of both open-ended questions and specific questions (when precise information is relevant). The questioning should be systematic, moving from one subject to another with smooth transitions. It should not, however, be so systematic as to keep the patient from expressing things that he or she wishes to tell you, nor should it resemble a cross-examination. Do not fail to follow significant leads given you by the patient.

The patient is free to digress, but you should avoid anything that would appear to the examiner like random questioning or jumping from one subject to another. Note changes in the patient's attitude during the examination and if you appear to be making him or her anxious or annoyed, modify your approach.

Use all of the time you have been allowed for the interview. Sometimes one may be certain of the diagnosis and the appropriate treatment within the first few minutes of an interview. However, when this is the case, the examiner will expect you to have made the best possible use of the remaining time so that you may better understand the patient as a person and the dynamics of the illness. Thank the patient when the session is terminated.

After you have completed examining the patient, the examiner will probably begin by asking what you observed about the patient and may then ask for a case formulation, after which he or she will ask about diagnosis. He or she may then inquire about the reasons that you asked certain questions or did not ask certain questions. There may be questions asked about further studies that you would obtain, differential diagnosis, and alternative treatment methods. Though the examiner may ask some questions that are only tangentially related to the interview (e.g., if you use a technical term you may be asked define it; if you mention a medication you may be asked its mode of action) questions will almost always be related in some way to the case. In fact, if you get a question that appears unrelated, it may give you a clue as to something you have missed.

When the examiner asks questions, do not hesitate to say, "I don't know." This is preferable to bluffing. If you are asked a question on an area in which you are weak, try to make your answer as brief and to the point as possible. It is better to get on to a question that you can answer well than to waste a great deal of time fumbling. If you do know the answer well you may want to answer at more length. If you think you know the answer, but you are not sure, it may be wise to qualify your answer to indicate your uncertainty.

If you are asked a question you do not understand, you may ask to have it repeated or ask for clarification (which may or may not be given). However, you should avoid quibbling with the examiners on the wording or specificity of questions. Aside from the fact that this may label you as defensive or contentious, it is likely to result in making the question more difficult. Choose for yourself the meaning of the question and answer it on the level that you can give the best response. If this is not what the examiner wants you will be asked another question.

Show a reasonable degree of humility and avoid arguing with the examiner; but do not allow yourself to be "led down the primrose path" by agreeing with incorrect or even absurd statements. You can always express what you have learned, read, or been taught in a way that is not argumentative. When asked a controversial question, give both sides and, if possible, give references. State your own opinion if asked to do so, indicating that it is based on what you have been taught and your experience to date, and may be subject to revision as you learn more. If you have a special basis for giving an expert opinion on the controversy (e.g., you have done significant research in the area) you may want to indicate this to the examiner.

In organizing your answer to a question, start and stop on strong points. For example, if you are asked to discuss five psychiatric syndromes which are associated with alcohol misuse, you will probably be asked to discuss one in detail. You may be interrupted at the beginning, but more likely you will be asked about the last or next to the last one you mention. Your own knowledge of interviewing techniques should tell you that an interviewer is most likely to go on from the point where the subject stops. Therefore, it is wise to stop on something upon which you can elaborate.

Do not expect to be able to answer all the questions you are asked. The examiner may possibly test the limits of your knowledge by asking you some very difficult questions. The examiner is also interested in how you handle frustration. Do not panic.

THE NATIONAL BOARD EXAMINATIONS

The National Board of Medical Examiners give a three-part examination. Some medical schools require that one pass these examinations; others require that one take them as a candidate, or noncandidate, and record a score on the first two parts; in others these examinations are optional.

National Boards Part I is a 2-day, multiple choice examination offered in June and September to American medical students who have completed, or nearly completed, the basic sciences. The mean of the examination is 500, with a standard deviation of 100. One needs an overall score of 380 on the seven sections (pathology, microbiology, biochemistry, anatomy, pharmacology, physiology, behavioral science) to pass (about 12 percent fail). The section which is in the psychiatric field is called behavioral science and includes an extremely broad range of subjects, e.g., sociology, psychology, statistics, child development, learning theory, etc. No single textbook is of much value in reviewing for this examination. For current information consult with your psychiatry department, since the material covered changes from year to year.

National Boards Part II is also a 2-day, multiple choice examination. It is offered in April or May to American medical students who are scheduled to graduate in May or June. It has the same mean (500) and standard deviation (100) as Part I (less than 3 percent fail). There are six sections in Part II, one of which is psychiatry. Knowledge of psychiatry is of benefit in between 20 and 30 percent of the questions in the other five sections (obstetrics-gynecology, internal medicine, pediatrics, preventive medicine and public health, and surgery). You will improve your Part II score most by learning the information in an introductory textbook of psychiatry and combining this knowledge with that obtainable in medical textbooks that encompass internal medicine, pediatrics, and obstetrics-gynecology.

Part III of National Boards is offered in the spring. You can take Parts I and II as a noncandidate, which means you do not get credit for your score(s) unless you pay for all three parts, or as a candidate, which means the score remains a permanent part of your academic record. To be eligible for Part III you have to complete medical school and pass both Parts I and II for credit. You can convert from a noncandidate to a candidate by paying for Parts I and II. You have to take Part III as a candidate (total cost is currently about $250). When you pass Part III, which is mostly clinical case histories with questions on patient management, you receive a certificate stating you are "certified by the National Board of Medical Examiners." Pass rate on Part III is very high (about 97+ percent). Knowledge of psychiatry helps some on Part III, but not as much as on Part II.

THE FLEX EXAMINATION

Though each state has its own licensing requirements, the Federation Licensing Examination, FLEX, provides a comprehensive examination for licensing purposes recognized by all licensing boards. The FLEX has been in use since 1968, but a "new, improved" FLEX (does this remind you of a detergent commercial?) is being introduced in June 1985. It will no longer be based exclusively on material developed for the National Board of Medical Examiners. It has two parts, each lasting $1\frac{1}{2}$ days. A State Board may require that these be taken sequentially or in one sitting. The first part covers basic science information with direct or indirect clinical relevance. The second part emphasizes internal medicine, pediatrics, general surgery, family practice, obstetrics/gynecology, psychiatry (child and adult), and preventive medicine. It also includes interdisciplinary topics (e.g., medical law, geriatrics).

The format is objective and in the second part will probably continue to use patient management questions. In these questions, a clinical history is presented and you are offered a number of options as to what to do. If you choose a statement you "erase" the answer. There are both errors of omission and commission in this type of examination, e.g., if you erase an answer you are not supposed to, it counts against you and if you do not erase an answer you should have, it also counts against you. The typical format is such that five or six of 10 responses should be erased; three or four of 10 responses should be left blank; and one of 10 responses is not scored. Note: The preceding comment refers to the entire examination, not just any group of 10 questions. The total number of patient-management questions in the "old" FLEX was at least 600.

EXAMINATIONS FOR FOREIGN MEDICAL GRADUATES

Graduates of foreign medical schools desiring to take advanced clinical training or to apply for licensure must first take the Foreign Medical Graduate Examination in the Medical Sciences (FMGEMS). This 2-day examination was introduced in July 1984. The Educational Council for Foreign Medical Graduates, ECFMG, English test is given with each examination. Passing these examinations meets visa requirements for entering a training program and the medical science examination requirement for ECFMG certification. The tests are objective. Questions on psychiatry and the behavioral sciences are expected to remain relatively simple and straightforward, but graduates of schools that offer limited instruction in psychiatry may need to devote some extra attention to preparation in the field.

THE AMERICAN BOARD OF PSYCHIATRY
AND NEUROLOGY EXAMINATIONS

The examinations in psychiatry given by the American Board of Psychiatry and Neurology consist of two parts, an objective written examination and an oral examination. For one to be "board eligible" one's credentials must be accepted by the American Board of Psychiatry and Neurology. One must have a medical degree and have completed an approved psychiatric residency (for possible exceptions to the latter requirement a person whose training and experience is atypical may correspond with the Board). Currently, approved residencies in psychiatry are 4-year programs. The first year, internship, must include at least 4 months' experience in the general medical care of children and/or adults.

The American Board of Psychiatry and Neurology allows house officers to apply for admission to examination during their last 6 months of house officer training. Before applying for the "Board" examination, one should check the material available through the Secretary of the American Board of Psychiatry and Neurology for any changes in the format which follow this publication. This information is published in the American Medical Association's (Matching Plan) book on Residencies and Internships and is revised each year. You may also wish to seek up-to-date information about the examinations, and suggestions for your review from: (1) the director of a house officer training program in psychiatry, (2) a chairperson of a department of psychiatry, and (3) colleagues who have recently taken the examination.

The Written Examination

The written examination requires 7 hours and includes questions in neurology and the behavioral sciences as well as in clinical psychiatry. Standard types of objective questions are used. However, some call for value judgments. Some questions are based on case histories. Some are based on reproductions of x-rays, EEG tracings, etc. Candidates report that the first sections tend to be the most difficult (a possible source of encouragement if one begins to feel overwhelmed early in the examination). Another source of encouragement is that over 70 percent of candidates pass the examination.

The Oral Examination

The oral examination for candidates for certification in psychiatry is open to those who have passed the written examination. It currently consists of two sections: a 1-hour examination in clinical psychiatry (audiovisual), and a 1-hour examination in clinical psychiatry (live patient), not necessarily in that order.

For the audiovisual examination in clinical psychiatry, one is shown a 30-minute tape of a patient interview and then is questioned orally for 30 minutes by an examiner. In watching the tape, as well as paying attention to the content of the interview, be sure to observe the patient carefully, noting appearance, grooming, mannerisms, outward signs of anxiety, facial expression, and nonverbal communication. You will be asked for your observations and will be asked to formulate the case, give the probable diagnosis, discuss differential diagnosis, and suggest a treatment plan (or plans) for the patient.

The quality of the tapes, and of the interviews they display, is variable. However, one should probably not criticize them unless asked to do so. After watching the tape one's first problem is likely to be one of reorganizing the interview material into a logical sequence. You will have a few minutes to do this and to review your observations before the questioning starts.

In the live patient examination in clinical psychiatry, you may be told that you will have 30 minutes to talk with the patient, but actually you may be given a few minutes less time than that. If you are in the habit of doing much longer initial interviews, as most of us are, you may want to practice some brief consultations so as to be able to use the shorter interviewing time effectively. If you are not in a setting that lends itself to this, perhaps you could arrange to do it at some nearby psychiatric hospital, and have a staff member observe your interview and review your findings with you afterward. Remember that your attitude toward the patient and the kind of rapport you establish are crucial.

After you have talked with the patient, you will be asked about your findings, diagnosis, and formulation. Questions may then focus on differential diagnosis, dynamics, or treatment. You may be asked about psychological tests or other procedures that might be indicated in the case and what you would expect them to show. Basic aspects will be emphasized.

You may need to practice case formulation (cf. Chapter 3). Make your formulation a complete biopsychosocial one. Do not merely repeat findings; organize them and draw inferences from them to explain the patient's condition. Near the end of the live patient interview, while you still have time, think of your working diagnosis and ask yourself if you have collected enough data for a biopsychosocial formulation for it. If the disorder is sometimes familial, have you asked about family history? Have you asked enough about childhood experiences and development to identify stages of psychosocial development that contribute to the patient's personality and/or illness? Have you asked enough about circumstances surrounding the onset of illness to identify stressors?

It is helpful to save time at the end of the interview to comment to the patient that you have asked a number of questions and to inquire if he or she feels that there is anything else you should know about him or her.

The American Board of Psychiatry and Neurology has attempted to make the grading of the oral examination as objective as possible. Grades include: pass, condition, and fail, but examiners also record comments on your performance. If you fail in either section, or condition in both, you will fail the examination. However, if you pass one section and condition in the other, the examiners' comments will be evaluated and you still may pass. In other words, excellent performance in one session may compensate for mediocre performance in the other. The five areas on which one is graded are:

1. Physician-patient interaction
2. Conduct of the clinical examination
3. Capacity to elicit clinical data
4. Case formulation, differential diagnosis, and prognosis
5. Therapeutic management and knowledge of therapies

One is graded on all five categories in the live patient hour and on numbers 4 and 5 in the clinical psychiatry audiovisual hour (but your ability to extract significant information from the interview you watch contributes heavily to your ability to cope with this examination).

During each section there will be two examiners asking questions and one or more others will observe portions. Do not attach any special significance to the number of observers or the length of time they are in the room.

Before grading your performance some examiners will use a check list, actually or mentally. This is likely to cover your interviewing skills; the quality of the history that you take; your ability to elicit and report mental status findings; the quality of your case presentation, discussion of differential diagnosis, and biopsychosocial case formulation; and the appropriateness of your treatment plans and prognosis.

The items scored in history-taking may present a problem. You will not have time to include them all. Be sure to include the ones that are relevant, and be aware of the ones you did not include. You must not try so hard to include everything that you sacrifice interviewing technique and rapport, but on the other hand, you do not want to get "hung up" on one part of the history. Common omissions in the history of the present illness include treatment history, which may be important, and questions about other disorders and problems, including nonpsychiatric illnesses and substance use. Family history should include information about the family of origin and the current family relationships. Past history should include an adequate developmental history and a chronological life history, including education, work, and military service as well as significant interpersonal relationships, sexual history, and difficulties with the law.

Your discussion of differential diagnosis should emphasize the most likely possibilities. You should mention diagnostic procedures that would be helpful.

In discussing treatment be sure to include appropriate alternatives, and just as your formulation should be psychobiosocial, your treatment plan should address all elements. Do not talk just about an appropriate medication if the patient also needs psychotherapy and other interventions (e.g., vocational counseling).

It helps to have reviewed current developments in psychiatry before taking the examination. These will be fresh in your examiners' minds and may be relevant to one of the cases. A review of articles that have appeared in the year before your examination in major journals may alert you to "hot" topics.

SELF-ASSESSMENT

Periodically the American Psychiatric Association offers a self-assessment examination. These are known by the acronym PSKAP (Psychiatric Skills and Knowledge Assessment Program). Interestingly, the scores of house officers have not varied significantly from those of psychiatrists in practice. Of course, no one ever said any of the examinations mentioned in this chapter even pretend to measure clinical skills. However, most examiners and a number of educators believe that there is a high positive correlation between the knowledge and problem-solving ability called for by this type of examination and one's clinical abilities. Certainly, it is reasonable to assume that without adequate knowledge, one cannot practice well. Even with adequate knowledge, one may not practice well. Probably only actual observation and some form of audit of one's day-to-day practice could actually reveal how well one's knowledge can be (and is) applied. The fact that the membership of the American Psychiatric Association is willing to participate in this self-assessment is, in itself, a step forward, since only about one-half of the psychiatrists in the United States are certified. We are entering an era of increased accountability in medicine. It is recognized that licensure and certification do not necessarily attest to current clinical competence. Relicensure, recertification, and required continuing education are increasingly likely to be mandated. You may never stop having to take tests!

FINAL COMMENTS

Practice is important for both oral and written examinations. In preparing for an oral examination, one should practice aloud; in practicing for a written examination, one should write; in practicing for the clinical type of examination, one should do actual examinations of appropriate length and have them critiqued by colleagues. Lists of sample questions and of review questions are available from various sources. Sometimes the organization giving an examination will furnish some sample questions to prospective candidates. Books containing review questions for various examinations are available and one can obtain some lists of questions that one's colleagues have used in reviewing or that they recall having been asked. Sometimes a person preparing for an examination by using review questions or actual questions from old examinations makes the mistake of simply drilling so as to memorize the answers. This is of limited value, though, of course, some questions are of such obvious importance that one should indeed memorize the answers. The two best uses of review questions are first, practice in answering the style of question used, and second, identifying those areas for which one needs further study. For example, if one were to go through the review questions at the end of each of the preceding chapters without rereading the chapters or looking for the answers, one would be able (after consulting references) to identify one's errors and also identify those questions which gave one some difficulty. The subjects that give one the most difficulty (making allowance for relative importance) are the general subjects for which the most additional review is likely to be necessary.

For most examinations in psychiatry it is best to remember that the examination is comprehensive, and extensive or esoteric knowledge of one subject will probably not be tested. It is best to cover everything to some degree rather than concentrate heavily in any one area.

Bear in mind that the scope of various examinations changes from time to time and that the type of questions used, and the way they are constructed and scored may also change. If you are going to take an examination, it is important to have up-to-date information about the examination itself as well as the subject on which you are being examined.

REVIEW QUESTIONS

1. How important do you think establishment of rapport with the patient is during the oral examination for certification in psychiatry? What would you do to enhance it if you were a candidate? If you were an examiner, how would you grade a candidate who did not relate well to the patient?
2. What do multiple-choice examinations evaluate?
3. What are the five areas on which one is evaluated when taking the oral examination for board certification in psychiatry?
4. A foreign medical graduate in a U.S. training program is having difficulty with examinations in various courses, though her knowledge of the subject matter appears adequate. What are the possible causes of her difficulty? Assuming you have identified the causes correctly, what can be done to help her?
5. You are taking an oral examination and your examiner makes a statement that is clearly incorrect. How do you handle the situation? What do you do if the examiner asks you if you agree?
6. If you were serving on the American Board of Psychiatry and Neurology, would you consider making all of the examinations objective (multiple choice)? Why? Why not?
7. Following observing a videotaped interview, you are asked to give a case formulation, but you feel that certain essential data for the formulation was not elicited. How do you handle this situation?
8. You are taking a "live patient" examination and find that your patient is practically mute (refuses to answer most questions). What do you do? What do you do if a patient insists on leaving the room after you have used about half of the allotted time for the interview?

SELECTED REFERENCES

1. American Medical Association: *Directory of Residency Training Programs Accredited by the Liaison Committee on Graduate Medical Education.* Chicago, American Medical Association, published annually.

2. Damlouji, Namir F.: *Psychiatry Specialty Board Review.* 3rd ed. New York, Medical Examination Publishing Company, 1983.

3. Davis, Richard E.: Changing examination answers: An educational myth? *J Med Ed* 50(7):685-687, 1975.

4. Easson, William M.: *Psychiatry Examination Review,* Third edition. New York, ARCO Publishing, 1983.

5. Levy, Maurice, and Richard E. Easton: Tips to help you score better. *Res Staff Physician* 25(10):13-15, 1979.

6. Maleson, Franklin G., Paul J. Fink, and Howard L. Field: Board certification anxiety. *Am J Psychiatry* 137(7):837–840, 1980.

7. McQuarrie, Howard G.: The transition task force answers questions about the new FLEX program. *Fed Bull* 71(4):117–121, 1984.

8. Napoliello, Michael J.: How to prepare for the psychiatry boards. *Res Staff Physician* 25(10):45–55, 1979.

9. Nelson, J. Craig, and David Greenfeld (Eds.): *Pretest psychiatry: Pretest Self-Assessment and Review.* 2nd ed. New York, McGraw-Hill, 1982.

10. Small, S. Mouchly: Evaluation methodology for the oral examination of the American Board of Psychiatry and Neurology. In: *Evaluation of Noncognitive Skills and Clinical Performance.* John S. Lloyd (Ed.). Chicago, American Board of Medical Specialties, 1982.

11. Talbott, John A.: Is the "live patient" interview on the boards necessary? *Am J Psychiatry* 140(7):890–893, 1983.

12. Val, Eduardo, and Suzanne Quick: Foreign medical graduates and board certification: Myths and realities. *Am J Psychiatry* 140(2):184–188, 1983.

INDEX